Horse and St[able] Management

incorporating

Horse Care

Omnibus (Third) Edition

Jeremy Houghton Brown
Vincent Powell-Smith
Sarah Pilliner

THE LIBRARY
FILTON COLLEGE
BRISTOL
BS12 7AT

Blackwell
Science

© Jeremy Houghton Brown and the Estate of
Powell-Smith 1984, 1994, 1997 and Blackwell
Science Ltd 1994, 1997

Blackwell Science Ltd
Editorial Offices:
Osney Mead, Oxford OX2 0EL
25 John Street, London WC1N 2BL
23 Ainslie Place, Edinburgh EH3 6AJ
350 Main Street, Malden
  MA 02148 5018, USA
54 University Street, Carlton
  Victoria 3053, Australia
10, rue Casimir Delavigne
  75006 Paris, France

Other Editorial Offices:

Blackwell Wissenschafts-Verlag GmbH
Kurfürstendamm 57
10707 Berlin, Germany

Blackwell Science KK
MG Kodenmacho Building
7–10 Kodenmacho Nihombashi
Chuo-ku, Tokyo 104, Japan

The right of the Author to be identified as the Author
of this Work has been asserted in accordance with
the Copyright, Designs and Patents Act 1988.

All rights reserved. No part of this publication
may be reproduced, stored in a retrieval
system, or transmitted, in any form or by any
means, electronic, mechanical, photocopying,
recording or otherwise, except as permitted by
the UK Copyright, Designs and Patents Act
1988, without the prior permission of the
publisher.

First published as *Horse and Stable
Management* first edition by Granada
Publishing 1984; reprinted by Collins
Professional Books 1985, 1986, 1987 (twice):
reprinted by BSP Professional Books 1987,
1988 (twice), 1989, 1990 (twice), 1991, 1992;
second edition by Blackwell Science 1994;
reprinted 1995 and *Horse Care* published by
Blackwell Science 1994.
Omnibus (third) edition published by
Blackwell Science 1997
Reprinted 1998 (twice)

Set in 11/13 pt Times
by DP Photosetting, Aylesbury, Bucks
Printed and bound in Great Britain at
the University Press, Cambridge

The Blackwell Science logo is a trade mark of
Blackwell Science Ltd, registered at the United
Kingdom Trade Marks Registry

For further information on
Blackwell Science, visit our
website:
www.blackwell-science@com

Book Services Ltd
PO Box 269
Abingdon
Oxon OX14 4YN
(*Orders*: Tel: 01235 465500
       Fax: 01235 465555)

USA
  Blackwell Science, Inc.
  Commerce Place
  350 Main Street
  Malden, MA 02148 5018
  (*Orders*: Tel: 800 759 6102
           781 388 8250
        Fax: 781 388 8255)

Canada
  Login Brothers Book Company
  324 Saulteaux Crescent
  Winnipeg, Manitoba R3J 3T2
  (*Orders*: Tel: 204 224-4068)

Australia
  Blackwell Science Pty Ltd
  54 University Street
  Carlton, Victoria 3053
  (*Orders*: Tel: 03 9347 0300
          Fax: 03 9347 5001)

A catalogue record for this title
is available from the British Library

ISBN 0-632-04152-8

Library of Congress
Cataloging-in-Publication Data
Brown, Jeremy Houghton.
    Horse and stable management
  incorporating Horse care/Jeremy
  Houghton Brown, Vincent Powell-Smith,
  Sarah Pilliner.—Omnibus (3rd.) ed.
      p.   cm.
    Rev. ed. of: Horse and stable
  management. 2nd ed. c1994 and Horse care.
  1994.
    Includes index.
    ISBN 0-632-04152-8
    1. Horses.   2. Horses—Psychology.
  3. Horses—Health.   4. Stables—
  Management.   I. Powell-Smith, Vincent.
  II. Pilliner, Sarah.   III. Brown, Jeremy
  Houghton.   Horse and stable
  management.   IV. Brown, Jeremy
  Houghton.   Horse care.   V. Title.
  SF285.3.B76   1996
  636.1′083—dc20   96-24285
                                        CIP

636.1

0020632

£17-99

19-10-98

Contents

Preface

In this book, the authors have combined their two standard texts, *Horse and Stable Management* and *Horse Care*, both of which are regarded as essential reading for every horse owner and student of the horse.

Horse and Stable Management has been acknowledged for over a decade as the definitive text on how horses function and thus how to manage them with understanding. Its companion volume, *Horse Care*, offered guidance on the practical skills needed for successful equine care. Combining the two books produces a comprehensive text that covers all aspects of horse knowledge and care and horse management in a single volume and is intended for all those who own or work with horses and ponies and who wish to learn more about them. It also provides all the information readers will require for a variety of horse courses and examinations.

It is recommended as a textbook for those taking examinations and assessments set by the British Horse Society, the National Pony Society and the Association of British Riding Schools, as well as those attempting Scottish and National Vocational Qualifications or on college horse courses.

The principle behind the book is that the horse is a complex of systems all of which are discussed. A problem in one system can have repercussions in others, and thus cause complications. If a sick horse is to be made well, the first and essential step is to identify the cause of the problem. Careful examination will reveal symptoms but it is pointless to treat them and ignore the cause. Only by understanding the systems can one really appreciate what may go wrong and when it is likely to do so. The good horsemaster, man or woman, understands and cares for the horse in such a way that all the systems co-ordinate and function efficiently and in this way the horse is able to give of its best. Good horse management means competently and pleasantly getting the best out of the horse in all seasons and on all occasions be it in the stable, at grass, in competition, at stud, in sickness, in health, in youth or in maturity.

The book is divided into six separate parts. The first two discuss the health and the various systems of the horse. The next three parts detail the principles of stable management and the practical skills required for horse mastership and the final part looks at stud management. Although the book discusses fitness and exercise it does not cover riding or teaching which are dealt with elsewhere. Those taking NVQs at levels three and four will find that the management of people and other practical management considerations are also dealt with in *Horse Business Management* by Jeremy Houghton Brown and Vincent Powell-Smith.

In the text there is a mixture of horseman's jargon and veterinary terminology, as well as discussion of some scientific concepts, but the accent is always on sound practical care. The methods described are not the only ones but they are safe, well proven and generally recommended.

We believe that the best horse care comes from understanding both the body and the mind of the horse and treating your animals accordingly.

Acknowledgement

The authors pay tribute to Jane Houghton Brown whose vision has been so influential in establishing education and training as key factors required for successful horse performance.

Jeremy Houghton Brown
Vincent Powell-Smith
Sarah Pilliner

Part I
The Horse in Sickness and Health

1   The Healthy Horse

Before horses were domesticated they lived in herds ranging over a wide area (see Fig. 1.1). They roamed as they pleased, eating herbage, grasses and bushes, this wide choice of plants supplying all their nutritional needs. They drank only once or twice a day because the food they were eating contained a high percentage of water. In fact they lived much as the herds of zebra do in Africa today, and one rarely sees a thin zebra!

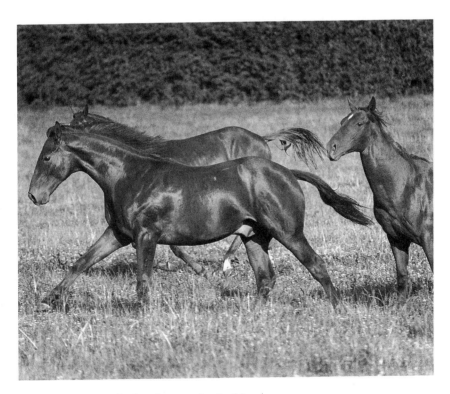

Fig. 1.1 Horses evolved as free-ranging herbivores.

3

Man's domestication of the horse has led to the horse being kept captive in paddocks or stables so that we can manipulate its exercise and feeding to suit our own purposes, be it producing a racehorse or a gymkhana pony. With captivity comes a moral responsibility; the horse is entirely dependent on us to provide adequate feed, water and exercise and to provide an environment which will keep the horse healthy. There are also economic considerations; horses are expensive to keep and a healthy, well-kept horse will be better at his job and have fewer costly vet bills.

In order to keep the horse healthy, both in body and in mind, the horsemaster should remember the natural habits of the horse and try to reproduce the same conditions as far as possible. Ideally the horse should be turned out to grass every day and the feeding programme should be arranged so that it covers as wide a period as possible and does not include long periods when food is not available.

The horsemaster's task is to keep the horse fit and healthy in an economical fashion, both in the stable and out at grass. In order to do this the horse must be provided with a clean and safe environment, fed and watered correctly and observed closely so that prompt action can be taken if signs of ill-health are noticed.

Describing the horse

In order to communicate effectively within the horse industry it is necessary to be familiar with a certain amount of 'horsey jargon'; being asked to catch 'the bay mare' may not be very helpful in a field of 20 horses. Describing a horse thoroughly involves identifying the horse's sex, height, colour, markings, age and type.

Sex
The following terms more accurately describe the sex of a horse:

- A *filly* is a female less than four years old.
- A *mare* is a female of four years old or more.
- A *colt* is an uncastrated male of three years old or less.
- As a four year old onwards he is known as a *stallion* or *entire*.
- A *gelding* is a castrated male.

Height
Horses are traditionally measured in hands with one hand being equivalent to four inches. The trend is now for ponies to be measured

Table 1.1 Horse measurement in hands and centimetres.

Hands	Centimetres	Hands	Centimetres
11.0	111.8	14.2	147.2
11.2	116.8	15.0	152.4
12.0	121.9	15.2	157.5
12.2	127.0	16.0	162.6
13.0	132.0	16.2	167.6
13.2	137.0	17.0	172.7
14.0	142.2	17.2	177.8

in centimetres as are horses in many other countries, with one hand being equivalent to 10.16 cm. The measurement is taken with the horse standing squarely on a smooth level surface. Measure from the highest point of the withers, using a measuring stick with a spirit level on the cross bar. Take 12 mm (½ in) off the height if the horse is shod.

Colour

The colour and markings of a horse are considered by some people to be significant with tradition suggesting, for example, that chestnut mares are more difficult than mares of other colours. The foal's colour at birth may not indicate the eventual colour with many grey horses, for instance, being born dark. Grey horses also become lighter grey as they get older. Some horses have a summer coat a different shade to their winter coat and may change again when clipped; the colour of the horse's muzzle is used to identify the true colour.

- The *bay* comes in three different shades: the light bay is a golden or reddish brown; the bright bay is a horse-chestnut colour; and the dark bay is a rich dark brown. Bay horses have a black mane, tail and lower leg; these parts of the animal are known as the 'points'.
- The *brown* horse is a darker brown than the dark bay and may appear black until you check the muzzle.
- The *black* horse is black with black points and a black muzzle.
- The *chestnut* also comes in many shades: a liver chestnut verges on brown and tends to have darkish points, but careful examination will show that these are not black; at the other end of the chestnut range comes the lighter chestnut and finally the palomino with its golden body and silvery mane and tail.
- The colour *grey* includes white through to iron grey and the horse

may be dappled to a varying degree. Flea-bitten greys have small flecks of dark hair scattered through the coat.

- A horse is described as *white* if it has a pink skin though more usually the coat is a light cream colour and the eyes may be an unusual bluish colour.
- A *roan* has a mix of white and other colours in the coat giving rise to strawberry (chestnut), red (bay) or blue (diluted black) roans.
- The *dun* may vary from blue, which is a diluted black, to yellow. The mane, tail and lower legs are black and there may be a dark dorsal stripe or 'list' running along the backbone.
- The *piebald* is black and white.
- The *skewbald* is generally brown and white, although it is correctly any colour other than black and white.

This list is not exhaustive and many breed societies have detailed descriptions of allowed colours.

Markings
The horse's markings, including scars, brands and acquired marks from saddle sores, etc., are recorded on veterinary certificates and registration forms.

On the head

- *Star* – a white mark on the forehead. Even if there are only a few hairs, these should be noted (see Fig. 1.2).
- *Stripe* – a narrow white mark down the face which may be a continuation of a star when it is described as a star and stripe (see Fig. 1.3).
- *Blaze* – a wide covering of white hair running down the face (see Fig. 1.4).
- *White face* – an exaggerated blaze covering much of the horse's forehead and face.
- *Snip* – a white mark between the nostrils (see Fig. 1.5).
- *White muzzle* – white skin covering both lips and the nostrils.
- *White upper/underlip* – white skin at the edge of the lips.
- *Wall eye* – the eye is a grey–blue colour; sight is not affected.

On the body

- *List, dorsal stripe* or *ray* – the dark line found along the backbone of dun horses and donkeys.

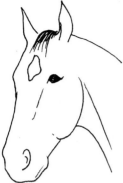

Fig. 1.2 Star.

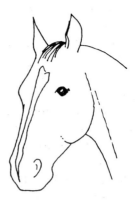

Fig. 1.3 Star and stripe.

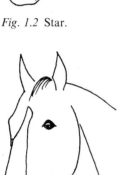

Fig. 1.4 Blaze.

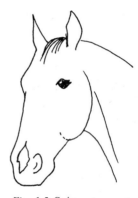

Fig. 1.5 Snip.

- *Zebra marks* – any stripes found on the body.
- *Whorls* – small areas formed by a change in the direction of hair growth, found, for example, on the forehead and crest of the neck. They are unique to each horse and are in effect the horse's 'fingerprint'.
- *Prophet's thumb mark* – an obvious indentation in the muscle on the neck or shoulder or hindquarters, said to be a sign of good luck.
- *Flesh marks* – patches of pink skin which grow white hair.

The horse may also be marked by scars or brands. Freeze brands resulting in white hair are a method of protecting horses against theft, each horse having its own number and being on a national register. Brands indicating breed or country of origin may be situated on the neck, shoulder or quarters. Identification brands may also be placed on the hooves or tattooed on the lips or gums.

Although not a marking in the traditional sense, it should be noted that horses can also be identified by inserting a microchip about the size of a grain of rice into the neck muscle; it is then reliably identified with a hand-held read-out meter.

On the legs

The terms *white sock*, *stocking* or *leg* are now only used for casual description and it is more correct to refer to the horse's anatomy (see Fig. 1.6). For example, right leg to just below the knee instead of stocking. Black spots on white marks are called *ermine marks*.

Any variation of the colour of the hooves should be noted. Hoof colour usually reflects the colour of the skin on the coronet.

Age

A description of a horse is not complete without including its age. As the biting surface of the incisor (front, cutting) teeth wears away, the pattern on the surface of the tooth changes so that, with experience, the age of the horse can be estimated by examining the teeth. This is described in detail in Chapter 8.

Type

A brief description of the type or breed (if known) of the horse is helpful. For example, fine horses are described as light-weight, those with a little more substance are middle-weight and the substantial weight-carrying horse is a heavy-weight. If the breed is not known but the horse has characteristics of a certain breed then it could be

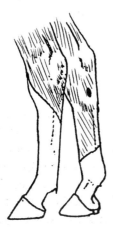

Fig. 1.6 White stockings. Left hind: white to lower hock, extending to mid hock. Right hind: white to lower cannon bone.

described, for example, as a Thoroughbred-type. The idea is to describe the horse in a concise manner, but as clearly as possible.

What is health?

In its natural state a horse strives to do three fundamental things: to survive, to nourish itself and to reproduce. When frightened it flees or, if cornered, it fights. It eats and drinks in response to hunger and thirst and thus grows to maturity and maintains its strength. In response to sexual desire it endeavours to reproduce and so continue its species. These three things are key points which are characteristic of a healthy horse. It has a good appetite and a digestive system that works well. It grows strong and fit for the work to which it is accustomed. It is alert and perceptive. If not interfered with, it is eager and able to breed. Thus, health is not merely freedom from disease; it is also a state of well-being and vigour. In practical terms, the healthy horse must be able to give of its best consistently, whether in terms of producing a foal yearly, or running races well, or of hunting three days a fortnight through the Season.

The key to maintaining health is to be observant and perceptive. Anyone who looks after animals must learn to develop that great gift, 'the stockman's eye'. This is the ability to note the normal look, feel and behaviour of an animal so that any difference is spotted at once. To keep a horse healthy it is vital to know how it looks and behaves normally. This is particularly important when the horse is undergoing change, as is the case with pregnant mares, foals, growing stock, horses just up from grass, horses being roughed off, those being fittened and those under the stress of competition.

Signs of health

Behaviour
A group of horses generally acts as a herd. An isolated horse or one uninterested in the behaviour of its fellows is abnormal. Mature horses in fields generally remain standing during the day and often have favourite spots for dozing. It is usual for horses to doze for about a third of the time. Each nap is generally of short duration. When they lie down, which happens more frequently in stables than in the open, horses go down front end first with bent front legs. They get up front

end first with straight front legs. Horses rest with the breast bone to one side and can only change sides by rolling their legs up and over or by getting up and lying down again.

The stabled horse is not free to roam and so his natural behaviour patterns have to change. Each individual horse will adapt to life in the stable in a different way and it is important to appreciate what is normal for each horse that you are looking after: some are more extrovert, approaching you as you enter the stable, demanding attention, while other, more introvert horses, keep to themselves. What the horseman has to be alert to is any deviation from the normal behaviour of that particular horse – it may be the first sign that a horse is off colour.

Appetite

When food is available continuously, the horse prefers to eat little and often. It is therefore normal for the horse at grass to graze inter-mittently day and night. The stabled horse normally goes straight to its short feed and eats it all. Some stabled horses are shy feeders and eat slowly when left in peace; others are anxious and eat best if the manger is hung on the door. After resting, foals normally get up and go straight to their mother for a drink. The vast majority of horses relish good food: any horse that does not must arouse suspicion about its health. Horses' drinking habits can also indicate their health, and because of this it is best not to use self-filling drinkers for off-colour horses.

Dung and urine

Dung should be green–brown to golden brown depending on the diet, it should be moist, and it should break slightly on hitting the ground. Adult horses normally excrete between eight and ten drop-pings per day and pass urine four to six times a day, producing from four to fifteen litres per day, depending on diet and water intake. Any changes from usual quantity, colour or pattern of behaviour should be noted.

Eyes and ears

The eye should be bright and wide open and the ears mobile. These organs give good indications of alertness and interest. Any failure to respond to sights or sounds may be an indication that something is wrong.

Membranes
The membranes of the eyes and gums should be a healthy salmon pink colour and free of any discharges.

Stance
It is quite normal for relaxed horses to rest alternate hind legs and they may occasionally shift the weight of their front feet. Any prolonged periods of resting a front foot, however, should be noted as this may indicate a problem.

Coat
The skin and coat are very good indicators of health; the skin should glide freely over the underlying bones and muscles and a pinch of skin picked up on the neck or shoulder should return smoothly and promptly into place. If the skin remains pinched up this indicates dehydration and/or a lack of subcutaneous fat. The horse's coat should be smooth to the touch and glossy to look at.

Body processes
Temperature, pulse and respiratory rate (TPR) are not obvious in a healthy horse at rest. If any one of these is unusually apparent, then the cause must be sought. When a horse is at rest the pulse rate, being a reflection of heart rate, will be at its slowest for that horse – nature's economy at work. The normal rates for an adult horse at rest are: temperature 38°C (100.5°F); pulse about 40 beats per minute; respiration about 12 breaths per minute.

The horse's temperature is taken in the rectum with a clinical thermometer. The procedure is as follows:

(1) Shake the thermometer so that it reads several degrees lower than normal.
(2) Lubricate the bulb with vaseline or saliva. Stand behind but to one side of the horse to avoid being kicked.
(3) Hold the horse's tail to one side and insert the bulb of the thermometer gently into the horse's anus, rotating it slightly as you do so. It should be inserted to half-way, at a slight angle to press the bulb against the side of the rectum.
(4) Leave in position for one minute.
(5) Withdraw and read the thermometer, taking care not to hold it at the bulb end. The mercury is most clearly seen if viewed through the apex which runs the full length of the thermometer.

(6)   Clean and disinfect the thermometer before returning it to its
      case.

Many horses have a temperature that is normally up to 1°C lower than
the book normal and the temperature may vary slightly between the
morning and the evening. Make sure that you take your horse's
temperature at the same time every day until you have established
what is normal for him. The temperature may safely vary half a degree
from normal, and in foals the norm can be as high as 38.6°C (101.5°F).

   The pulse can be taken by pressing the fingers against an artery
passing over a bone close to the surface, e.g. the facial artery on the
inside edge of the lower jaw (see Fig. 1.7) or on the radial artery inside
the foreleg, level with the elbow. Some people like to take the pulse
under the dock while taking the temperature. The simplest method of
taking the pulse is to use a stethoscope just behind the horse's left
elbow; however, after the horse has worked, even a flat hand lightly
placed there may feel the heart beat. The importance of monitoring

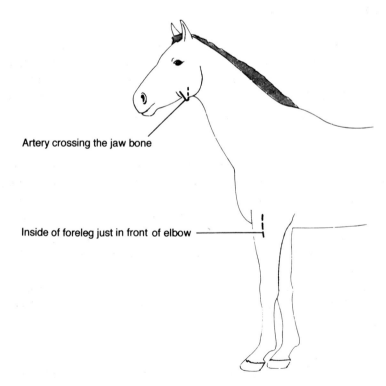

Artery crossing the jaw bone

Inside of foreleg just in front of elbow

Fig. 1.7 Positions for feeling the pulse with the fingertips resting lightly on the artery.

pulse in such sports as long-distance riding has brought the use of the stethoscope into the range of the layman. The pulse rate of individual horses varies: a rate of between 35 to 45 a minute may be normal for a particular horse at rest but a very fit horse may have a resting pulse rate that is considerably lower than this. A rate of 50 to 100 a minute is normal for a foal.

To observe respiration, the horse must be standing still and undisturbed. Watch the horse's flanks from the side. Each complete rise and fall is one breath. On a chilly day, respiration can be observed at the nostrils as condensation in the air. A range of 8 to 16 breaths a minute is acceptable in the adult horse at rest; 20 to 30 breaths a minute is acceptable in the foal. It is important to monitor the temperature, pulse and respiration (TPR) of a new arrival in the stable, doing so at the same time each day (preferably first thing in the morning) for several days, so that one knows what is normal for that individual.

Maintaining health

Domestication has deprived horses of some of their natural means of staying healthy. The wandering, grazing herd gets steady exercise, intake of a widely mixed diet little and often, ready access to water, and freedom from mental and physical stress. Some aspects of maintaining health merit individual consideration at this stage.

Air
Hot, stuffy, stale or limited air all predispose to respiratory problems. Horses must have plenty of fresh air at all times, but they dislike draughts. They do not mind the air being cold. In racing stables, the practice of shutting top doors at certain times is to ensure peace and quiet to each horse; each of these stables must have independent air access. Even those stables warmed by infra-red lamps need access for plenty of fresh air.

Current research indicates that all the air in the stable (total air exchange) should be changed 6–8 times each hour; the higher figure if the hay or straw is dusty.

Exercise and rest
In the wild the horse takes exercise gently but steadily throughout the day. In a field, the horse is able to wander as it grazes and this exercise

is sufficient to aid digestion and circulation. Ideally, the stabled horse should have a period in the field every day, but in larger establishments this would pose too many problems and risks. The alternative is daily exercise, ridden or in hand. When horses spend even one day a week in the box, this can lead to the so-called 'Monday morning diseases' such as azoturia and lymphangitis.

When hard work is in progress, blood is in great demand in the muscles and is therefore drawn away from the digestive system. Fast work also calls for greater use of the diaphragm to assist in the maximum intake of air. Since the stomach presses against the diaphragm, it is important that it is relatively empty when the horse is working. It is therefore usual not to do work for at least an hour after feeding.

Exercise must be built up slowly so that the horse can cope efficiently with the demands without 'running up light' or getting 'tucked up'. (These terms are explained later in the chapter.) Each horse has its own physical limits and special talents. It is up to the owner to get the greatest benefit from each individual animal.

The horse must get proper rest as well as exercise. This principle is well understood in racing yards, with their afternoon 'siesta' period of quiet in the yard. Stabled horses generally enjoy a rest during the day. A comfortable bed and a peaceful and orderly yard will encourage this. The natural pattern of about three hours' grazing, followed by a rest of up to two hours, is the ideal for good digestion and food utilisation.

Protection

The wild horse has natural grease in its coat to protect it from the weather, and it can seek shelter from the prevailing wind and from flies. In a field, the horse either has the grease left in its coat or is provided with at least a New Zealand rug to keep out the wet. It may also be provided with a field shelter. The stabled horse is not free to wander, and if there is a draught in the stable the horse cannot escape it. Inadequate bedding will cause the horse to bruise itself and get cold and damp when it lies down. A stabled horse that feels chilly or stiff cannot take exercise to stimulate the circulation, ease the joints and keep itself warm. If its circulation is sluggish and its legs start to fill, the stabled horse relies on its keeper for its exercise. The horse owner must accept full responsibility for his or her animal's exercise, warmth and protection.

Peace of mind

In order to maintain health in the horse, its peace of mind must be considered. This subject is not yet well documented or researched, but common sense and consideration are the keynotes.

The horse is a herd animal which seeks refuge in flight. The herd has natural leaders who insist on discipline and obedience, and within the herd the mares will require these things of their foals. By observing horses, the owner can learn how best to treat them.

The horse tends to do better with company, regular routine, fair punishment when it does wrong, and reward when it does right, with consistency being the most important factor.

Feeding

In order for a horse to remain healthy it is vital that he receives adequate amounts of a balanced diet and free access to clean, fresh water. The domesticated horse is entirely dependent on us for all his nutrition and we must ensure that we provide what he needs. Feeding and nutrition are discussed in more detail in Chapters 8, 18 and 19.

Routine preventive medicine

The artificial lifestyle of modern horses has made them vulnerable to large internal parasite burdens and exposed them to infectious and contagious diseases that would not otherwise affect them. Part of keeping horses healthy is to protect them against these conditions by following well-planned worming and vaccination programmes. In the UK horses should be vaccinated against equine influenza and tetanus; tetanus toxoid is given by intramuscular injection in two doses four to six weeks apart, followed by revaccination after one year and subsequently every one to three years. Mares should receive a booster one month before foaling to help protect the foal. The foal should then be inoculated with toxoid at about two, three and six months of age and boosted after one year. If the vaccination history of an injured horse is not known tetanus antitoxin should be given to prevent infection.

Many competitions demand that participating horses have evidence of an up-to-date vaccination programme against equine influenza; the basic programme is an initial injection, followed by a booster at about four to six weeks and a further booster at six months, followed by annual injections. This protects horses to a large degree and helps prevent 'flu epidemics.

Conformation

Conformation is the horse's inherited structure. Beauty is said to be 'in the eye of the beholder' and some people watching the judging of a show class may wonder if conformation is equally difficult to define. Conformation is certainly a matter of opinion, but if we agree on what is meant by conformation, then the horseman can build up mental pictures and a list of criteria.

Conformation has two main aspects. The first is the shape of the horse and is called *static conformation*. The second aspect is the way the horse moves, and is called *dynamic conformation*. The horse's performance, in terms of speed, endurance, jumping ability, agility, and so on, is not generally included in conformation. Temperament factors, such as obedience, kindness and generosity, are taken into slight consideration when assessing dynamic conformation. The important factor is that the horse should conform to a pattern proved over the years to produce the best performance, and not be predisposed to weakness, illness or disease. Consideration of conformation is thus an essential part of the attention given to maintaining a healthy horse.

'Good conformation' in various types of horse can be seen in the show ring. First impressions are very important and, although turnout can help, the discerning eye will concentrate on the shape of the skeleton and of the muscle clothing it.

Static conformation

The head
The head must be in proportion to the size of the horse. If it is too big, the horse will always tend to be on its forehand. The rounded convex profile of a Roman nose may indicate common blood and a dished profile may be a sign of Arab blood. The lower and upper jaws should meet evenly at the front, so the lips should be drawn back to check. If the upper jaw is too long, the horse is said to be 'parrot mouthed', and this is an unsoundness. Conversely it may be 'sow mouthed', when the lower jaw is too long. The terms 'overshot' and 'undershot' are confused in some textbooks and so are best avoided. In either case the fault will affect the horse's ability to bite food such as grass, but not its ability to chew.

Experience suggests that a bold eye indicates a generous spirit and a small 'piggy' eye may indicate meanness. The eyes should be set well out at the side of the head, and be clear, large and prominent. An excess of white in the eye suggests the possibility of an excitable and ill-tempered nature. Lop ears are not a fault, although such horses may need more encouragement.

Next to size, the most important aspect of the head is the way it is set on to the neck. There must be adequate clearance between the wing of the top bone in the neck and the branch of the lower jaw. This clearance should be sufficient to take two fingers when the horse's head is raised, and it must not restrict the flexion at the poll when it is brought into a position where the front of the face runs vertically, as in the collected gaits. The horse must not be fleshy around the jowl. The muzzle should be fine, with thin lips and sound and regular incisor teeth. The nostrils should be large.

The neck

A long neck goes with elegance, and a shorter, heavily muscled one with strength. From the rider's point of view it is not comfortable to have 'the horse's head in one's lap', and the judge of a ridden horse assesses the horse's 'front' as much from the saddle as from the side. If the neck dips down in front of the withers, the horse is 'ewe-necked', and this makes it more difficult to achieve the desirable steady head carriage, with flexion at the poll and a relaxed lower jaw. There should be an unbroken curve from the poll to the withers.

The withers

The withers should be of good height and well defined. Withers which are too high can make fitting a saddle very difficult, while low thick withers are associated with deficient action and poor mobility of the shoulder and problems with keeping the saddle in place.

The shoulder

The shoulder starts at the withers with the cartilage extension of the shoulder blade or scapula, which runs forward to the point of the shoulder (see Fig. 1.8). The line from the withers to the point of the shoulder is known as the slope of the shoulder. The slope of the shoulder and the angle made by the pastern to the ground should be about the same. Thus a horse with a slightly upright shoulder would be expected to have rather upright pasterns; this helps evenly distribute the forces down the limb. An upright shoulder gives a short stride and the front legs will show wear more quickly. A good sloping shoulder is necessary. From the point of the shoulder the upper arm

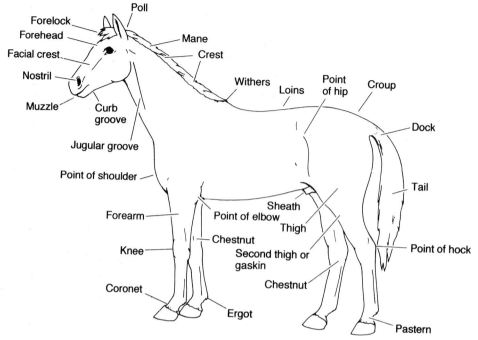

Fig. 1.8 Points of the horse.

bone or humerus runs down and back to the elbow. In the riding horse the whole shoulder should be well muscled and yet without heaviness.

The front legs
The forearm should be well muscled from the elbow, and length is required for speed. The knee is a box of bones, each separated by shock-absorbing cartilage. Knees should be broad and flat in front. (See Fig. 1.9) The fault of 'calf knees' means they are shallow from front to back. The leg should not appear to be 'tied in' as if the horse were wearing tight stockings restricting the tendons below the knee.

The measurement around the leg just below the knee is used to define the amount of 'bone' the animal has. This measurement includes the tendons. Common-bred horses will have more bone. The normal aim is to combine quality with good bone. As a rough guide, in a horse of 16.2 hands there should be over 20 cm (8 in) of bone for a lightweight and over 23 cm (9 in) for a heavyweight.

When viewed from the front and side, the knee joint should be straight. Viewed from the side, if the knee is slightly forward of the line

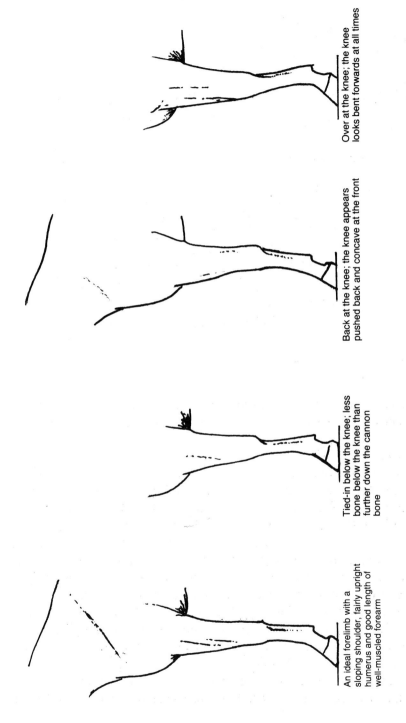

An ideal forelimb with a sloping shoulder, fairly upright humerus and good length of well-muscled forearm

Tied-in below the knee; less bone below the knee than further down the cannon bone

Back at the knee; the knee appears pushed back and concave at the front

Over at the knee; the knee looks bent forwards at all times

Fig. 1.9 The front leg (side view) showing the ideal and three less than ideal examples – tied in below the knee, back at the knee and over at the knee.

from the elbow to the top of the pastern, the horse is 'over at the knee'. The reverse case of 'back at the knee' is to be avoided as the strain on the tendons may prove too great.

The cannon bones should be rather short and flat in front, with the tendons standing out cleanly at the back. This ensures that the tendons are short and less liable to damage. The slope of the pastern is important: too much slope puts too great a strain on the tendons, and too little creates excess concussion and leads to foot troubles (see Fig. 1.10).

The feet must be good. 'No foot no horse' is a true adage. Upright feet are called 'boxy' and are to be avoided. Flat feet are equally undesirable. The angle of the hoof wall should be such that it continues the line of the pastern. There should be a good frog on the underside of the foot, and the bars and the heel of the hoof must be wide and deep. Any irregularity of the feet may cause or be the result of foot trouble. The front legs should be checked from the front to see

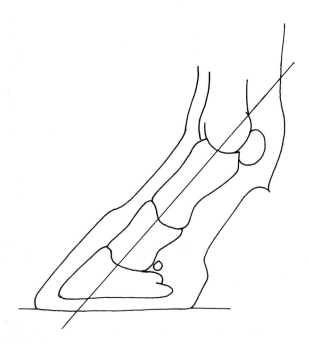

Fig. 1.10 Good hoof-pastern angle. The pedal, long pastern and short pastern bones are correctly aligned and run parallel to the hoof wall and heel.

if they are upright and straight from the body right into the feet. The horse must not be knock-kneed or bandy. The feet should face the front and not be turned in ('pigeon toed'), turned out or be 'splay footed' (see Fig. 1.11).

The chest and barrel

A deep, full chest with long, 'well-sprung' ribs is essential to provide good lung- and heart-room. (See Fig. 1.12.) A horse with flat ribs is 'slab sided'. A horse of 16 hands or more should have a girth that exceeds 1.83 m (6 ft). The front legs must have clear space between

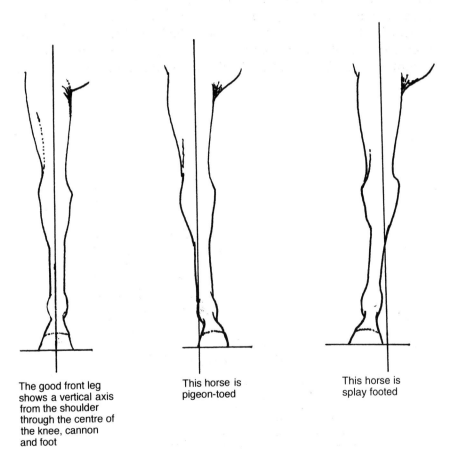

The good front leg shows a vertical axis from the shoulder through the centre of the knee, cannon and foot

This horse is pigeon-toed

This horse is splay footed

Fig. 1.11 The front leg (front view) showing a good front leg, pigeon toes and splay footed. It should be noted that poor alignment and turning in or out are *not* the same; a horse's leg can have good alignment yet a toe turned in or out with the rotation starting at any joint.

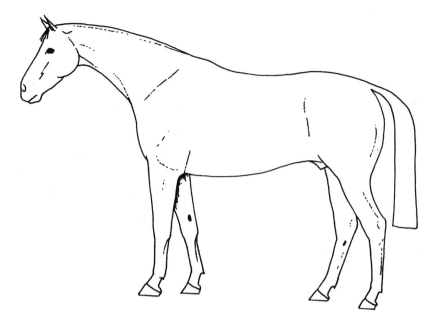

Fig. 1.12 A well-defined wither and a strong back supported by a deep chest and well-sprung ribs.

them and not 'come out of one hole'. On the other hand, if the chest is too wide, it may produce a rolling action.

The back may be dipped or hollow from old age or from lack of good conformation. A 'roach back' is one curved upwards and might make saddle-fitting difficult (see Fig. 1.13). The back should also be checked with a saddle to see whether the horse sinks under the rider's weight when first mounted or even when girthing up. Such a horse is said to be 'cold backed'.

Good lung- and heart-room is the first essential of the body, which must not be weak over the loins. The first eight pairs of ribs connect up to the breast bone and are called 'true ribs'. The next ten pairs of ribs are connected by long cartilage extensions to the breast bone and they are known as 'false ribs'. Some horses have a nineteenth rib on one or both sides. The rearmost ribs must come close to the point of hip so that the horse is 'well ribbed up'. A wide distance between the last rib and the point of hip makes a horse 'slack in the loins', and such a horse is sometimes described as 'short of a rib'.

It is a weakness when the underline of the horse slopes up from front to back (described as being 'herring gutted') (see Fig. 1.14). This

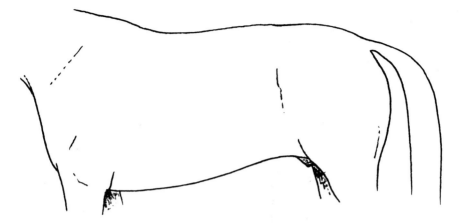

Fig. 1.13 A roach back.

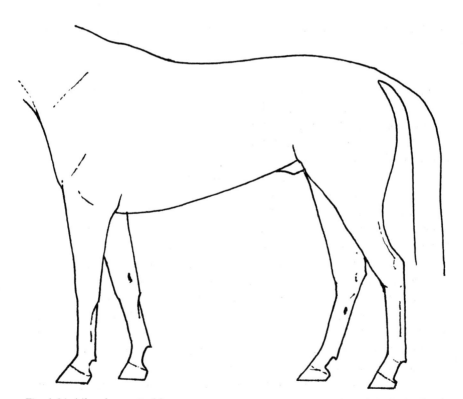

Fig. 1.14 A herring-gutted horse.

fault may cause the girth to slip back. The underline of the horse may also vary according to the diet and degree of fitness. A horse at grass normally has a very full gut and may even be 'pot-bellied'. After stress, there may be a tightening of the abdominal muscles for several hours and the horse is accurately described as 'tucked up'. This is not the same as 'run up light', which denotes the overall leanness which may go with hard training, hard work or lack of food.

The top line of the horse should be such that, once the horse is fully grown, the withers are higher than the croup. In a young horse the croup is often higher, but if this persists into maturity, the horse will ride 'down hill' and tend to be on its forehand.

The hindquarters
The powerhouse of the horse lies behind the saddle and so one looks on the quarters for good flat muscle which reaches well down into the hind leg (see Fig. 1.15). A high croup is called a 'jumping bump'. A 'goose rump' is one with the tail set low down and the quarters drooping downwards (see Fig. 1.16). Horses with 'goose rumps' are thought to lack speed. Good speed is expected from horses with plenty of length from the point of hip to the hocks; thus one may refer to 'well-let-down hocks'. The horse must not appear split up the middle when viewed from behind; the thigh muscles of the hind legs must be well developed on the inside of these limbs. The human knee joint is the equivalent of the horse's stifle joint: both have a patella or kneecap. With a human runner we note good muscle development above and below the knee; so with the horse we look for good development of the gaskin or second thigh muscles, which run from the stifle to the hock.

Hocks must not point towards each other (a fault described as being 'cow hocked') nor must they be 'bowed out' (see Fig. 1.17). They must not be over bent so that the cannon bones slant ('sickle hocked'). The hock joint should be large but not fleshy. The line from the point of hock down the back of the leg should be vertical and should not bulge outwards over the hock joint. A bulge of this sort is called a 'curb' and is usually caused by strain on the tendon at the back of the hock. The bulge could also be caused by enlarged heads of the splint bones and is then called a 'false curb'. Curbs are considered a sign of weakness, but generally give little trouble once they have formed on the young horse. The vertical line below the hock should, when the horse is standing squarely, line up with the rearmost part of its quarters (point of the buttock). The comments concerning the lower forelimb apply equally to the lower hindlimb.

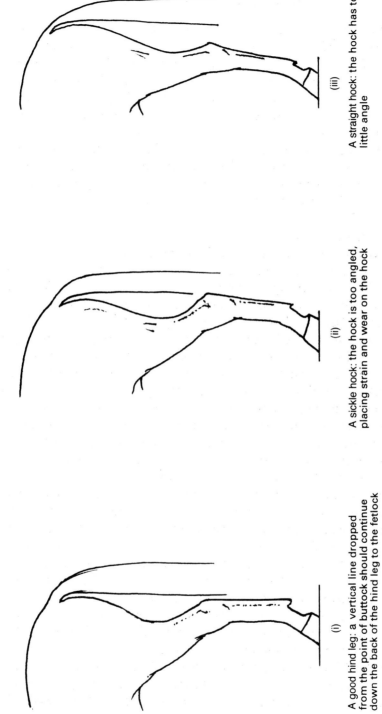

(i)

A good hind leg: a vertical line dropped
from the point of buttock should continue
down the back of the hind leg to the fetlock

(ii)

A sickle hock: the hock is too angled,
placing strain and wear on the hock

(iii)

A straight hock: the hock has too
little angle

Fig. 1.15 The hindquarters viewed from the side. (i) A good hind leg. (ii) A sickle hock. (iii) A straight hock.

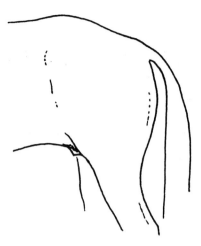

Fig. 1.16 A goose rump.

Dynamic conformation
The walk and trot should be checked both in hand and under saddle.

The walk
The walk is a symmetrical gait with a four time beat. The horse's feet follow one another in the following sequence: off hind, off fore, near hind, near fore (see Fig. 1.18). Regular steps of even length are required. The footprint of the front foot should be studied to see whether the back foot comes on to it (tracking up), or, correctly, goes beyond it (overtracking). The amount by which it overtracks should be noted. A good walker will give the impression that it is going somewhere in a purposeful manner. The walk is a difficult pace to improve. A good walker is generally a good galloper. The way the shoes are worn gives clues as to how the horse uses its feet.

The trot
The trot is a two-time gait with the legs moving in diagonal pairs (near hind, off fore and off hind and near fore), and when there is any extension there is a moment of suspension between each beat (see Fig. 1.19). The horse should be trotted towards the observer, then on past and away from him or her. The action of the front legs should be noted. A straight action is best. To swing the feet out from the knee or fetlock joint is called 'dishing' and is unsightly and energy wasting although it is not harmful. Any action that brings one foot up too close to the other leg, which could result in 'brushing' or, if higher, in

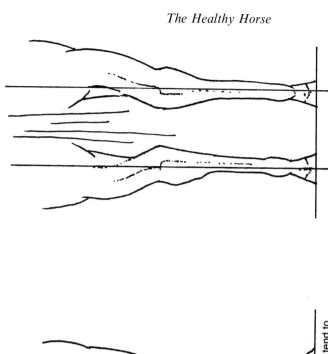

In a good hind limb a vertical line dropped from the point of buttock passes through the centre of the hock, cannon bone, fetlock and foot

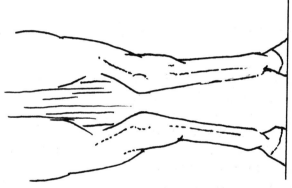

Cow hocks turn in and the feet tend to turn out

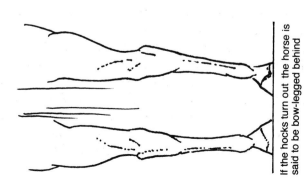

If the hocks turn out the horse is said to be bow-legged behind

Fig. 1.17 The hocks viewed from behind.

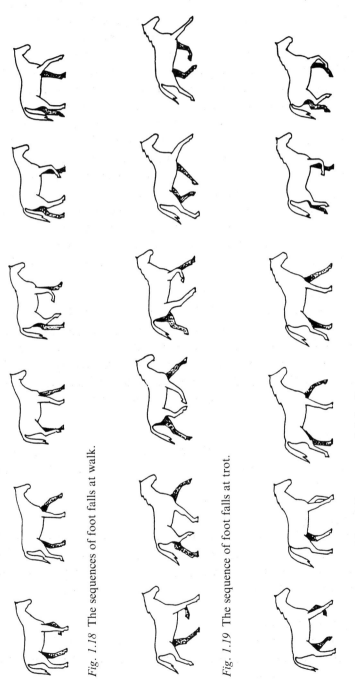

Fig. 1.18 The sequences of foot falls at walk.

Fig. 1.19 The sequence of foot falls at trot.

Fig. 1.20 The sequence of foot falls at canter (left lead).

'speedy cutting', is to be avoided. The hind feet often pass close by each other and one can check the hair on the inside of the hind fetlock joints. If it is rubbed, the horse may require Yorkshire boots or other protection. When the horse trots, any tendency to 'forge' should be listened for. Forging is the hind shoe striking the fore shoe. Both forging and over-reaching can be helped by shoeing. Viewed from the side, the strides of the left diagonal, near fore and off hind, should be the same length as the right diagonal. The amount of knee action required depends on fashion and use. However, where knee action is required (as with some driving and draught horses), the animal must still cover the ground well. The show horse tends to push its foot out a long way, and then drops it vertically down the last few inches. A good riding horse will push its toe out well without any exaggeration of movement. It will not land heavily on its heels. A free moving shoulder with no sign of cramped or restricted movement when the horse is asked to lengthen the trot is desirable. A supple back and well-engaged hindquarters, with freely, evenly flexing hocks, are needed.

The canter
This gait is in three time, followed by a moment of suspension (see Fig. 1.20). If cantering to the right, the sequence of footfalls is left hind, left fore and right hind together and right fore. Balance comes from the hind legs coming well under the horse. The young or newly broken horse may find it difficult to canter in a confined area. At the canter one can also listen for soundness of the wind.

The gallop
Some horses achieve the rhythm of the gallop but seem to be 'going into the ground'. Look for the horse that achieves both speed and lightness.

The step back
When checking soundness, the horse is asked by its handler to step back on the ground and also to turn in tight circles to left and right. These movements may reveal any stiffness or other problems. Conformation and soundness are relative to each other.

Legal unsoundness
Unsoundness is a question of usefulness and not of disease. The position in English law was stated in the 19th century case of *Coates* v. *Stephens* in this way:

The rule as to unsoundness is, if at the time of sale or examination, the horse has any disease, which either actually does diminish the natural usefulness of the animal, so as to make him less capable of work of any description, or which in its ordinary course will diminish its natural usefulness; or if that horse has, either from disease (whether such disease be congenital, or arising subsequently to birth) or from accident has undergone any alteration of structure that either does at the time or in its ordinary course will diminish the natural usefulness of the horse, such horse is unsound.

Despite the antique flavour of the judicial language, this is still the legal position today.

The Royal College of Veterinary Surgeons and the British Veterinary Association try to discourage their members from using the word 'sound'. This is because the veterinary profession had become increasingly anxious over the years at the way in which Baron Parkes' famous definition of soundness was being interpreted by the courts. It is one thing to ascertain if a horse has, at the present time, a disease or a defect which diminishes its natural usefulness. It is quite another to be certain whether it has some latent or minor defect or disease condition which, in its ordinary progress, will diminish its natural usefulness in the future.

Moreover, with all the sophisticated diagnostic aids available today, it is an open question as to the lengths in effort, time and expense to which the vet must go in order to discover the presence of some defect or disease condition which is not ascertainable on an ordinary clinical examination.

As a result, vets now have a recommended form of examination of a horse for a purchaser, after which they are advised to conclude that the horse is or is not suitable for purchase for a particular use, e.g. as a child's pony, an eventer or whatever. The vet's certificate is given to the intending purchaser, and not to the vendor – and is related to the purchaser's specific intentions regarding the horse's use.

The most suitable horse or pony

After considering all the aspects of conformation, both static and dynamic, one must put all the factors into the balance to make a judgement. A buyer will certainly consider price. One guide to the potential of a young horse is the achievement of both parents and even grandparents, but the performance record of siblings (brothers and sisters) and other progeny of either parent should also be taken into consideration.

Most important of all, however, in choosing a competition horse will be two factors – athleticism and good character.

2   The Sick Horse

There are four main types of ill health. The first has *physical causes*, e.g. an injury resulting from an accident. The second type has *physiological causes*, e.g. the improper function of one part of the body. The third type of disorder arises from *nutritional causes*, which may be due to a deficiency in diet or to the ingestion of a poison, such as contaminated food or a poisonous plant. The fourth type of ill health is caused by an *invasion* of the horse's body by a living organism.

The invaders

The invaders of the horse can be broadly divided into two groups: micro-organisms (Fig. 2.1) and parasites, both internal and external (Fig. 2.2). The infection of a horse by one of these invaders leads to a battle between two sides – the micro-organisms or parasites and the horse. The reactions of the horse to the presence of the infecting agent are the symptoms of the disease. Early recognition of these symptoms is important so that the vet can be called in time for treatment to be effective. It is also helpful to understand the way in which these organisms invade the horse so that logical and effective control measures can be taken.

Microbial infection

Infectious diseases are caused by tiny living organisms, called micro-organisms because we need a microscope to be able to see them. The micro-organisms capable of causing disease are said to be pathogenic. Bacteria are micro-organisms and many are pathogenic, however, there are millions of bacteria within the horse's gut which play an important role in digestion and are beneficial to the horse.

Invasions by micro-organisms tend to follow a similar pattern, the organism enters the body through the mouth (by being swallowed),

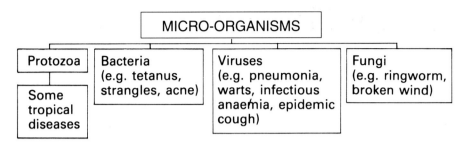

Fig. 2.1 Micro-organisms that invade the horse.

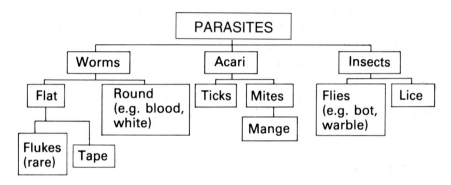

Fig. 2.2 Parasites that invade the horse.

through the nostrils (by being inhaled) through the skin, along the urinary tract, via the genitals or through the eyes. When these organisms enter the body, each cell divides and subdivides until there are millions of germs entrenched in the host. Only then do they make their presence felt and produce symptoms of disease. The time between infection and development of symptoms is called *the incubation period*: it may be a few hours or several months.

Some of these micro-organisms may find themselves in unsuitable circumstances; they then grow a thick protective coat and become spores. These are very hard to kill and can exist for years waiting for a suitable host. Once inside the host some micro-organisms invade the whole body; others stay localised in one organ. They vary in their ability to invade, persist and multiply, and this ability is called their *virulence*. Bacteria with a low virulence will cause a local infection such as an abscess, whereas one with a high virulence may invade the bloodstream and cause septicaemia (blood poisoning). Horses will be susceptible to certain micro-organisms but not to others; for example, horses cannot catch flu from humans.

Many bacteria and viruses produce poisons, called *toxins*, and these may spread through the body. When attacked, the host starts its defence programme against both the invaders and the toxins. The animal is said to suffer an *acute attack* when its defences are inadequate and the disease is severe. If the defence is slow to react and merely holds the disease without overcoming it, the disease is *chronic*, i.e. longer lasting at a lower level.

The skin is the first line of defence. The second line of defence is the white blood cells, which engulf bacteria and destroy them. This defence programme may cause inflammation and the production of pus, which is formed from the dead combatants. In addition to white cells, the body can develop other defence agents, called *antibodies* which can combat only one type of invader. These are produced by the animal only when it encounters that particular micro-organism. Further defence agents, called *antitoxins*, are produced to cope with the toxins produced by the invading micro-organisms. An animal is said to be *immune* to a disease when it has suffered it and has produced the specific defence agents to combat that disease. Such acquired immunity is of variable duration; in some cases it may be life-long.

Some disease-causing micro-organisms can be cultivated in a laboratory and then killed and let into the host, which acquires immunity once it has produced the necessary antibodies. The dead micro-organisms are prepared as a *vaccine*; being dead, they cannot multiply and thus they are easily overcome by the host, causing only minor symptoms.

For some diseases, dead micro-organisms will not achieve the desired effect, so the vaccine is prepared with live micro-organisms which have been weakened. In some cases, it may be necessary to repeat the process of vaccination initially after a short interval and then at regular, long-term intervals thereafter.

The vaccine may be injected or inoculated by scratching the skin, according to type. For some diseases, modified toxins are used in vaccines. The host takes time to develop immunity after vaccination, and so if immediate protection is needed, blood serum will be injected. This will have been taken from an animal with a very strong built-up immunity so that the serum contains antibodies specific to the disease. The protection from this *hyperimmune serum* is only temporary. Foals acquire a similar temporary immunity from their mothers through colostrum.

Sometimes a situation demands both an immediate and a longer-lasting protection. This can be provided by a dose containing both hyperimmune serum and vaccine.

The invaders can be attacked externally by the use of both disinfectants and antiseptics. Disinfectants tend to be stronger and more aggressive and thus are usually used to destroy micro-organisms on equipment or housing, as opposed to the body of the horse. The term 'antiseptics' tends to be reserved for products that may only stop micro-organisms multiplying, but they can safely be used on infected wounds as they will not inhibit healing.

An antibiotic is a chemical substance, such as penicillin, which kills bacteria or stops them multiplying. Sulpha drugs may also be used to

Table 2.1 (a) Invasion by micro-organisms, (b) animal invaders.

(a) Invasion by micro-organisms.

Disease	Cause	Symptoms
Ringworm	Ringworm fungus	Circular patches of raised hair, going bald
Broken wind	Fungus (an allergic reaction)	Cough, respiratory problems
Fungal abortion	Fungus	Abortion
Lockjaw	Tetanus bacterial toxin	Spasms, stretched-out stance
Strangles	Specific bacteria	Nasal discharge and abscesses between jaw bones and in neck glands
Poll evil and fistulous withers	Brucellosis bacteria	Infection of the relevant areas
Acne	Bacteria	Roughened skin with sores
Contagious equine metritis (CEM)	Contagious equine metritis bacillus	Discharge from the vulva
Pneumonia	Bacterial and viral infections	Inflamed lungs, fever
Influenza (epidemic cough)	A specific influenza virus with three main strains identified	Cough, loss of appetite, nasal discharge and fever
Cold	Cold viruses	Cough and running nose
Swamp fever (infectious anaemia)	Specific virus	Fever, debilitation (*Note*: horses for export may have to be checked by Coggins test)
Warts	Papova virus	Small skin growths
Angleberries (sarcoids)	Papova virus	Nasty growths which tend to spread and bleed
Spots or pox (coital exanthema)	Herpes virus	Sores on vulva or penis

(b) Animal invaders.

Disease	Cause	Symptoms
Ticks	Ticks	Irriation
Mange	Mites	Intense itching, scabs and loss of hair
Ear mange	Ear mites	Head shaking and restlessness
Autumn itching	Harvest mites	Restlessness, stamping, scabby legs
Lice	Lice (lice eggs = nits)	Irritation, possible hair loss, unthriftiness
Bots	Bot flies	Unthriftiness
Warbles	Warble flies	Swellings on the back in early summer
Fluke	Liver fluke	Unthriftiness, lack of growth, anaemia
Tapeworm	Tapeworm	Unthriftiness
Whiteworms	*Ascarids*	Lack of growth and lung damage in foals.
Seatworms	*Oxyuris*	Irritation causing tail rubbing
Lungworms	*Dictyocaulus*	Coughing
Bloodworms	Redworms (*Strongylus*)	Colic, unthriftiness, anaemia, poor coat

inhibit the activity of bacteria and are used to treat some bacterial infections. It is important to use specific antibiotics at the correct dose and for a prescribed length of time to avoid bacteria becoming resistant to common antibiotics. Viruses are not affected by antibiotics and viral diseases can prove very difficult to control.

Table 2.1(a) shows that disease may be caused not only by bacteria and viruses but also by fungi. These may be on the surface of the skin, e.g. ringworm, or elsewhere, e.g. on the lining of the lungs or other parts of the respiratory tract, or in the genital tract.

Animal invasion
Parasites come mainly from the animal kingdom and include acari (such as ticks and mites), together with insects (such as lice). Because these attack the outside of the horse they are called *ectoparasites*. Flies come within the insect group. They lay eggs on horses and the eggs hatch into larvae which continue their life cycle within the horse as *endoparasites*. The horse is also troubled with worms, including flatworms (such as liver fluke and tapeworms), and roundworms, the latter being the horse's greatest enemy.

Symptoms of disease

A symptom is an indication that something is wrong. It is a warning sign that should prompt investigation.

Behaviour
The first sign of disease is often a change in behaviour – anything which is different to that horse's normal pattern. The person in charge of the horse must ask himself the cause for the horse's change in behaviour. Is this attributable to external events, or to something in the creature's body or mind?

A mare about to foal, or a horse with colic, may display similar symptoms. Any abnormal activities should be noticed. The horse is normally alert and interested: any dullness or lack of zest should be regarded as a warning sign. It may be an indication of pain or of something else.

Appetite
A horse that does not hurry to the manger or finish a meal should always be regarded with suspicion. The horse may chew the food and let some slip back out, or it may have difficulty in swallowing. The cause may be in the food or in the manger, but it may be in the horse's mouth or in its digestive system. A stabled horse that drinks more or less water than usual should be similarly regarded, although it is to be expected that a horse will feel more thirsty on hot days or after sweating.

Action
When the horse is free in the field or turning round in the stable, or being ridden or driven, telltale signs may be evident. For example, the ears may suddenly flick back or the tail may be clamped down. The horse may grunt when mounted or be unwilling to go forward. Its stride may be uneven or it may be lame. It may rest a leg when standing in the stable but this is generally suspicious only if it is a front leg.

When the horse resists going forward, it is one of the most difficult decisions that the horseman has to make as to whether the animal is being stubborn or nappy, or whether it is in pain for some reason, or finds movement physically difficult or frightening. The horseman's great dilemma is to know when to punish and when to be understanding; when to encourage and when to be firm.

Coat

A harsh, 'staring', dull, tight coat is unnatural and is usually a sign that something is wrong. The coat should be soft and move freely over the muscles. Except when the horse is cold, the hairs should lie flat and the coat should gleam. Rough or raised patches, rubbed hair or any local differences in one area should be watched out for. The horse should also be checked for cuts, wounds, splinters and bruises.

Respiration

Changes in respiration may be noticed in the stable or the field. The respiration rate will rise during fever and infection. Respiration type is also significant; shallow and rapid breathing is characteristic of infections of the respiratory tract. Respiration rate will be affected by the environment, rising in hotter and more humid conditions.

There may be a cough when the horse is feeding or working, and it is important that the circumstances and type of cough should be noted to assist in the diagnosis. The horse may make a noise when galloping. It is important to note if the noise is made by air going into or coming out of the lungs, as explained in Chapter 6.

Temperature

Whenever the horse is thought to be unwell, its temperature should be taken as this gives one of the most useful guides. An above-normal temperature accompanies all cases of acute disease to a greater or lesser extent. It will also indicate fever, a local infection, such as an abscess or one caused by the presence of a thorn, and pain, whether acute or general.

A fall in temperature is characteristic of loss of blood, starvation, collapse, coma, hypothermia and some chronic diseases. An abnormal temperature indicates that the vet should be called.

Pulse

The pulse rate is a useful aid to diagnosis and to help determine fitness. The pulse rate at rest rises in cases of fever and acute pain; it falls in debilitating diseases.

Dung and urine

If the faeces are too hard, or too soft, strong smelling or slimy, all is not well within the digestive tract. Urine of unusual colour, cloudiness or smell may be a sign that problems are developing.

Eyes

A dull eye or one that is half closed is an indication that the horse may be feeling unwell. A special watch should be kept for damage to the eye. The inner side of the eyelid is a useful membrane to study, as it will change colour according to the condition of the blood. The gums may also be studied similarly. Healthy horses must be examined regularly so that any changes become apparent quickly.

Lumps, bumps and swellings

It is easy to find swellings on horses when grooming them; it is much harder to notice such things on animals in the field.

Swellings by the jaw bone may indicate glandular disorder. The inside of the mouth should be checked occasionally for ulcers and sores. When unaccustomed tack or clothing comes into use, particular care should be taken until the skin has hardened. A sore or rub is more easily dealt with if detected in the early stages. Where there is swelling, it should be checked for heat, and bruising, strains, thorns and infection should be considered.

A watchful eye should be kept on the legs; the tendons that go down the back of each lower leg should stand out clearly. Slight filling, or puffiness round the fetlock joint, is a danger sign which must not be ignored. The cause might be a knock the day before, a strain, exercise on hard ground, or being shut in the stable too long. The first essential is to note the symptom; the second essential is to realise its significance.

Discharges

A runny nose is the common first symptom of a cough or cold but it may have other meanings, particularly if only one nostril is affected. Discharges may appear at any of the body's other orifices: eyes, ears, anus, vulva, sheath or teats. Each discharge will have its own particular meaning.

First aid

If the problem is of a minor nature, it may well be dealt with using the equipment kept in the stable yard. With this in mind a complete and readily accessible first aid kit should always be available. When preparing a first aid kit bear in mind that its main role is to deal with minor injuries such as superficial cuts and grazes, kicks, thorns, overreaches and wire cuts or to care for the horse before the vet arrives.

First-aid kit

The best place to keep a first-aid kit is in the tack or feed room on top of the medicine chest, which should be kept locked. A second kit may be needed for travelling. As the human first-aid kit could to advantage stand beside it, the container for the horse's kit should be clearly marked, for example, 'First Aid – Horse'.

A clean bowl is often required, and so a useful container for the first-aid kit is a large plastic bowl with a well-fitting lid. The vet's name and telephone number should be clearly written on the inside of the lid. A clean cloth serves as a cover-all inside the bowl and is useful for covering a small table or straw bale when the contents are laid out. The kit might include the following, which should conveniently fill the bowl:

- Bowl for antiseptic solution.
- Cloth upon which the kit can be laid.
- Antiseptics for cleaning wounds, e.g. Savlon, Pevidine. A ready diluted antiseptic solution is useful in the travelling kit.
- Wound powder or spray for use if the wound is left open. These prevent infection and dry wound. Examples are Acrimide, which is antibacterial, and Aureomycin, which is antibiotic. In summer a fly-repellent powder is useful.
- Antiseptic ointment for cracked heels and mud fever and a healing cream, e.g. Dermisol, to put on the dressing before bandaging a wound.
- Clean crepe bandages for support and slight pressure and adhesive bandages to hold dressings in place.
- Sterile non-adherent dressings to place over a wound before bandaging.
- Cotton wool for cleaning wounds.
- Curved, blunt-ended scissors for cutting hair from the wound and straight scissors for cutting tapes and bandages.
- Ready-to-use poultice in sealed pack, e.g. Animalintex.
- Veterinary thermometer and Vaseline.
- Forceps or tweezers to remove thorns and splinters from wounds.
- The travelling kit should also contain money for a telephone call.

Expendable items must be replaced as used. The contents must be kept scrupulously clean. Many of these items may be purchased from the vet.

As well as the first-aid kit there should be a medicine cupboard. Its contents are largely a matter of personal preference but the following list may be helpful:

- Cling film or plastic bags as backing to poultices.
- Gamgee for padding under bandage (but baby's nappy roll is just as effective and less expensive).
- Antiseptic or 'purple spray', coloured with gentian violet which has antifungal properties. If it contains antibiotics the shelf life will be limited. Use with care as the horse may take fright or kick at the noise.
- Udder cream to protect heels.
- Wormers.
- Cooling lotion, gel or clay.
- Prepared poultice dressing pack.
- Icepack.
- Fly repellant.
- Stable bandages and crepe bandages.
- Eye ointment and bottle of human eye wash.
- Germicidal shampoo or soap for skin infections.
- Hoof care preparation.
- Witch hazel lotion or gel.
- Salt to clean wounds.
- Liniment or cream rub for sore muscles.

Types of wound
Horses are very prone to injury through falls, kicks, bites, hitting jumps and getting tangled in fences. The wound sustained may be classified as open or closed: open wounds involve skin damage while closed wounds include bruises, sprains or ruptures.

Open wounds can be further classified as incised wounds, lacerated wounds, puncture wounds or abrasions.

Incised wounds
These wounds have clean straight edges and often bleed freely. Usually there is little bruising and they normally heal quite quickly. Incised wounds are caused by surgical incisions or cuts by metal or glass.

Lacerations and tears

These wounds have torn edges and an irregular shape, with some bruising. The amount of bleeding will be variable depending on the position of the wound. Frequently there are torn flaps of skin which will probably die before the wound heals. Lacerated wounds are caused by barbed wire, protruding nails and other hazards.

Puncture wounds

These wounds tend to be more serious than they look; the skin opening may be small but the flesh can be penetrated to a varying depth. Puncture wounds are caused by bites, stakes and treading on nails and splinters; bacteria are carried deep into the wound, leading to infection. The skin wound may be so small that it is overlooked. If you are not sure of the horse's vaccination status the horse should be given an antitetanus injection by the vet. The wound must be treated so that it heals from the inside out, which usually involves poulticing the wound to draw out any infection.

Abrasions

These are very superficial skin wounds, such as saddle sores or grazes from falling.

Closed wounds

These include injuries such as bruises, sprains, muscle damage and tendon strain. There is usually internal bleeding without breaking the skin, leading to swelling, heat and pain. The area should be immobilised as much as possible and treated with cold hosing or ice packs. Once the heat has gone from the area heat treatments can be used to absorb excess fluid.

First-aid procedure

Safety

The horse must be controlled quietly but firmly. It is best to have it held by someone else and if it becomes fractious a bridle should be fitted for greater control. A restraining influence may be obtained by holding up a front leg. When examining a hind leg, it sometimes helps to hold the horse's tail firmly downwards. A horse may also be restrained by grasping a fold of skin on its neck. There is no point in either the horse or a handler being hurt, and if necessary a twitch should be used on the upper lip.

Simple methods of restraint are described in Chapter 10.

Calm

The attendants should talk reassuringly to the horse, pat and stroke it and work without fuss or bother. This will maintain a calm atmosphere. Thoroughness is more important than speed.

Blood control

There are three types of bleeding or haemorrhage. First, there is the blood around a cut from the tiny capillaries in the flesh; this is not serious. The second type flows gently and is dark red; it comes from the veins and is called venous bleeding. The third type is bright red and comes from an artery; the blood runs freely and may spurt out under pressure from the heartbeat. An injury involving bleeding of the first type can wait for treatment until return to the horse transport or stable. However, an injury involving venous and arterial bleeding calls for immediate treatment.

Venous bleeding can be controlled with a clean pad such as a folded handkerchief placed on the wound, and then securing the pad firmly over the wound using a bandage, tie, stock or belt. Slight bleeding actually helps clean the wound and a little blood goes a long way, so try not to panic.

Where arterial bleeding is dominant, the blood flow is more difficult to stop and veterinary attention is needed. While you are waiting for the vet to arrive apply very firm pressure by pressing a clean dressing to the wound. If the wound is on the horse's leg put a pressure bandage on over several layers of gamgee but take care that the bandage does not act as a tourniquet and cut off the blood supply. The bandage should be removed as soon as the bleeding stops. If the wound is not on a leg, it may be necessary to hold the pressure pad in place until help can be obtained. The horse should be kept warm and quiet until it is taken home for treatment. If the need arises, help must be summoned or the horse led to the nearest house, where transport can be arranged. If any doubt exists, the vet should be called as the wound may need suturing, and antitetanus protection may be required.

Cleanliness

A dirty wound should first be washed under a cold hose, although care must be taken not to frighten the horse. Hair is then cut away from the region of the wound. A piece of cotton wool soaked in antiseptic solution is applied, taking care to wipe dirt out and not rub it in. Each swab should be used once only, and should not be put back into the disinfectant solution. When the wound is clear, it is dried with a dry piece of cotton wool. Wound powder is then 'puffed on' lightly. Antiseptic cream is useful for sores and grazes. Where a dressing is required to keep out dirt, the wound is covered with gauze, preferably medicated, and a cotton wool pad is bandaged gently in place.

Healing

The healing process starts immediately after the injury has occurred; wounds can heal differently, depending on the site and the type of injury. Healing by first intention only occurs in non-contaminated incised wounds where the edges of the wound can be brought together and held closely with stitches or sutures. The stitches usually stay in for a minimum of ten days and should be protected with a bandage if possible.

Healing by second intention occurs in lacerated wounds and involves the wound contracting and the cells of the skin multiplying and migrating across the wound to form a scab and new tissue. Wounds on the body cause little scarring as the skin is loose and the wound can contract so that a minimum of new tissue has to be formed. The horse's limbs have little or no loose flesh and the new skin cells multiply excessively to form granulation tissue or proud flesh. This inhibits healing as the proud flesh prevents new skin from covering the wound. Proud flesh formation can be prevented by pressure bandaging and immobilising the wound as much as possible. Once proud flesh has formed it is removed by surgery or using caustic solutions.

Drugs

The vet may give the horse antibiotics, anti-inflammatories or painkillers depending on the severity and type of wound.

Choke

First aid is concerned principally with preventing death from loss of blood or, in rare cases, from failure to obtain air, which is called asphyxia; for example, a horse breathing very deeply after severe exertion is given food, which gets stuck in its larynx thus causing rapid death. If a horse is choking, it will appear distressed and keep trying to swallow; saliva will run from its mouth or nose. In such circumstances asphyxia is unlikely. The first task is to identify where the obstruction is. If it is lower than the pharynx, at the back of the throat, it will not greatly interfere with air intake. It may be possible to feel the obstruction in the gullet on the left side of the neck just behind the windpipe, which is the tube down the front of the throat. Massage may be effective in moving the obstruction. The horse should not be drenched, or it will be drowned by the fluid going into the lungs. If the obstruction is at the back of the throat, by holding the tongue out to the side it may be possible to put a hand into the mouth and remove the obstruction, although there is a risk of being bitten. In other cases the vet should be called.

Fractures
Where there is a suspected fracture of a leg, the horse should be restrained. A horse with a broken leg can be a very distressing sight, and while a vet is being summoned onlookers should be kept back and something used to screen the horse from view.

Principles of nursing

General
The first essential is to keep the horse comfortable and relaxed. If the horse is not getting exercise, the diet must be cut right back and should be such that it keeps the bowels working well. Cut grass can usefully be included in the feed, as can damp bran and other slightly laxative foods. Oats and barley should be avoided, but carrots and apples are beneficial. The horse should be kept warm with deep bedding, leg bandages and rugs as necessary, but with ample fresh air, without draughts.

If the horse breaks out into a sweat, it should be dried with an old towel and its ears should be 'stripped' by grasping them gently round the base and sliding the hand to the tip, working on each ear alternately.

The horse's drinking should be monitored and an automatic drinker should not be used. At feeding time, the sick horse should be dealt with last to avoid carrying infection. The horse's legs may fill if it is not being walked out. A thorough twice-daily massage to the legs will relieve this. Rubbing should be towards the heart, and stable bandages should then be applied immediately, bandaging upwards over padding. Provided its condition allows, the horse should be well groomed. A very sick horse may prefer a quick wipe over with a damp cloth, including nostrils, eyes, sheath and dock. When grooming, care should be taken not to let the horse get chilled. The top door may be shut and in winter an infra-red heat lamp may be used. However, it must always be remembered that fresh air and adequate ventilation are vital.

The instructions on all medications should be read with care and followed exactly. The vet's instructions should be carried out correctly too, so they should be carefully noted to avoid mistakes. As in hospital, a TPR chart with clinical notes should be kept.

Hygiene is important at all times, but especially so for the sick horse. The grooming kit and feed containers must be kept scrupulously clean and should not be used for any other horse. The coat and feet should receive 'better than ever' attention. All things used in connection with a sick animal should be kept away from the equipment for the other horses. It is also wise to wear a clean smock or work-coat when working with the sick horse.

The sick box, like a foaling box, should be designed so that it can be cleaned and disinfected regularly and thoroughly. Sun and wind will disinfect, and so the sick box should be left open when not in use. Before disinfecting with chemicals, the building must be completely clean; it is then scrubbed with warm disinfectant solution. A useful disinfectant for concrete floors is a hot solution of washing soda. At least a day should be allowed before the disinfectant is washed off with clean water. Kit which is soaked in a disinfectant solution should be immersed for at least six hours. In 'disease-free' areas, great importance is always attached to clean footwear, so it is a sound idea to have a boot-wash situated where mud can be washed off rubber boots. There should also be provision for the attendants to wash their hands. To maintain hygiene unpainted wood may be dressed with creosote, when applying, safety glasses and rubber gloves must be worn.

Isolation

All diseases associated with micro-organisms are infections. The passage of the disease from one animal to the next can be made less likely by isolation procedures. There are two forms of isolation: within the yard for a contagious disease (one carried by contact), or outside the yard for airborne infection. The contact that spreads a contagious disease need not be direct. For example, a horse with a skin infection may be ridden under saddle, after which the saddle may be placed temporarily on a saddle horse. Later another saddle is rested on the saddle horse and may well pick up the germs and carry them on. Mildly contagious diseases can be kept under control by careful application of the principles outlined here.

Some diseases can be carried in the air. When a horse coughs, it releases germs which may float down wind. Birds and flies also carry germs. With more highly infectious diseases, the ideal is an isolation box sited about 400 m (around a quarter of a mile) down wind of the stable yard. This gives a better chance of keeping a disease out of the yard itself. Such a box can also be used for visiting horses and, for the first fortnight, for new arrivals in a yard.

Treatment of injury

Cold hosing

Where there is any bruising or tearing of the tissues, cold applications will shrink the blood vessels. To control swelling after injury, cold and pressure may be needed for the first day, but then heat is required to aid healing. Cold is easily applied by running cold water. While an assistant holds the horse using a bridle, the hose should be run very gently, first on the ground and then on the foot; it is then worked gradually up the leg. This should continue for ten minutes, and several sessions per day are needed, using pressure bandages between sessions. If the horse can be stood in a suitable stall, such as in a horsebox or trailer, the horse can be allowed to eat from a hay net and the hose can be bandaged to its leg. Alternatives to cold hosing include standing or walking in the river or the sea.

Cold bandages, massage and astringents

An ice pack can be made by crushing some ice cubes in a cloth with a hammer or rolling pin, and then transferring this crushed ice to a polythene bag which may be bandaged on to the leg over a thin layer of gamgee to prevent skin scald. Methods of bandaging are shown in Fig. 2.3.

In addition to using cold bandages, some swellings – particularly those involving filling of the legs – respond well to massage. The legs should be rubbed upwards, towards the heart. To reduce friction, it may help to use soapy water, baby lotion or oil. Alternating hot and cold applications also produces a massaging effect.

Some horses, particularly those that have to gallop or jump on hard ground, tend to get filled legs after work. This condition may be helped by using a cooling lotion after work, or by rubbing a diluted astringent into the lower leg in the evening. As a general rule, bandages should not be applied over these liniments or the skin may be

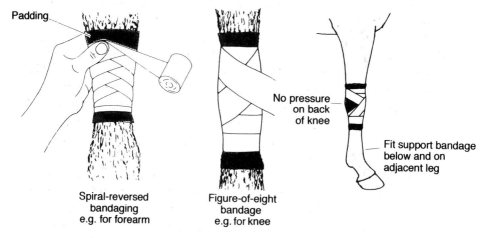

Spiral-reversed
bandaging
e.g. for forearm

Figure-of-eight
bandage
e.g. for knee

Fig. 2.3 Bandaging.

blistered. As a preventative measure against legs filling, an astringent paste may be used. The hair is wetted, then the paste is applied, first against and then with the lie of the hair. The paste sets so the horse can be worked at home with the paste on. The paste can be washed off when the horse is required to be tidy.

Poulticing

Where there is damaged tissue, the application of heat will stimulate the blood supply to the area and this will help repair the damage. A poultice also has a drawing effect, which will help any pus form into an abscess. It is thus often useful for a wound, whereas an ice pack is useful for a bruise, and an astringent for reducing swelling.

Impregnated padding can be purchased ready for use, complete with instructions on the pack. Alternatively, a kaolin poultice may be used. The procedure is simple. The lid of the tin is loosened and the tin is then placed in a pan of boiling water for several minutes, until the paste is as hot as can be borne on the back of the hand. Paste is then put on a piece of lint, and covered with gauze, and is then applied. The poultice is then covered with a polythene sheet so that it draws from the wound and not from the air. The next cover is a piece of gamgee or similar padding, to retain the heat, and finally it is bandaged in place. The dressing is usually changed morning and evening. Alternatively the cold paste can be applied to the lint and put in the microwave for 30 seconds. It is then covered with gauze, the temperature tested on the hand and the poultice applied.

If the wound or sore is in the sole of the foot, some people like to use a bran poultice. Boiling water is mixed with antiseptic and poured on to bran until a crumbly consistency is obtained: if the bran is squeezed, there should be no excess moisture. The mixture is allowed to cool until it can be tolerated by the palm of the hand and then it is placed in polythene inside sacking. The foot is stood in the bran and the wrapping secured around padding on the leg. It is tidier to finish off with a stable bandage. The poultice should be renewed night and morning. The antiseptic will mask the smell of the bran so that the horse will not try to eat it.

A puncture wound is sometimes poulticed with a mixture of Epsom salts (magnesium sulphate) and glycerine. This has the advantage of not being edible and not making the sole hard as does kaolin.

Irrespective of the type of poultice in use, there is one situation which demands particular care. If an open wound lies over a joint, there is a possibility that the joint capsule may be damaged and a poultice could draw out the joint oil. A poultice should never be used in such cases.

Where the horse is taking more weight on the sound leg than on the injured one, this should be bandaged for support.

Fomentations

Fomentations are a useful way of applying heat to an area which is not easily poulticed. They should be repeated several times a day and continued for about 20 minutes on each occasion. A bucket and a container of hot water should be taken to the horse. Hot and cold water should then be mixed to a temperature which can just be tolerated by the human elbow. A double handful of Epsom salts may be added. A cloth, such as an old towel, is then soaked in the water, wrung out and applied to the area for a couple of minutes. This procedure is repeated, keeping the water as hot as can be tolerated.

Tubbing

Open wounds in the foot may call for regular applications of heat; this can be achieved by tubbing. The preparations are similar to fomentations but a non-metal bucket or tub is used. Some antiseptic may be added to the water and as much Epsom salts as will dissolve, thus making a saturated solution. The horse's foot is placed firmly in the tub or bucket. The water may be hotter if the water level does not come above the top of the hoof. Generally, however, it is easier to have the water hand-hot. If the horse is reluctant to immerse its foot, hot water should be splashed gently over the leg until the horse is willing to lower it into the bucket. Tubbing should last about 20 minutes and should be repeated at least twice a day.

Physiotherapy

Today's horse must be fit enough to perform considerable feats and is thus exposed to the risk of injury. Physiotherapy is widely used during the training of human athletes, both to prevent injury and to aid recovery after it. These techniques are now being successfully adapted for use with the 'equine athlete' such as the hunter or competition horse. Obviously, it is more complicated to diagnose the exact site and type of pain in a horse and to gain its co-operation during treatment.

Traditionally, rest has been the treatment for the many athletic problems associated with horses. Now there are a number of techniques which, when used by competent people under veterinary supervision, lead to faster recovery, often of a more permanent nature.

A number of sophisticated medical appliances have been adapted to treat various equine athletic conditions. Some of these, such as faradism and ultrasound, obtain their effect by applying energy sources directly to the horse.

Muscles give stability as well as function to joints. Deterioration of joint function can be the result of a previous slight injury which may not have been noticed. The horse cannot control or operate the joint as well as before, but is not lame. If not noticed, the next time the joint is stressed it may malfunction and sustain a serious injury. Permanent damage may perhaps result, or the horse may show poor form due to discomfort. This could be the start of a nappy horse.

Faradism
Faradism can be used for both diagnostic and therapeutic work. It consists of the application of an intermittent alternating electrical current, allowing the muscle in question to contract and relax, thus preventing atrophy. The artificial stimulation applied by faradic current induces circulation to the injured parts without any damaging effect, so giving an ample supply of blood carrying nutrients and oxygen just when and where they are most needed. Faradism can reduce adhesions and promote the interchange of fluids within the body with beneficial results. It can also be of great assistance in correcting muscle imbalance and releasing long-term muscle tension.

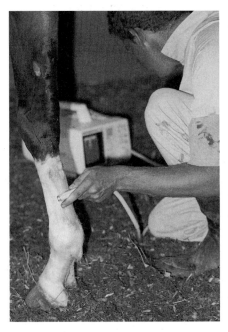

Fig. 2.4 A proper education concerning both the horse and the techniques is essential before attempting physiotherapy.

Faradism is not well tolerated by some horses and it has generally been superseded by more effective stimulation techniques.

Ultrasonic therapy

This consists of ultra-high-frequency sound waves above the normal range of hearing. These waves are produced by conversion of high-frequency electrical energy waves to sound waves by the crystal in the head of the instrument.

Ultrasound can penetrate to a depth of between 5 and 10 cm (2–4 in) and affects the tissue in different ways. The resistance met in the tissues by the sound waves induces heat, a mechanical vibration is produced and the waves stimulate a chemical reaction. All three assist in the dissipation of swelling and inflammation, the removal of harmful breakdown products, the reduction of swollen tendons, and the breakdown of adhesions.

Vibration and massage

The therapeutic value of massage and vibration has been known for many years. Their greatest value is in producing complete relaxation and dispersing muscle tension. Muscles cannot develop if they suffer from constant tension. Horses are generally exposed to unnatural ways of living and working which can induce muscle tension. The temperament of the individual horse is of importance in its attitude to its work and to its owner/trainer. Muscle tension can prevent the horse from relaxing mentally and physically as muscles held in undue tension become exhausted. In this state they cannot develop and this may lead to muscle imbalance or incorrect development in shape or form. The elimination of undesirable muscle tension as soon as it is observed enables the trainer to progress with the horse's training programme and helps to preserve the animal's co-operation.

Remedial exercises

Injury can reduce the range of movement in joints, and by reduction of ligament suppleness or painful adhesions it can cause limitations.

Specific exercises can build up joint suppleness, help to break down adhesions slowly and to restore the horse's confidence in the use of the joint, and remedy muscle imbalance resulting from previous injury or use.

A combination of therapy and exercise is known as rehabilitation and the equine sports therapist will design a programme for an injured horse that aims to restore the horse to its full athletic potential.

Heat treatment

Heat in therapy can be used in three forms: radiant, conductive and conversive. The physiological effects of the three methods are basically the same and range from superficial to deep. Radiant heat is applied by means of infra-red light. Conductive heat is applied by hot-water bottles, electric heating pads, hot fomentations and poultices. Conversive heat is developed in the tissues by resistance to high-frequency electrical energy.

Heat promotes circulation in the area, which aids healing and also helps to alleviate pain; thus it relaxes and soothes the patient.

Generally speaking cold therapy is used in the acute stages of an injury – applying heat to a new injury may be harmful. After the cold therapy has reduced the inflammation hot and cold may be alternated to great benefit.

Hydrotherapy

Generally the application of water is a means of applying cold.

However, equine swimming pools allow the heart and lungs to be kept fit without any weight on the legs.

Remember that swimming horses should only be carried out by experienced professional people as poor swimming technique can be detrimental to a horse's development. Other forms of hydrotherapy include water treadmills and jacuzzis.

Nursing

Care and attention to detail has a psychological as well as a physical benefit. As with people, horses respond in a happy relaxed atmosphere with a positive attitude, gain confidence and becoming willing patients.

Giving medicine

Steaming the head

Where there is considerable discharge from the nostrils, the head may be steamed. To prepare for the treatment, a handful of hay is placed in a plastic bucket in the bottom of an old sack. This is then sprinkled with friar's balsam or oil of eucalyptus. Boiling water is poured over the hay so that it steams. The horse's head is put into the entrance of the sack and kept there for several minutes. More hot water is then poured over the hay and the procedure repeated. From time to time the horse will need a break. For heavy catarrh it may be necessary to steam the head twice daily.

In cases of pneumonia the sack should not be used as it limits fresh air. After the steaming process, the hay will be contaminated with nasal discharge and should be burned. The bucket and bag must be scalded to sterilise them.

Horses being steamed are best fed at ground level to encourage discharge. A little ointment containing menthol, oil of eucalyptus or something similar may be placed in the outer nostril. If the discharge tends to create a sore, the skin should be protected with petroleum jelly or nappy-rash cream.

Electuary

This old-fashioned paste still provides a useful aid to soothing a cough. It is usual to draw out the horse's tongue and, using the flat handle of a spatula, place the paste on the tongue. The treatment is repeated at least twice a day.

Drenching
Giving a horse liquid medicine can prove to be a difficult business. Some horses accept a drench quite easily, but others are not so co-operative, so it is wise to take precautions. The horse's head should be raised so that the liquid can be poured down its throat. This is not difficult with a small pony but most people find their arms are too short to treat a horse this way. A rope should be attached to the middle front of the noseband of the head collar and the rope is passed over a beam. Extra height is gained by standing on a straw bale or two. This is essential if a beam is not available. An assistant can then control the horse and raise and lower its head as required. The drench is best placed in a plastic bottle. If a glass bottle is used, then the neck of the bottle must be bandaged in case the glass is broken by the horse's teeth. The animal's head is raised gently and the neck of the bottle is placed in the corner of the mouth. Gentle pouring may then commence. When one mouthful has been swallowed, another may be given. If the horse coughs, lower the head at once. If the medicine goes down 'the wrong way', it will end up in the lungs and may give the horse pneumonia. *Drenching should be done only by someone competent because of the risks involved.*

Other methods of giving medicines
Some powders and granules may be added to the food, but the horse has a sensitive nose and palate and may easily detect these additions and be put off. The meal should therefore be made particularly tempting by the addition of apples or carrots. If the horse fails to eat all of the prepared meal, the value of the medicine might be lost. Some medicines can be poured straight into the water bucket.

A useful way to ensure that the horse receives the appropriate medicine dosage is to make up a paste with icing sugar to which the medicine is added. Using a large syringe, without a needle, the mixture is squirted into the horse's mouth towards the back of the cheek. Some drugs are now supplied as a paste in a syringe for use in this way.

Some treatments require administration to the skin, and for some of these, rubber gloves are required. In every case the great essential is to read the instructions or to follow the vet's directions.

Injections
It is now common for stockmen to inject certain classes of stock. The horse is not easy to inject as it has a tough hide and also sometimes produces a reaction to the injection. Furthermore, if the injection is not done smoothly and at the first attempt, the horse is apt to become

fractious and be difficult on the next occasion when injection is attempted.

Injections may be given intravenously (into the vein), and this is certainly a job for the vet. They may also be given intramuscularly. If the vet approves of an experienced person giving intramuscular injections, then he can demonstrate the proper technique.

Enemas and back-raking

It is sometimes helpful to the passage of faeces through the rectum to flush or lubricate this part of the bowel with a fluid. There are several other reasons for giving an enema, and different fluids are used for different causes. The normal procedure is to lubricate the rounded end of a special tube and pass it through the anus into the rectum. Then, soapy warm water or liquid paraffin is passed down the tube. When dealing with a foal, gravity is often used, but in the case of a horse, a pump may help to pass the fluid along the tube. The giving of an enema is usually a task for the vet.

Back-raking is the removal of faeces, or of meconium in the case of newborn foals. In the horse or pony, a well-lubricated hand is used, but for a foal a small, smooth, well-lubricated finger is all that there is room for without causing inflammation. Generally, back-raking is best left to the vet.

Treatments using tubes

A stomach tube is used to place either a large quantity of fluid, or a small quantity without wastage, into the stomach. The tube is about 3 m (10 ft) long and about 12 mm (around half an inch) in diameter. It is passed up one nostril and goes down the gullet (oesophagus) towards the stomach. If the tube should accidentally go the wrong way at the pharynx, then it would pass into the trachea, and unless immediately remedied, the fluid would pass into the lungs. *The stomach tube is only used by a vet.* Occasionally, there will be minimal bleeding at the nostril, but this is of little consequence.

Where it is necessary to empty the bladder, and the horse seems unable to oblige, the vet will pass a thin tube up the urethra into the bladder and thus allow the urine to escape. Such a tube is called a catheter.

Tooth care

Until the horse is four years old the teeth should be examined twice a year to make sure that the milk (deciduous) teeth are not getting in the way of the permanent teeth. After the age of four the teeth should be examined once or twice a year for sharp edges. To examine the molar teeth, it is easier to use a gag as the horse has sufficient power to damage a finger should the grip on the tongue be lost. However, care must be taken not to get the horse alarmed or excited. Sharp edges on both the top and bottom molars need to be rasped off with a long-handled tooth rasp. Most horses do not mind this operation, which can be done by an experienced operator instead of the vet, provided that the correct equipment is available, that reasonable care is taken and that the operator makes sure that the desired result is achieved. Rasping is a two-person job. The horse, in a head collar, is backed into a corner to face the light, and the assistant, standing on the opposite side to the person doing the rasping, steadies the head and may be required to hold the tongue. The rasp must be dipped into water at regular intervals to keep the cutting edges clean.

Aids to diagnosis

A nerve block is effected by a vet injecting anaesthetic over a nerve to achieve a loss of sensation in the area covered by that nerve. This process can be used to achieve local anaesthesia for treating a wound or it can be used to help diagnosis. If a lame horse cannot feel its near fore foot and yet still limps, the seat of lameness is not in that foot.

Radiation is sometimes used to check inflammation and treat skin diseases. It is most often used to provide X-ray plates (radiographs), which are particularly useful in helping diagnosis of leg and foot problems. X-ray units with sufficient power to produce a satisfactory plate of the horse's body are only found at major equine research and teaching centres.

When a vet is diagnosing the cause of a problem, he may refer to the horse using terminology that indicates the aspect with which he is concerned. The terminologies used in the equitation and veterinary contexts are explained in Fig. 2.5.

Minor operations

Castration is carried out either by giving a sedative and a local anaesthetic, which leaves the horse standing, or under a general anaesthetic, which collapses the horse on to suitable clean soft ground. When a horse goes down from a general anaesthetic, it is helpful to have a strong assistant to hold the leadrope and steady the horse. When the horse comes round, it may be easily upset and it is left alone to struggle in peace, but the surroundings must be soft so that it does not hurt itself. After castration, there will be some swelling. However, the wound is free draining so, as long as the patient continues to eat well, there is usually no cause for concern.

Another common minor operation is Caslick's or 'stitching a mare'. When a breeding mare has poor conformation of the vulva, this may allow air and germs to enter the genital tract. This operation involves sealing the top half of the vulva under local anaesthetic by making two cuts and sewing them together. In spite of the adjacent position of the anus as a source of infection, this operation is usually trouble free.

Another simple routine operation is the removal of a tooth. Deciduous or milk teeth which have failed to clear out of the way for the permanent teeth are easily removed. To remove wolf teeth (see Chapter 8), a local anaesthetic may sometimes be needed. For a large tooth it might be necessary to give a general anaesthetic. Horses vary considerably in the amount of interference they will tolerate without sedatives. It is helpful if those who are accustomed to the horse can advise the vet concerning its temperament and any relevant idiosyncrasies.

Treatment for lameness

Lameness due to soft tissue may first be treated by the application of cold to reduce swelling, and later this may be interspersed with heat to draw blood to the area to aid healing. Heat may come from poultices, fomentations or ultrasonic therapy. Once the initial swelling has gone, it may be thought advisable to produce further inflammation by the use of counter-irritants. The simplest of these are known as 'blisters'. The first task is to clip the coat over the area. The blister is then applied according to the directions on the container. When blistering a tendon, the rear lower part of the leg should be covered with petroleum jelly or lard so that the blister does not run down the leg and inflame the heels. When blistering a joint, its inside angle should be avoided. The horse will need a cradle put on its neck so that it cannot nibble or lick the blister. Similarly, if the hocks are blistered, the tail must be kept bandaged up double so that it cannot swish over the blister and carry it to the flanks. The horse must be put on a very light laxative diet before the operation and for a few days afterwards.

Less severe treatment is given by the use of 'working blisters'; these do not always need the hair to be clipped. Generally, they are rubbed in with a soft toothbrush each day until the skin becomes scaly. A working blister is normally to be found in most medicine chests, whereas the use of a full blister is a matter for the vet, who will advise on current thinking of its value.

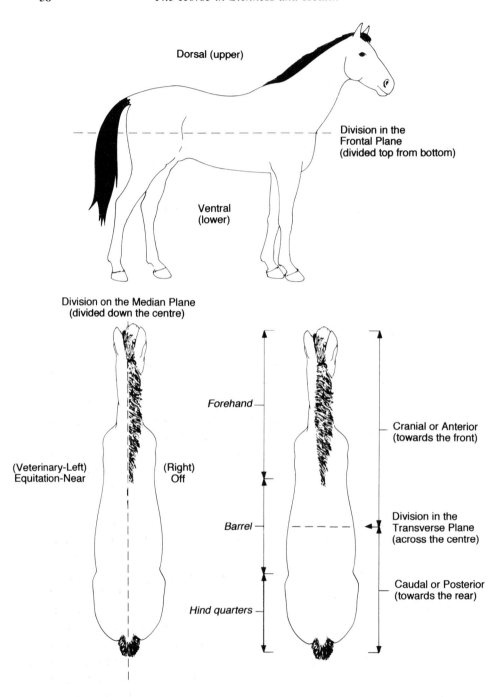

Fig. 2.5 Terminology.

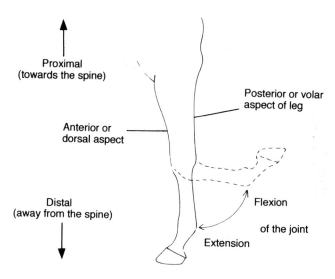

Fig. 2.5 contd.

The practice of 'firing' damaged tendons by applying electrically heated irons to the skin of the horse's legs is rarely carried out now. The technique of wounding tendons in a 'split tendon operation' to gain extra support tissue has also come under attack, but the use of 'carbon-fibre implants' appears to be successful in some cases. The most popular treatment for tendon strain is box rest and cold treatment during the acute phase of the injury, followed by physiotherapy and controlled exercise until the horse is sound. Best results are obtained if the horse is then rested in the field to allow full recovery.

Whatever method is used to strengthen the legs, it is important to remember that the horse kept in the stable without exercise needs a light laxative diet, and that the sound leg, on the other side to the damaged one, will be taking extra weight and so will need support bandages. Eventually, and it may be after several months, the horse is turned out to grass. It will tend to gallop about and may reinjure the damaged leg. The front shoes should be left on for a front-leg injury but the back shoes can be taken off and the feet cut back so that the horse is very footsore behind and thus not inclined even to trot. Drugs can provide an alternative restraint, which can be used for the first few days. It is essential that the horse be left out at grass for some months, as complete rest is the best cure for such injuries.

Diagnosis of lameness

The first task in the diagnosis of lameness is to decide which leg is the lame one. Lameness may be due to back problems, but generally the cause is in the lower leg.

The horse should be observed in the stable. If it points a fore leg, then that is probably the limb giving pain. The horse should be turned to left and right; if it drops on one side, then it is trying to favour the other side. The horse is then walked up and back and then is trotted up and back on a level surface. Its head jerks up when the lame front leg carries weight. The horse should be equally balanced so that at the walk and trot the weight should move evenly, with each limb taking an equal proportion to its neighbour. If the horse tries to save one limb so that it carries less weight, it may do so by using the head and neck as a counterbalance. To favour a leg means to reduce its work load by transferring weight off it quickly.

If both front legs are lame, the stride will be short and inhibited as the horse will try to take a shorter stride on an unsound limb. Less commonly, a back leg is the seat of trouble and is more difficult to diagnose. A left (near) hind causes the horse to carry its left hip up high but the head will drop as the lame hind limb takes the weight. Next, the horse should be worked on the soft to see if it runs up more sound. As shown in Table 2.2, a number of tests will help locate the lameness.

Once a decision has been made as to which leg is the lame one, it must be inspected more carefully. Good light is needed. The knee should be pressed gently all round (palpated). Then the leg is picked

Table 2.2   Tests to locate lameness.

Location	Tests and symptoms
Foot	Points at rest, warmer than the others, more lame on hard ground, heat at coronet
Tendon	More lame on soft ground, swelling and tenderness over tendon
Splint	Lameness comes on at exercise, lamer on hard ground
Knee	Swelling, heat, pain on flexion, followed by increased lameness
Shoulder	Move the leg and watch for pain symptoms
Hock	Limps on turning, lamer on hard ground. Hold up hind leg to belly for 30 seconds and then release, trot horse away and look for lameness. This is called the 'spavin test'
Stifle	Leg rested forwards, reacts to manipulation
Hip	Reacts to movement of the leg

up. The area down the length of each splint bone must be squeezed firmly but evenly. Following this, the same treatment is given to each major tendon and ligament, working carefully from knee to fetlock joint. If the horse lays back its ears, pulls its leg away, flinches or reacts in any other way, then it may be that the trouble is in that area. Until the trouble is located, the search must proceed, using sight as well as feel. The fetlock must be examined and then the heels. Heat or a sore place may be the only clue. Infection may enter through a tiny scrape. Every test must be compared with the same test on the neighbouring leg.

The foot must be examined, but it must first be picked clean and scrubbed with water. Observation may reveal damage on the sole. Each nail should be tapped with a hammer and pressure applied to the seat of corn. Shoeing history may be relevant. If the cause is not found, then it could be that the wrong leg was selected or that the problem lies above the knee.

Diagnosis of lameness is difficult and the experience of the vet may be needed; however, good observations may aid his task. *'No leg, no horse.' This is not a matter to be treated lightly.*

Part II
The Systems of the Horse

3 Systems of Support and Movement

It is a characteristic of the higher orders of the Animal Kingdom to have a framework that gives structure and form to the body. The parts of a horse's body are fixed to a frame, the skeleton, which is built of bone and cartilage for strength. The main supporting member of the frame is the backbone which, together with the skull, affords protection to the central nervous system. The ribs also give some protection to the vital organs. There are also joints, bonded by ligaments, and muscles attached at one end by tendons to the bones in order to move them. The most vulnerable part of the system is the lower leg and foot, which occupies all of the attention of the farrier and much of the vet's equine practice. The task of these systems is to provide support, protection and movement – particularly locomotion.

Bones and cartilage

The horse's skeleton consists of over 200 bones. These are so arranged that they can be used as rigid supports or become freely movable when the joints are brought into play, thus acting as levers to provide movement. Bones also store minerals and contain the marrow which is responsible for the formation of blood cells.

Bones are living structures with blood vessels. They are made of protein, (giving them strength) and mineral matter (which makes them hard and strong). There is less mineral matter in the bones of young animals, whose bones are softer in consequence. The mineral matter consists largely of calcium and phosphorous and this is why it is important to look closely at the ratio of these two minerals in the horse's diet.

Typically, a long bone, e.g., the cannon bone, is made of compact dense bone on the outside, forming the cortex. Within the cortex is the medullary cavity composed of spongy (cancellous) bone forming a

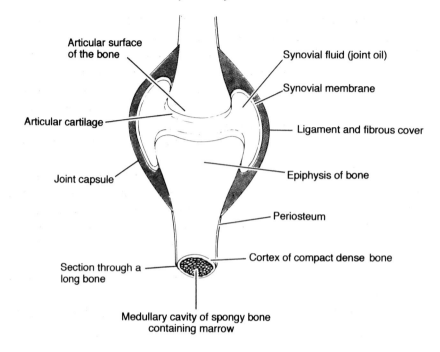

Articular surface
of the bone

Synovial fluid (joint oil)

Synovial membrane

Articular cartilage

Ligament and fibrous cover

Joint capsule

Epiphysis of bone

Periosteum

Section through a
long bone

Cortex of compact dense bone

Medullary cavity of spongy bone
containing marrow

Fig. 3.1 Bone and joint.

porous network containing marrow. The bone is surrounded by a
sheath of tissue called the periosteum, the cells of which are responsible for the formation of new bone material when young bones are
increasing in girth. Bones grow in length at the epiphyses, which are
areas just behind the end surfaces of the bone. The end surfaces where
one bone meets another are called articulatory surfaces, and they are
covered in cartilage.

Cartilage has a firm but slightly flexible consistency, providing a
very smooth surface. When it is found in meat it is called gristle. Non-
articular cartilage can be converted to bone by laying down minerals
within the tissue, a process called ossification.

Joints

Bones meet at joints (see Fig. 3.1), which are of three types:

(1) *Immovable joints*, e.g. the junctions of the bones in the skull.

(2) *Slightly movable joints*, e.g. the junction between bones forming the spinal column or backbone.

(3) *Freely movable joints*, which take various forms: there are *hinge-type* joints, such as the fetlock; *plane-type* joints, such as the knee, where bones with flat surfaces glide over each other; *pivot joints*, which allow turning, e.g. the joint between the top bone in the neck (the atlas vertebra) and the second bone in the neck (the axis vertebra); there are also *ball-and-socket* joints, such as the hip.

Each freely movable joint is enclosed in a capsule, the lining of which is the synovial membrane. This secretes synovial fluid or 'joint oil', which acts as a lubricant. The outer cover of the capsule is fibrous and acts like a ligament, holding the joint together. There are similar capsules on prominent bone ends (such as the elbow), and these are called bursae (singular, bursa).

Ligaments are strong connective bands of tissue holding joints together. Some are within the joint capsule itself, but most are outside it, connecting the two bones on the sides, front and back of the joint.

Skeleton

The horse's skeleton is made up of bones, cartilage, joints and ligaments. It consists of the axial portion, made up of skull, back-bones and ribs, and the appendicular portion, which is made up of the legs.

The axial skeleton
The axial skeleton is shown in Fig. 3.2. *The skull* consists of many small bones fused together to form protection for the brain, optic nerves, inner ears and nasal passages. One of the largest bones in the horse is the lower jaw-bone or mandible, which is hinged between the eye and the base of the ear. The skull also contains the teeth. The back of the skull is formed by the occipital bone, which has a junction with the top bones of the neck.

The neck contains the atlas, the axis and five other cervical vertebrae. The bones of the backbone or vertebral column are called vertebrae (singular, vertebra).

The chest part of the vertebral column contains 18 thoracic vertebrae to which are attached the 18 pairs of ribs. There are eight pairs of 'true' ribs attached directly to the breast bone or sternum. In

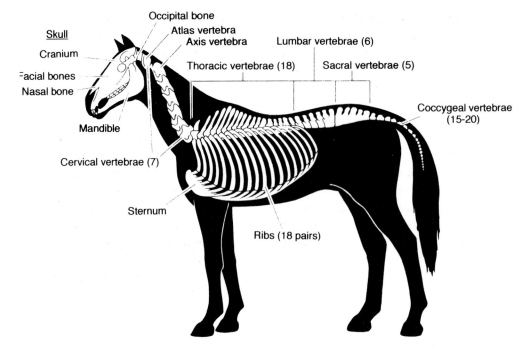

Fig. 3.2 Axial skeleton.

addition there are ten pairs of 'false' ribs, attached to the breast bone by long cartilage extensions. The horse has no collar bone.

The next part of the vertebral column consists of six lumbar vertebrae forming the loins. Behind the loins are the five sacral vertebrae fused together as a firm base for the pelvis and forming the croup. There are also some 15 to 20 bones called the coccygeal vertebrae, which go down into the dock of the tail.

The neck and tail vertebrae are freely jointed to provide a wide range of movement, but little movement is possible through the thoracic and lumbar vertebrae. When we speak of a horse 'bending its back', most of the movement is in fact occurring in the neck. The apparent lateral bending is effectively a combination of neck, shoulder and limb alignment, the backbone remaining almost straight. The ribs limit movement through the barrel of the horse, and so any movement is confined to the region of the loins.

The vertebrae have vertical and transverse processes which aid muscle attachment. There is a canal or channel through the centre of the vertebrae housing the spinal cord. This is the continuation from the brain down the backbone. Occasionally, vertebrae seem to get slightly out of alignment and in some cases manipulation appears to help. Sometimes vertebrae will fuse together at their extremities. This can cause pain and reduced performance until the fusion is complete. Given time, however, the horse appears none the worse when the fusion is complete.

The appendicular skeleton

Figure 3.3 show the bones that comprise the appendicular skeleton. The front legs are not joined by any bony attachment to the horse's axial skeleton. Thus, the weight of the horse is taken at the front by muscles, tendons and ligaments from the two front legs, so forming a sling in which the body is carried. This arrangement is part of the shock-absorbing mechanism built into the front legs. The other parts of this mechanism are the angles in the shoulders and fetlocks, the many bones of the knee, and the design of the foot itself.

The fore leg starts with the scapula or shoulder blade, the top part of which consists of cartilage. The scapula forms the shoulder joint

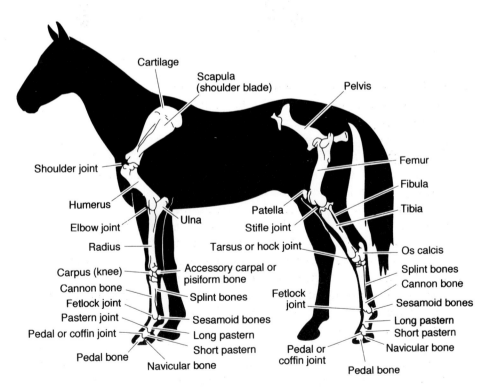

Fig. 3.3 Appendicular skeleton: the limbs.

with the humerus or upper arm bone. The front of the humerus is known as the point of the shoulder. The rear or distal (lower) end of the humerus forms the elbow joint together with the radius and ulna, which are fused together to form the forearm. The radius is the main weight carrier of the two bones, and the ulna reaches up to form the point of the elbow (olecranon process). Below the forearm comes the knee or carpus, which is the equivalent of the human wrist. It is made up of two rows of small bones with a small extra bone at the back, called the accessory carpal or pisiform bone. This little bone makes the tendon pull at an angle to bend the knee.

Below the knee are the three metacarpal bones; the central large one is the cannon bone, and the two small bones on either side of it are the splint bones. The cannon and splint bones are the equivalent to the three bones running across the back of the human hand (see Fig. 3.4). The bones equivalent to those of the little finger and thumb have disappeared through evolution.

The cannon bone meets the digit at the fetlock joint. This digit is equivalent to the human middle finger. It consists of three principal bones (the phalanges): the long pastern (first phalanx), the short pastern (second phalanx) and the coffin or pedal bone (third phalanx).

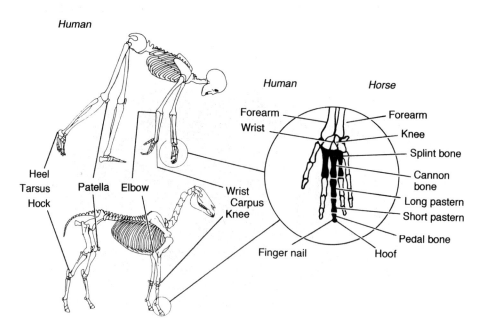

Fig. 3.4 Comparison of equine and human skeletons.

The joint of the long and short pastern bones is the pastern joint. That between the short pastern bones and the pedal bone is the coffin joint.

At the back of the fetlock joint there are two small bones designed to gain mechanical advantage in bending the joint; these are the sesamoid bones (proximal sesamoids). At the back of the coffin joint is another sesamoid-type bone called the navicular bone (distal sesamoid).

The hind leg starts with the pelvic girdle (see Fig. 3.5). This is made up from the fused sacral vertebrae and the two hip or pelvic bones (os coxae), which meet underneath at the symphysis. Each hip bone is formed from three bones fused together: the ilium, the ischium and the pubis. The ilium joins the sacrum on either side at the sacro-iliac joint. The front end of the ilium has the point of croup (tuber sacralae) near the sacrum and the point of hip (tuber coxae) on the outer side. The ilium unites with the ischium at the hip joint. The ischium has a rearward projection called the seatbone or point of buttock (tuber ischii). The pubis also meets at the hip joint, and the pubis, together with the lower part of the ischium, form the floor of the pelvis. Thus, the pelvis forms a complete hoop of bones protecting the vital parts of the horse's body. A long flat pelvis is said to be best for high speeds.

The thigh bone (femur) comes from the hip joint and runs down to the stifle joint. At the stifle there is another sesamoid bone called the

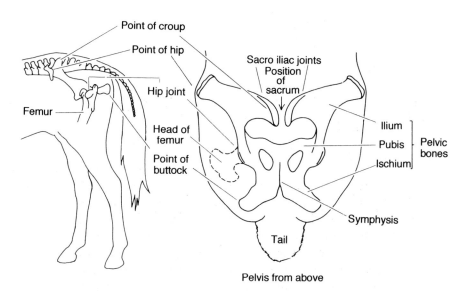

Pelvis from above

Fig. 3.5 The pelvis.

patella, which corresponds to the human kneecap. The femur meets the tibia, which is within the second thigh or gaskin. In human beings, beside the tibia is the fibula; the fibula in the horse is only a vestigial remnant, sometimes no more than 10 cm (4 in) long. The tibia goes to the hock (tarsus), which, like the knee, consists of several small bones. The hock equates to the human ankle. At the back of the hock is a bone called the calcaneus or point of hock (fibular tarsal), which acts as a lever to extend the leg. It forms the heel in man. Below the hock, the bones are similar to those below the knee.

Muscles

There are three main types of muscle in horses:

(1) *Cardiac* muscle, which is found in the heart.
(2) *Smooth or involuntary* muscle, which is generally found in automatic systems such as the walls of the digestive tract.
(3) *Skeletal* muscle, the flesh of the horse, which is like the red meat that we eat.

Each fibre of a muscle is controlled by a branch from a nerve. These muscle fibres are arranged in bundles surrounded by connective tissue. When stimulated, muscles reduce in length, thus exerting a pull. The more muscle fibres involved, the stronger is the pull. Thus, for extra strength the horse must build extra muscle. Muscles are arranged in sheets and bands, and in herring-bone and spindle-like groups according to their function.

Each muscle has an origin where it is attached to a stable part of the skeleton. At the other end it has an insertion into the part of the skeleton which it moves. Where the bone to be moved is distant from the muscle, there is a dense fibrous connection between them called a tendon. Tendons are usually cord or band shaped, but some are flat like sheets. They have little elasticity and are poorly supplied with blood. They also take considerable strain and, because of these factors, take a long time to heal when injured.

Just as a joint has a covering that supplies lubrication to help the moving parts, each tendon has a sheath where it passes over a joint, which protects and lubricates it. Similarly, just as a prominent bone end has a protective capsule (bursa), there are tendon bursae to help tendons pass over bones at a joint.

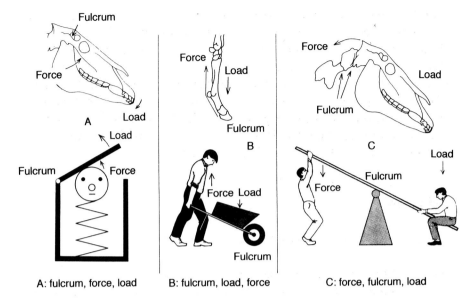

A: fulcrum, force, load   B: fulcrum, load, force   C: force, fulcrum, load

Fig. 3.6 Bones as levers.

If a joint is to be bent, flexor muscles pull and extensor muscles allow. Other muscles (fixator or synergic muscles) steady the rest of the body. When the joint is to be straightened, the extensors are directly responsible muscles (agonists or activators) and the flexors (antagonists) allow or give while the limb is steadied by the other muscles.

When a muscle acts through a tendon on a bone to operate a joint, it gains mechanical advantage in different ways, as shown in Fig. 3.6.

The muscles of the horse's body are too complex to name and separate in a simple study. This is because there are many overlapping layers and the shape of the outer, superficial muscles is partly dependent on the deeper muscles. Some of the main muscles of interest to horse-owners are as follows and as shown in Fig. 3.7.

Trapezius, the muscle on either side of the withers. It lies over the rhomboideus and splenius muscles. In some horses these muscles are poorly developed, which gives them prominent withers and 'ewe necks'.

Brachiocephalicus, the muscle which pulls the shoulder forward and is attached at its front end to the back of the head. This is why it is easier for a horse to jump well using its shoulders if it is given sufficient length of rein to extend the neck and head in flight. Similarly, at the

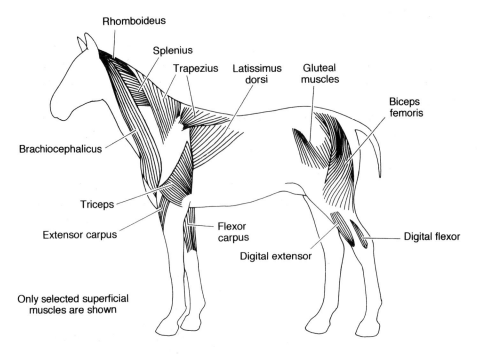

Fig. 3.7 Muscles.

collected paces where elevation of the steps is required, this muscle helps to carry the neck high and not stretched out, thus raising the shoulder.

Latissimus dorsi, the muscles from the shoulder blade to the back. Those running along the back are the *longissimus dorsi*. These are the muscles on which the rider sits.

The elbow has extensor muscles called *triceps* and flexor muscles called *biceps*. The lower joints also have paired muscles, but in order to keep the lower leg light they are kept in the upper leg. This is advantageous for high speed. The extensor muscles acting on the hip are known as the hamstring muscles. These pass up the back of the hindquarters and attach to the croup. On fit horses these muscles stand out clearly with divisions between them.

By removing a minute portion of tissue (in a biopsy), laboratory analysis has shown fast-twitch and slow-twitch muscle fibres. The mix of these in a racehorse has bearing on its sprinting or staying ability.

The lower leg and foot

A man wearing heavy boots is slower than a man in lightweight running shoes. Evolution favours the fast-running horse to escape from its enemies, and similarly selects the horse with lightweight lower legs and feet. The remote ancestor of the horse had several toes; the modern horse has only one, which takes all the strain and is sometimes the weakest link. This is particularly so in the front leg, which takes all the strain on landing from a jump and which normally carries about 60% of the horse's weight.

The main strain is taken by the suspensory ligament (see Fig. 3.8) coming from the back of the knee and running against the cannon bone down the back of the leg to the fetlock. Part of the suspensory

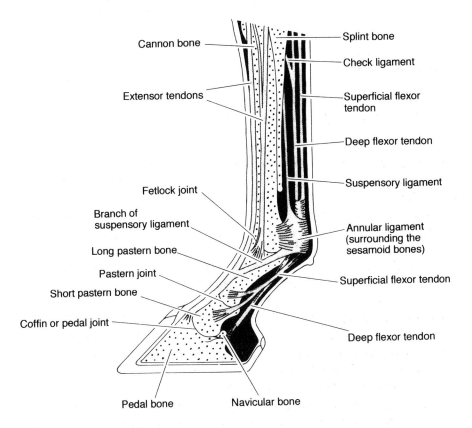

Cannon bone

Extensor tendons

Fetlock joint

Branch of
suspensory ligament

Long pastern bone

Pastern joint

Short pastern bone

Coffin or pedal joint

Splint bone

Check ligament

Superficial flexor
tendon

Deep flexor tendon

Suspensory ligament

Annular ligament
(surrounding the
sesamoid bones)

Superficial flexor tendon

Deep flexor tendon

Pedal bone   Navicular bone

Fig. 3.8 The lower leg.

ligament is then attached to the sesamoid bones and part divides into two and comes round the pastern from each side.

The two tendons running down the back of the lower leg are together called the superficial flexor tendon and under it is the deep flexor tendon, which has a check ligament. This takes some of the strain from the muscles situated above the knee in the forearm, or above the hock in the second thigh. The deep flexor tendon runs over the sesamoid bones down to the pastern, into the hoof, and round the navicular bone. It is attached to the coffin or pedal bone. The superficial flexor tendon divides into two branches at the fetlock: these attach on both sides to both pastern bones.

The extensor tendons run down the front of the leg. As they take no weight, they are slim and generally trouble-free.

There is a band of tissue at the coronet called the coronary band. This creates horn and so produces the hoof. The outer layer of the hoof, called the periople, serves to control the movement of moisture in and out of the hoof. There is next a horny layer and inside that the insensitive laminae. These mesh with the sensitive laminae that surround the pedal bone, and in this way the pedal bone is firmly held in the foot.

The lower surface of the foot is composed of the sole and the raised frog and bars (Fig. 3.10), which act like the treads on the wheels of a tractor, to help grip the ground. The shape of the underside of the foot is slightly concave, so aiding grip.

Under the back of the pedal bone is the pedal (plantar) cushion, which takes and spreads some of the weight from the short pastern bone; it does this by pushing wide the lateral cartilages, two wings of

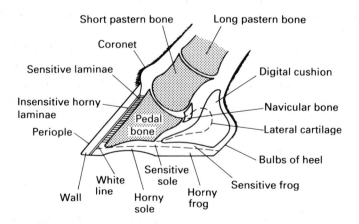

Fig. 3.9 Foot structure.

cartilage attached to the pedal bone, so spreading the heel and pressing the frog against the ground. Much of the concussion of normal working is thus absorbed within the foot. The foot is well supplied with blood and the action of the pedal cushion being compressed at every step is like a small pump helping the circulation.

Figure 3.9 shows the structure of the foot.

Farriery

A normal hind foot is longer than the fore foot (Fig. 3.10). When the horse is working under stress, it is important to keep the toe of the fore foot short, the frog in contact with the ground and the heels wide. This helps the foot to work most efficiently.

The rate of the growth of horn varies according to food, environment and exercise, and is greater at the front of the foot than at the heel. Wild ponies normally walk far enough and live in sufficiently rough conditions to keep their feet correctly worn. An unshod horse in a field may need its feet rasping every six weeks, as will a shod horse, although in the latter case wear of the shoe may dictate more frequent treatment.

If the farrier is attempting to alter action by trimming the foot, this must be done only a little at a time, as it will alter the angle of wear on the joints. The foot is usually trimmed so that the angle of the pastern to the ground is the same as the angle of the foot (see Fig. 3.11). When rasping, it is harder work to take down the front of the foot and there is a tendency to take off too much at the heels or to reduce the bars, which may lead to contracted heels.

The preparation of the hoof for the reception of a shoe consists of removing loose particles of sole and tidying ragged pieces of frog. The bearing surface of the wall must be made level with the outer edge of the sole.

Although a shoe may not be worn out, it must be refitted every four to six weeks, otherwise it will be carried forwards by hoof growth. The weight of the horse borne by the shoe should not be far in front of the line down through the centre of the cannon bone, otherwise damage to hooves, joints and tendons will occur.

What to look for in the well shod foot

- The shoe should have been made to fit the foot, not the foot to fit the shoe.
- The type and weight of shoe should be suitable for the horse and the work required.

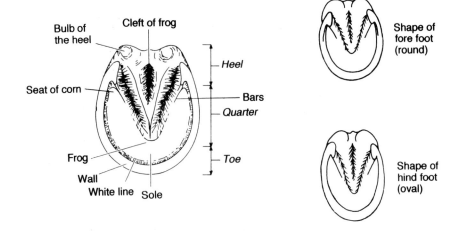

Fig. 3.10 Feet.

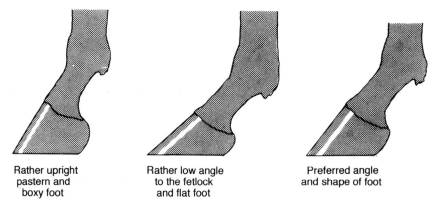

| Rather upright pastern and boxy foot | Rather low angle to the fetlock and flat foot | Preferred angle and shape of foot |

Fig. 3.11 Although not all ideal these feet are all in balance, with an unbroken hoof-pastern angle.

- The hoof pastern angle should be maintained as in Fig. 3.11 and Fig. 3.12 and the foot trimmed evenly on the inside and the outside.
- The sole and frog should not be excessively trimmed.
- The frog should be in contact with the ground.
- Sufficient nails should have been used and they should be of the right size and well driven home to fill the nail holes.
- Clenches should be well formed, not too low and all in line.
- No daylight should show between the shoe and the foot, particularly at the heel.

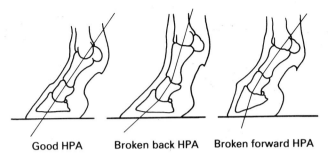

Good HPA   Broken back HPA   Broken forward HPA

Fig. 3.12 The hoof-pastern angle (HPA) should be unbroken in the balanced foot.

- The heels of the shoe should not be short and put pressure on the seat of corn.
- The place for the clip should have been neatly cut and the clip well fitted.

Basic corrective shoeing

Navicular disease
The front shoes are thick at the heels and gradually thinned to a rolled toe.

Three-quarter shoe for corn
The web of a shoe is cut out over the region of the corn and prevents pressure on the corn while allowing the heels to take the weight.

Over-reaching
Over-reaching occurs when a horse is galloping and jumping and the bulb of the heel of the fore foot is struck by the inner border of the toe of the hind shoe. The heels of the fore shoes should be raised and the toes rolled to enable the quick getaway of the fore feet. The toes of the hind shoes should be set back and may be lowered at the heel.

Brushing
In many cases a shoe rasped on the inside ground surface, smoothed off and fitted close to the inside wall is all that is required. However, feather-edged shoes may be used; there are varieties adapted to correct various types of brushing and the part of the shoe that is causing the trouble must be located first.

Disorders of the skeletal, articular and muscular systems

The main disorders (Fig. 3.13) of the systems of support and movement are as follows.

Abscess in the foot
Symptoms: Lameness caused by pus in the foot. Heat and tenderness. (Gravel is a similar condition.)
Causes: A penetrating wound or a bruise.
Treatment: A hole must be cut to allow the pus to drain. Tub the foot, and poultice twice daily until the condition is cleared. The hole must then be plugged securely.

Arthritis
Symptoms: Heat, swelling and pain at a joint.
Causes: Inflammation of a joint from any cause, e.g. an infection, a blow or a sprain.
Treatment: Rest, together with treatment of any infection. (*Note:* the use of drugs such as phenylbutazone ('Bute') may mask the pain. Such drugs are anti-inflammatory.)

Bruises in the foot
Symptoms: Lameness and pointing or resting the foot. Pus may break out at the heel from a septic corn. The horse flinches from pressure or when the area is tapped. Corns – at the seat of the corn. Bruised frog, sole or heel.

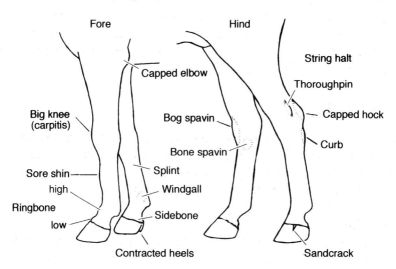

Fig. 3.13 Leg problems.

Causes: A sharp stone, etc., or, for a corn, a badly fitting shoe.

Treatment: For a corn remove the shoe. Thin the sole or seat of the corn, cutting down towards the reddened area. Tub the foot, and poultice, repeating twice daily for two or three days. Re-shoe with care, possibly using a seated-out or three-quarter shoe if there is a corn.

Bursitis

Symptoms: Soft swelling at the bursa, sometimes with initial heat and pain. This condition is called *synovitis* if a tendon sheath is involved.

Causes: A knock, e.g. through travelling in too short a space, may cause a capped hock. Using too little bedding may cause a capped elbow, which may also be caused by a knock from the heel of a front shoe. A knock from a jump pole may cause a big knee (*carpitis*). Bursitis at the poll may result from a knock on a low roof. Going over backwards or a poorly fitting saddle may cause bursitis at the withers. *Bog spavin*, which is a soft swelling at the front of the hock, may be caused by a strain or injury. Concussion, e.g. too much ''ammer, 'ammer, 'ammer' on the hard road, may cause *windgalls. Thoroughpins* may be caused by a strain, e.g. jumping an unfit horse in deep going.

Treatment: If a capped elbow is caused by the heel of a shoe, then a protective ring, called a 'sausage boot' is put on the pastern at night. This protects the elbow while it heals itself. Pressure bandages may help windgalls, as may the regular use of an embrocation or even a working blister to tighten the skin. Cold hosing combined with pressure stockings will generally help a big knee. A bursa may be drained and some of the fluid replaced with cortisone but this is a task for the vet. Any bursitis may prove unsightly and difficult to get rid of but is often harmless; however, at the poll or withers, problems such as poll evil and fistulous withers may develop.

Contracted heels

Symptoms: The horse may go lame.

Causes: Excessive paring of the bars and heels and leaving the toe too long. *Thrush* (see below) reducing the frog is an alternative cause.

Treatment: Keep the toe short; this method takes several months. A pad or bar may also be used to induce extra frog pressure.

Dislocation

A partial dislocation is called *subluxation*. These are both very rare in the horse. The more common bone location problem is upward fixation of the patella.

Symptoms: The affected hind leg is stretched out and back.

Causes: A weakness in conformation may predispose towards this problem. It is more common in young horses and they may well grow out of it.

Treatment: The condition may right itself if the hose is made to step forwards or back or turn. In other cases manipulation of the patella and leg may be needed. It may be necessary for the horse to wear a higher-heeled shoe.

Exostoses

Symptoms: The growth of excess new bone, forming a bony enlargement, following a tear of the periosteum or a bruise. The horse may first go lame and there may be heat, but eventually, when the bony growth has settled, the horse will usually go sound. However, flexion of a joint may be reduced. X-rays (radiographs) may help diagnosis.

There are many examples of exostoses, e.g. high ringbone, on the front of a pastern joint; low ringbone, on the front of the coffin joint; and false ringbone, not on the joint (non-articular). Other examples are osselets on the front of the lower cannon and upper long pastern; splints on the splint bone; bone spavin at the front of the hock; and occult spavin on the articular surfaces of the hock.

Causes: There may first be inflammation of the bone (*ostitis*) or inflammation of the periosteum (the skin around the bone). This is called *periostitis*. There may be a fracture, and this is one possible cause of a splint. Exostoses of the sesamoid bones may follow inflammation (due either to strain at the ligament/bone junction or to fracture). This is known as *sesamoiditis*. Upright joints and too much roadwork may predispose the horse to various forms of exostoses of the lower leg. Some people consider that ringbone is hereditary.

Treatment: A mild blister is sometimes used. Phenylbutazone eases the pain, as in arthritis. De-nerving is carried out in extreme cases. Rest is often prescribed, but walking exercise has proved beneficial. Improved nutrition and physiotherapy may both help.

Fractures (a break in bone or cartilage)

Symptoms: There may be an incomplete break as in the 'greenstick' fracture of a youngster. The fracture may be simple, crushed (comminuted), compound or open, with the outer skin broken. It may be only a hairline fracture going a little way into the bone, as found, for example, in sore or bucked shins. The break may be heard and may be seen. The horse will be lame and in great pain.

Causes: The lower leg may break under stress during exercise; the cannon may break during jumping. The pelvis may fracture if the horse slips up on the road and lands heavily on its hip. Any bone may break from the trauma of a severe blow.

Treatment: Immediate immobility is essential. The decision must be made as to whether treatment is realistic or whether the animal should be put down. Poulticing will provide helpful heat for sore shins.

Laminitis (founder)

Symptoms: Hot feet in which the laminae are inflamed. The horse stands leaning backwards with the hindlegs well engaged and the fore feet toes not taking weight. The animal is in pain and shows it. The foot may have rings of growth caused by previous attacks.

Causes: Rich pasture, too long feet and lack of work leading to overweight all combine to give fat ponies laminitis. Any horse or pony which breaks into the food store or is on fast-growing grass may get a sudden excess of starch or sugar, which creates toxin formation in the intestines; these poisons circulate and damage blood vessels, especially in the hoof. Similarly, a retained afterbirth or severe inflammation of the gut will both produce inflammatory toxins.

Treatment: Call the vet. Apply ice packs to the feet or cold-hose for five minutes every half hour while you are waiting for the vet. It is now thought best not to force the horse to walk as this can push the pedal bone through the sole of the foot. The horse should be stabled and allowed to lie down if he wants to. The horse's diet will have to be reduced but must be kept balanced in terms of energy, protein, minerals and vitamins – starving fat ponies can cause further problems. After the vet has given initial treatment he will advise special trimming and shoeing of the front feet; this is a case for close co-operation between the vet, owner, groom and farrier.

Pony-type laminitis is avoided by allowing such animals limited grazing by tethering or leaving in a yard where they get straw, cut grass or hay plus one hour's grazing daily. Spring grass is the worst offender, but the extra moisture in late summer and autumn may produce a second flush of grass. Keep the animal's feet well trimmed.

If the wall of the foot separates from the sole at the toe, this is called seedy toe. The crumbling horn must be cut away and the cavity packed with antiseptic paste. Such feet will need rocker shoes. Acute laminitis may lead to rotation of the pedal bone and a dropped sole.

Navicular syndrome and pedal osteitis (ostitis)

Symptoms: Shorter stride; slight lameness on the day after work; resting a front foot in the stable; stumbling; pivoting on the front feet when turned in its own length; heat; pain from pressure on the sole; lameness, reducing with work.

Causes: Bruised or punctured sole or the result of too much work on the hard with flat, thin-soled feet may all cause pedal osteitis. Navicular disease is now considered to be a syndrome with many causative agents. There are probably several causes of pain in the navicular bone which give rise to a variety of changes in the area and result in similar signs.

Treatment: The foot should be nerve blocked to establish that the source of pain is in the foot. Subsequent X-ray examination will help to show which of the two bones is involved. The farrier may fit shoes with rolled toes to reduce stumbling. He may fit wedges to raise the heels and lessen the angle of the deep flexor tendon over the navicular bone. The horse may be worked on pain-killing drugs as a short-term expedient. Blood-thinning drugs (such as Warfarin) or blood vessel dilatory drugs (such as isoxsuprine hydrochloride) may help circulation to such an extent that damaged areas may even be replaced by new bone. As a last resort, the foot may be de-nerved. This makes the horse legally 'unsound' and must be disclosed upon sale.

Abscess at the coronet

Symptoms: A sore swelling above the coronet, caused by pus in the foot, breaking out at the top of the foot.

Causes: Gravel; foreign matter gaining access to the foot at the white line. Pricked sole (either a nail driven wrong by the farrier or a sharp object, which may still be embedded). Binding nail (a shoeing nail driven too close to the sensitive laminae). Quittor (damage to top of lateral cartilage). (A tread – another foot bruises the coronet – may appear similar.)

Treatment: Treat the cause of infection in the foot. If necessary, a hole may be cut in the sole by the vet or farrier to let the poison out. This may be assisted by poulticing. Keep the sore at the coronet open and free-draining to let pus out. Pack the holes with antiseptic on cotton wool and cover with clean bandage. Always make sure that the animal is protected against tetanus.

Sand cracks

Symptoms: A split running downwards, from the coronary band, in the wall of the hoof.

Causes: Treads (see below) or blows to the coronet.

Treatment: The farrier may put a groove across the hoof at the bottom of the crack to stop it running down. Alternatively, he may insert a clench, a special staple to hold the horn together. If the crack runs to the bottom of the foot, the farrier should seat out the shoe under the crack. Feed biotin and/or methionine (gelatine).

Self-inflicted damage

This may take several forms, treads, over-reaches, speedy cuts and brushing.

Symptoms. Cuts or sore places caused by the horse's own feet, located as follows:

Treads – coronet, often cause by other horses.

Over-reach – heels or back of tendon on front legs.

Speedy cuts – inside cannon.

Brushing – inside fetlock or coronet.

Causes: Tired animals or those with poor conformation moving on poor going or in crowded conditions.

Treatment: Treat as for a wound. Corrective farriery as needed.

(*Note:* prevention is better than cure. Protective clothing, such as over-reach boots, brushing boots and Yorkshire boots, may be used. Exercise bandages will also protect from brushing.)

Sidebones

Symptoms: Ossification of the lateral cartilages which can cause lameness while the bone is forming. Sidebones may be felt as hard areas in the bulb of the heel and forwards from that area.

Causes: The Horse Breeding Act 1918 lists sidebones as hereditary and an unsoundness. However, ossification of this cartilage is normal, and premature ossification with temporary lameness is probably due only to excessive roadwork.

Treatment: Temporary rest.

Sprains and strains

These are synonymous and especially affect the front leg.

Symptoms: Pain giving rise to lameness; heat and swelling.

Causes: Sudden stress on a tendon or ligament beyond its normal limits, causing torn fibres. Upright pastern or 'back at the knee' may be a predisposing cause as may deterioration in the conformation of the foot, or lameness from some other cause. The toe landing on a stone or the heel hitting softer ground when the horse is stressed and exhausted, e.g. the last run of the day when hunting, may also cause strains and sprains.

Treatment: Immediate application of cold to control swelling and of a pressure bandage over padding to give support. The horse should be boxed home and given complete rest until the heat and swelling subside. Walking exercise, cold hosing and regular massage form the later stages of treatment. Muscles may respond well to ultrasonic or similar treatments. Carbon implant and split-tendon operations all have their supporters, but repair is slow and difficult. Time is the greatest healer.

Thrush

Symptoms: A smelly frog with moisture in the cleft. There is sometimes lameness.

Causes: Standing in dirty bedding and failure to pick out the feet regularly.

Treatment: Keep both bedding and feet clean. Clean the feet using a stiff brush and disinfectant solution. Trim the cleft of the frog to allow access of air. Treat the area regularly with an antiseptic dressing or Stockholm tar.

Sore shins

Symptoms: Occurs mainly in young racehorses in training; usually affects forelimbs with swelling over the front of the cannon bone and a shuffling gait and/or lameness.

Causes: Working horses with immature bones on hard ground; exact cause of pain not known but may be due to tiny stress fractures of the bone.

Treatment: Avoid overworking on hard ground. Rest and physiotherapy.

4 Systems of Information and Control

Information and control are provided by the nervous and sensory systems and the ductless glands. The nervous system governs reasoned and co-ordinated movement. It stores information, evaluates situations against experience and instinct, makes decisions, and also sends commands to the muscles. The sensory systems act as an information service about matters both inside and outside the body. The sensory organs are the ears (hearing), the eyes (sight), the nose (smell), the mouth (taste), and the skin (feel of heat, pressure and pain). The ductless glands are small centres that receive information and control some aspects of the body in a way quite different from the nervous system. Their efficiency is vital to the well-being of the horse, but as yet they are imperfectly understood.

A knowledge and understanding of these systems will help to answer many questions that horsemasters may ask themselves about the horse, such as 'Why does the horse do it?', 'What will it do next time?', 'How did it know?'.

The nervous systems

The horse reacts to changes in the world about it. Each change, be it of light, temperature or any other stimulus, produces a reaction in the horse. The change or stimulus is first received and then conducted to a central control system, which interprets the message and causes appropriate action to be taken. This is the central nervous system (CNS, see Fig. 4.1) and consists of the brain and the spinal cord.

Central nervous system (CNS)
The brain is placed for safety in the horse's skull. It receives all messages from the senses, via the sensory nerves, and puts this information together to form an understanding of its immediate environment.

87

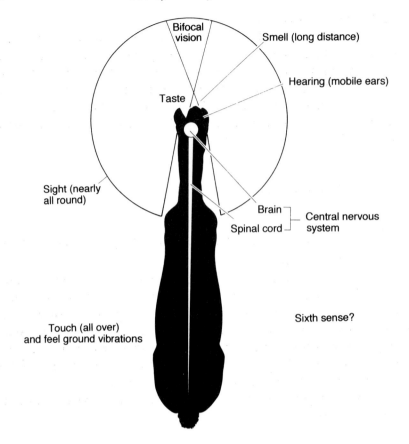

Fig. 4.1 Central nervous system and senses.

This information can be stored as experiences. Thus, the horse can learn and can associate a past experience with a present happening and thus anticipate the next event.

Although it has well-developed senses and an adequate memory, the horse lacks the powers of imagination or foresight. While the horse has an inborn instinct for self-preservation, it has no conception of death. It cannot cast its mind forward in tackling a situation. However, the horse may be influenced by its natural instincts and appetites.

Based on the horse's decision about its next action, the brain sends out messages to the body through cranial nerves in the skull and through the spinal cord which runs down the centre of the spinal column ('backbone') and on through spinal nerves that emerge between the vertebrae to go to all parts of the body.

Peripheral nervous system

This includes the cranial and spinal nerves, plus the autonomic nervous system that controls the digestive system, much of the urinogenital system, the movement of blood by the heart and some of the activities of the glands. The peripheral nervous system also includes the motor and sensory nerves. The job of the motor nerves is to transmit instructions to the muscles, while the sensory nerves receive stimuli and relay these back to the CNS.

Aspects of behaviour

Instinct

Instinct is inherent or innate ability. A foal will get up, feed, drink and walk without instruction. It also learns as it progresses. A foal moves unevenly when compared with an adult horse, but it acquires greater skill rapidly. When a woman in high-heeled shoes walks, her ankle makes small adjusting movements continuously; this is an acquired skill. A thoroughbred horse has been bred to make similar compensating movements better than any other horse. One aspect of training horses is to teach them to move better and thus be more skilful in terms of movement than they are in the natural state.

The instincts guide the horse in its attempts to survive, to nourish itself and to reproduce.

Behaviour

Behaviour may be group or individual. Each horse is a distinct personality with a different temperament from its fellows. Temperament varies from horse to horse and can be observed not only in its actions but also in its facial expressions. Horses soon learn to recognise different situations and people. They can be nervous, happy, sensible, brave, cowardly or stupid – as can human beings!

As a group, horses tend to be nervous, responding quickly and violently to changes in environment. A horse is made this way because that is how it escapes from its enemies. It is not its nature to fight, except over food or sex. In a group, horses will establish a 'pecking order'. A horse (which need not be a male) will put others in their place, and within the group this order runs all down the line. Thus, when feeding hay in a field, it is essential to so place it that each horse can feed without being threatened by its fellows.

In the breeding situation, males will fight from about two years of age and upwards. Generally mares will not fight, but they will have only a limited period when they will receive a stallion.

Reflex action
This is an automatic or unconscious response of a muscle or a gland to a stimulus. It is an immediate and involuntary response, such as coughing. Another example of a reflex action is the postural reflex, which allows a horse to sleep standing up. Its auditory reflex makes it turn its head towards a new sound. Happily for the horsemaster, the tonic neck reflex makes it less likely that a horse will kick or buck if its head is raised.

Inaction
Inaction may be caused by lack of either feeling or of the ability to move. Lack of feeling may be induced by anaesthetics, which are chemicals or drugs that prevent the passage of nerve impulses. A local anaesthetic is used to deaden a particular area, and a general anaesthetic affects the central nervous system, thus causing unconsciousness. If used in excess, a general anaesthetic will cause death by depressing the vital reflex centres in the brain.

Lack of the ability to move can be caused by paralysis, which in turn is caused by nerve damage. Damaged nerves may recover, but dead ones cannot do so. However, they may be replaced to some extent by other nerves taking over their duties if given sufficient time.

Sensory systems

The senses are the five faculties of sight, hearing, smell, taste and touch. Through these senses the horse perceives the external world.

Sight
The eye (Fig. 4.2) is the organ of sight. An image enters through the lens and is focused on the retina at the back of the eyeball, just as in a camera the picture is focused on the film. In comparison with other animals, the muscles that change the shape of the lens are poorly developed in the case of the horse. This could create difficulties in focusing, but it is thought that the horse can compensate for this by viewing objects at distances on different parts of the retina.

It has been suggested that the distance from the lens to the retina varies very slightly from top to bottom. However, there does not

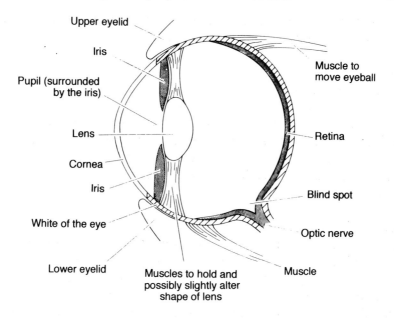

Fig. 4.2 The eye.

appear to be any *post mortem* evidence to support this claim. The theory is that to help focus on close objects, the horse can raise its muzzle and form the picture at the top of the retina. To look at distant objects it can tuck in its muzzle and view the object at the bottom of the retina. Thus, when the horse is grazing, the grass (viewed down its nose) is in focus, as are distant objects viewed under its brow. Horses probably suffer from astigmatism so that part of the picture they view is a little blurred.

The arrangement of the horse's eyes (set at the side of its head) enables it to be on the watch for enemies coming from any direction. Within this wide panoramic view, however, the horse probably has a poor definition of distance. To get a better idea of an object, the horse will turn its head and focus both eyes on it, probably concentrating on the object to the virtual exclusion of the rest of the picture.

When the horse is jumping, it needs to alter the angle of its head to keep the obstacle in focus until about the moment of take-off, when it loses sight of the obstacle itself.

It is believed that the horse has poor colour definition. Horses may well see colours differently to humans. As it has no imagination, the horse probably cannot distinguish stationary objects far from it. Possibly, too, the horse adjusts more slowly than humans to changes

in light intensity and so may hesitate before going willingly from light
to shade.

Although it is hard to be certain about such matters, the horse can
probably only see about 150 m (around 500 ft) and only achieves
recognition at about 60 m (200 ft). The horse apparently looking into
the distance may well be receiving information through other senses.

Hearing

The ear (Fig. 4.3) is the organ of hearing. The ears of a healthy horse
are always on the move. Horses have a keen sense of hearing – far
better than that of humans – and by turning their ears towards a
sound they can pinpoint accurately the direction from which it is
coming. This is an evolved protective mechanism.

The horse can convey a certain amount of meaning with its voice,
from the gentle whickers and whinnies of a mare to her foal, through
the neigh of a horse turned into a strange paddock, to the wild shriek
of an angry stallion. The horse also expresses meaning by snorting.
The interpretation of sound is aided by behaviour and situation. By

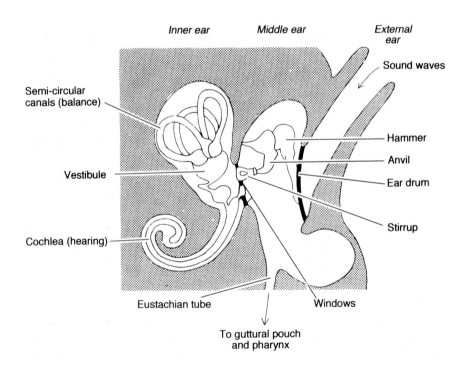

Fig. 4.3 The ear.

constant repetition, the horse can be taught to understand a short range of human verbal commands.

The ear is divided into three parts. The external ear is the mobile part which turns to catch sounds and can also denote mood. It continues into the head as far as the ear drum (tympanic membrane). The middle ear is a cavity behind the ear drum, and to maintain an equal pressure with the outside air it connects to the back of the throat (pharynx) by the Eustachian tubes, one on each side. The middle ear contains the three little bones that have the same 'horsey' names in all animals. They are the hammer (malleus), anvil (incus) and stirrup (stapes). These bones provide direct mechanical linkage from the ear drum to the oval window of the inner ear, the last of the three parts. This is tucked into a cavity within the skull. It has two parts: the cochlea receives the sound as fluid movement detected by hairs; the other part consists of a vestibule and three semi-circular canals, which are concerned with the balance of the horse. One of these is long-itudinal, one transverse and the third at right angles to give three-dimensional balance.

Smell

The nose is the organ of smell. A horse breathes in only through its nose and not through its mouth. Smell is a very important sense to the horse. In feeding, the horse blows into its feed bowl to test the smell and it may refuse food which has an unfamiliar smell. Stallions can detect an 'in-season' mare by smell at 200 m (660 ft).

Some people blow up a horse's nostrils to communicate friendship, just as horses do to each other. Interesting-smelling compounds may also entice a horse, e.g. ginger.

The horse has nostrils which it can dilate. These lead into the nasal chamber, which is long and contains coiled bones covered with moist membranes well supplied with blood. The olfactory or smell nerve cells are sited in these mucous membranes, which have tiny hairs over their surface. It is these hairs that contain the sensory cells that detect the smell as it goes into solution on the moisture of the membranes.

Taste

The mouth contains the organs of taste, which consist of taste buds. These are little groups of cells which are found at the end of each taste nerve fibre. They are found mostly on the tongue, but also on the palate and in the throat. The information about taste is fed to the brain as degrees of salt/sweet/bitter/sour. This taste information is received with information on smell and texture to give a composite impression.

Horses like saltiness and sweetness but they dislike bitterness or sourness. It is because of this that most worm powders are sugar-based, and some people rub salt on their hands before examining a horse's mouth or teeth.

Preparations designed to stop horses chewing wood are bitter tasting, but horses like to chew fence rails cured with preservative salts. Usually, horses are very fussy feeders and will reject unaccustomed tastes. Similarly, they will generally reject fats and meats, but on occasions will eat such things as acorns and yew leaves, which are bitter tasting to humans and may in fact be poisonous.

Feel

The horse's skin has specialist nerve endings to receive feel, which may be divided into the five sensations of touch, pressure, cold, heat and pain. These nerve endings are limited in number in most areas, and therefore an injection can miss a nerve by chance and be completely painless. On the other hand, nerve endings are densely grouped in the muzzle. Some sensations of feel – such as gut pain in colic – can come from internal parts of the body.

There is another sense like feel, which is that of 'awareness' of the body. This muscle sense or proprioception enables the horse to know what its limbs are doing and how they are responding to the muscle contractions that control movement.

A third sensation of a similar nature is the organic group. This group of sensations indicates conditions of bodily need, such as hunger, thirst, need to urinate (relieve the bladder) or copulate.

A further sensation of feel is the horse's awareness of ground vibrations. Thus, often before it can see or hear someone approaching, the horse will show its awareness of the approach.

The horse is receptive to rubbing, scratching and nibbling on certain areas. A pony that refuses to be caught and turns its quarters towards the would-be catcher may be caught by scratching its rump, though one should watch the ears for signs of intent to kick. The head-shy horse may be relaxed by scratching its withers and the crest of its neck prior to touching the head.

Sensitive areas can be dulled by misuse. The bars of the mouth become insensitive with hard hands and sharp bits. The horse's sides become dulled with constant kicking.

Sixth sense

Horses can detect certain things that human beings cannot. For example, horses will not go near radioactive material and also seem to be aware of approaching weather. Some people go so far as to suggest that horses are sensitive to 'psychic vibrations'. Horses certainly seem to be aware of the state of mind of humans with whom they have contact. Just as lie detectors attached to a person's skin can detect changes in thought patterns, so some animals appear to receive similar signals. Possibly it is for this reason that certain people have 'a way with animals'.

Although horses have no imagination, experience soon teaches them to associate. Thus a stranger smelling of surgical spirit tends to mean a sharp prick from a hypodermic needle! Being plaited-up means going hunting or to a show. This is so exciting to some horses that they will not eat breakfast. Thus, not everything to which we attribute sixth sense is beyond comprehension, but there are some things about the horse's awareness of its environment which are not yet understood.

Endocrine system

The endocrine system (ductless glands; see Fig. 4.4) controls the horse's patterns of behaviour. The system consists of a series of glands, which secrete hormones directly into the blood or lymph streams. A gland is an organ secreting chemical substances for use in the body. Those with which we are here concerned are called endocrine glands, in contrast to exocrine glands which secrete through ducts to the outside or to the digestive tract. The endocrine glands produce hormones, which travel in the blood or lymph streams to parts of the body often far removed from the gland itself and which exert a specific effect on certain tissues. The word 'hormone' comes from the Greek *hormon*, which means 'to stir up' or 'to arouse activity'. In some cases, the presence of a hormone in the blood system produces a concerted effect on the body, creating a specific state or condition. These glands control conception, gestation, parturition, metabolism, growth, puberty, ageing, aggression, passion, and so on.

Along with the nervous system the endocrine system allows comprehensive communication within the body. There are, however, several differences which allow the two systems to complement each other:

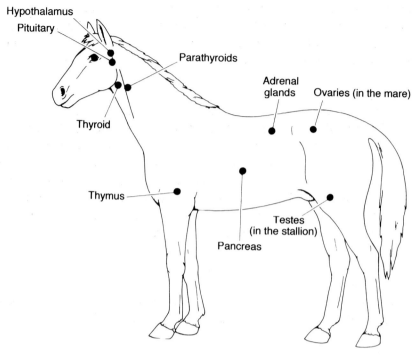

Fig. 4.4 Ductless (endocrine) glands.

- The messages sent by the nervous system are more rapid.
- Hormones can reach all of the body via the blood stream while nerves only go to specific points.
- Thus a hormonal response can be widespread while nervous responses may be localised.
- Hormonal responses can continue over long periods of time but nervous responses are rapid and short-lived.

The usual classification of the endocrine glands is as follows.

Hypothalamus

The hypothalamus is a nerve control centre at the base of the brain, and is concerned with hunger, thirst and other autonomic functions. It also releases factors that control the all-important pituitary gland.

Pituitary

This is attached by a stalk to the base of the brain and has been called 'the master endocrine gland'. It is the leader of the endocrine orchestra. The pituitary gland consists of two lobes, the anterior and the posterior. The anterior lobe produces follicle stimulating hormone

(FSH), and luteinising hormone (LH), which both act on the ovaries in the female. It also affects the testes of the male, and the thyroid and adrenal glands of both sexes. The posterior lobe produces hormones affecting the kidney, the uterus and the mammary glands.

Thyroid

This gland is situated on either side of the larynx and produces hormones dependent on iodine. A shortage of this chemical thus affects the operation of the thyroid. The thyroid gland controls metabolism and growth. An underactive thyroid results in a lack of energy and a tendency to overweight. If this gland is overactive, the reverse occurs. The thyroid gland has been likened to a blacksmith's bellows governing the fires of life. In normal function it has an automatic self-righting mechanism so that any excess hormone will act to shut off the pituitary stimulus.

Parathyroids

These are a group of four small glands situated near the thyroid and control calcium and phosphorus metabolism in the body.

Adrenal glands

These are located close to the kidneys and produce two hormones, cortisol and adrenalin. Cortisol has a variety of effects, including the control of inflammation. Adrenalin is a stimulant in response to stress: it increases the heart rate and blood pressure. It prepares the body for fight or flight.

Pancreas

The pancreas is situated behind the stomach in a loop of the small intestine and secretes insulin, which controls the level of blood sugar. This gland also produces digestive juices.

Thymus

The thymus is just under the breastbone between the lungs. 'Sweetbreads' as sold by the butcher are the thymus glands of calves. This gland is particularly large and active in foals because it is concerned with immunity. It is also a source of blood lymphocytes.

Other ductless glands

In the female, the uterus acts as a ductless gland to produce prostaglandin, which affects the body in many ways, particularly in bringing the mare into season (see Chapter 27). The ovaries, in addition to producing eggs, secrete oestrogen and progesterone. Oestrogen is responsible for the mare's behaviour and changes in her sex cycle, and progesterone, which is also produced in the placenta and adrenal glands, also has an important part to play in the mare's cycle (Chapter 9). The testes produce the male sex hormone, testosterone, which is responsible for the male characteristics and development.

Disorders of the systems of information and control

This section concentrates on those disorders and malfunctions commonly met in practice. In fact, the senses generally give little trouble, with the exception of the eye, where the commonest problem is injury. The nervous system also generally functions normally throughout the life of the horse, but occasional nervous diseases and conditions may be encountered. There are also nervous habits which are regarded as vices and which cause considerable concern to the horsemaster. Glandular disorders are comparatively rare.

Ailments of the eye

Bruising
Symptoms: Swollen eyelids, but without damage to the eyeball.
Causes: A blow is the most common cause, e.g. from a branch when riding through a wood.
Treatment: Hot fomentation, using a teaspoon of kitchen salt in half a litre of boiled cooled water. Any lacerations to the eyelids must be stitched at once by the vet.

Cataract
Symptoms: Jumpiness, because the horse has areas of partial blindness within his total field of vision. The condition can only be diagnosed through the use of an ophthalmoscope, which reveals an area of opacity in the lens.
Causes: It may be present at birth or may be caused by an injury or infection.
Treatment: A small cataract found on veterinary examination will not generally affect the horse. The condition may deteriorate.

Conjunctivitis
Symptoms: Inflammation of the membrane inside the eyelid: the eye itself may look bloodshot. The eyelids will be swollen and there may be tears and a mucus discharge from the eye.
Causes: Injury or a foreign body, and also irritation, cold, allergy or infection. Also associated with blocked tear ducts.
Treatment: Remove any foreign body present. Wash with warm water which has been boiled and allowed to cool. Flush with a cool mixture of a teaspoon of boracic acid or Epsom salts to 0.5 litre (about a pint) of boiled water several times a day. If discharge continues, an ophthalmic ointment from the vet is needed.

Entropion
Symptoms: An ingrowing eyelid. Irritation.
Cause: A foal may be born with this condition.
Treatment: It is essential that it be spotted and treated at a very early stage by the vet, who will probably stitch back the ingrowing eyelid for a short time, thus effecting a cure.

Keratitis
Symptoms: Inflammation of the cornea (the eye's transparent front covering) with tightly closed eyelids.
Causes: A blow, a foreign body, turned-in eyelids or an infection.
Treatment: Call the vet.

Periodic ophthalmia (moon blindness)
Symptoms: Generally, only one eyeball is affected. The eye undergoes progressive inflammatory changes and after a few weeks there is a tendency to partial recovery. The symptoms later recur.
Cause: The cause seems to be unknown but the ailment is possibly bacterial or viral in origin.
Treatment: Keep the horse stabled in relatively dark conditions and consult the vet.

Photosensitisation
Symptoms: Head shaking.
Cause: Bright sunlight.
Treatment: Discuss this condition with the vet. However, as he or she will advise, this is not the only possible reason for head shaking.

Nervous disorders

Concussion
Symptoms: Loss of or reduced consciousness; dilated pupils; laboured and irregular breathing.
Cause: A severe bang on the head.
Treatment: Give the horse space and quiet. The head and spine may be cooled by sponging with cold water. Send for the vet.

Shivering
Symptoms: Involuntary and spasmodic muscular contractions, usually of the hind leg and without pain.
Cause: Although this may follow serious illness or a bad fall, it is a progressive nervous disease.
Treatment: None known.

Staggers
Symptoms: Loss of equilibrium.
Causes: An infection of the brain, grass sickness, or possibly poisoning.
Treatment: The vet must be consulted.

Stringhalt
Symptoms: An upward jerking of one or both hind legs due to the excessive flexion of the hock. It may not occur on every step.
Cause: Not known but it is listed as a hereditary disease by the Horse Breeding Act 1918.
Treatment: Nothing need be done about it, but eventually the condition will get worse. However, for many years the horse can be used as normal and its effectiveness in galloping and jumping is not impaired. Nevertheless, it must be declared as an unsoundness. There is an operation for this problem.

Wobbler syndrome
Symptoms: Unco-ordinated movement, particularly of the hind limbs, causing a weak, wobbling gait. Onset can be sudden and severe or gradual and insidious.
Causes: Compression of the spinal cord in the neck, occurring most commonly in young, rapidly growing horses but it can occur in older horses of all types.

Treatment: The condition is generally thought to be incurable and may or may not get worse. Surgery can achieve limited success as can some 'alternative medicine' treatments.

Nervous habits (stable vices)

These may be caused by boredom or idleness, are difficult to cure, and a horse with such a habit is classified as unsound.

Crib-biting
Symptoms: The upper teeth may be unnaturally worn and on discreet observation the horse will be seen to grab hold of the manger (the crib) or the top of the door or anything handy, drawing air in through the mouth and swallowing it down to its stomach. This causes indigestion and unthriftiness.
Cause: Not known (neither copying another horse nor boredom will explain many cases). Chewing rails in the paddock or stable wood-work should be discouraged lest they lead to this vice.
Treatment: Turn out by day. Give regular work. Remove anything movable on which he can crib, and creosote all woodwork. Cover any remaining edges with a specially-made preparation.

Weaving
Symptoms: Swinging the head and neck from side to side, especially when placed in a strange stable. In the advanced form, the horse will rock from one fore foot to the other.
Causes: The horse may catch the habit by watching other horses. Boredom, nervous tension.
Treatment: Turn out by day and give regular exercise. A full grid may be fitted in the top door, but some horses will weave behind this. An antiweaving grid is probably the best solution and may effect a cure. Alternative treatments include hanging a brick on a string in the centre of the door or tying up for the afternoon. Offering a little fresh-cut gorse is a useful distraction, but an unpleasant chore in the gathering.

Wind-sucking
Symptoms: The horse arches his neck and swallows air without catching hold of anything. Some horses will only do this when left alone, and so it may be hard to observe. Like crib-biting, it may cause indigestion and unthriftiness.

Cause: May develop out of crib-biting.
Treatment: Fit a 'cribbing strap', which buckles around the top of the neck and catches the horse in the throat if it tries to arch its neck. Turn out by day and work regularly.

Stress

The horse encounters many forms of stress. Some physical stress is good because it allows the animal to develop strength and endurance. Other stresses can lead to distress. Anything causing stress is called a stressor, and the pressure may arise from a situation or a physical cause. Stress is the reaction to the stressor. It may be a physical breakdown, e.g. a stress fracture, or it may show as a syndrome of adaptive responses. These responses may be physiological (such as the release of adrenalin) or they may be psychological or behavioural.

The horse's responses are designed to cope with the problem and put an end to it. The trouble in stress is serious if the stressor continues or recurs so that the responses continue. The body is not designed to cope with such never-ending responses.

There are four main groups of stressors: equine psychology, human psychology, physical causes and situation causes.

Equine psychology
Physical conflict is common in the wild, but mental conflict creates greater stress. Common conflicts – for example, a horse that is frightened by an obstacle but is coerced by its rider – can give rise to later problems if they are mishandled. Uncertainty also creates mental pressures and confuses the horse, which then shows signs of its dilemma. It may stale or defaecate and such habits become repetitive.

Boredom is another stressor and is manifest by chewed wooden stables, fence rails and so on. It is possible that many vices such as wind-sucking and weaving are initiated by boredom.

The horse's temperament is an important factor. Temperament is probably governed most strongly by heredity, but is also affected by physical condition and mental development. In the short term, feeding is probably the most significant factor, e.g. a horse which is 'oated-up'.

Instinct is significant and must be taken into account. It is instinctive for the horse to get a predator off its back. In a moment of crisis it may do the same to its rider! The horse is gregarious by nature

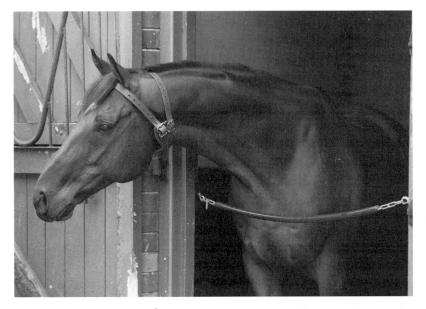

Fig. 4.5 Equine mental stress may be detected by 'bad habits' such as crib-biting and windsucking.

and can find loneliness a stressor. The right companions help the horse to relax.

Human psychology

The psychology of human beings is an important stressor to the horse. This may range from 'killing with kindness' to sheer neglect. Fear is a dilemma for any rider, but presents a far worse dilemma for the horse. The bonds of trust are broken. A rider who is out of control may be terrified and 'saw' at the reins, causing pain to the horse. The horse forgets its training and reacts to the pain: a bolting horse is certainly reacting to stress.

Physical causes

Many people thinking of stress consider only the physical aspect, and sometimes limit their horizons to stress that leads to fracture or other physical damage. There are many other physical causes of stress. Thus, speed, duration and weight of rider are all factors leading to exhaustion and fatigue, and it is the tired horse which fails to react quickly enough to protect itself at every footfall.

Environment is also important. Each horse is an individual in all respects, and environmental stresses vary with breed, age and condition. But there are certain basic rules. In light, airy stables with a good yard routine, the horse will lie down and relax during the day to a greater extent than in poky, dull and unpredictable yards.

Pain and ill health are clearly aspects where horses are at a disadvantage when compared with human beings. Diagnosis may locate the source, but it may be that many pains are unidentified.

Situation causes

Birth is obviously the first stressful experience for any animal, and it is probable that early experiences affect subsequent events.

There are many artificial situation causes. Breaking, selling, or a change of home are obvious stressors. Hunting and competing – where the work is often hard – is very stressful and usually manifests itself in physical causes. Conversely, some horses are never happier than when working at high level. The key is in understanding the particular horse.

5 Circulatory System

The body is a complex structure consisting of many cells, each with requirements which must receive attention on demand. Within the body, therefore, there must be a transport system which functions with unfailing efficiency.

The body's transport department is based on the heart. Essentials are carried to the point where they are needed, defence forces move along looking out for trouble and ready to summon help when necessary. Heat is evenly distributed throughout the body to meet the animal's needs. Waste products are collected and carried to disposal points.

Tasks of the system

The circulatory system carries the following essentials:

(1) *Oxygen* from the lungs to all of the body cells, especially muscles.
(2) *Carbon dioxide* from the body cells, especially muscles, to the lungs.
(3) *Water* and *nutrients* from the gut to the body cells.
(4) *Waste* from body tissues to the kidneys.
(5) *Messages* (hormones) from the endocrine glands to other organs.
(6) *Defence forces* to sites of attack.
(7) *Heat* from the centre of the body to its surface, as required.

Additionally, the system bathes the body cells in a uniform environment, and it resists leakage by virtue of the blood's ability to clot.

Blood

The constituents of the blood can be summarised as follows:

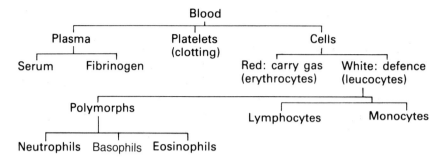

When a horse is off colour with no clear symptoms of disease, the vet may take a blood sample and produce a report showing the analysis of the blood. The vet will put some comment on the report, but it aids understanding to have some knowledge of blood itself.

Blood consists of a fluid called plasma, in which there are red and white blood cells or corpuscles of which red are the more numerous and give blood its characteristic colour. Blood is normally fluid during life and when freshly drawn from the body, but it clots or solidifies rapidly on exposure to air.

Plasma

Plasma contains fibrinogen (which aids the clotting of blood, together with platelets). The remainder of the plasma is called serum and this contains water, proteins, glucose, lipids, amino acids, salts, enzymes, hormones, antigens, antibodies and urea. It is this fluid which bathes the cells of the body. Plasma consists of about 90% water and its content is influenced principally by food and water from the gut, the requirements of the body, and the action of the kidneys.

Blood cells

The study of blood cells is called haematology. Blood cells are either red or white. Red blood cells originate in the bone marrow; they are also known as erythrocytes, and have the power of absorbing oxygen. White blood cells (leucocytes) defend against disease by attacking and destroying harmful germs, and are subdivided into two broad categories, the granulocytes (or polymorphs) and the agranulocytes, which are again subdivided into lymphocytes and monocytes, both of which originate in the lymphatic system (as discussed later). In contrast polymorphs originate in the bone marrow and are subdivided into neutrophils, which engulf bacteria to form pus; basophils, which help control inflammation; and eosinophils, which detoxify foreign proteins.

The red blood cells contain haemoglobin. This substance has the ability to combine with oxygen and carry it as oxyhaemoglobin from the lungs to the muscles. Haemoglobin also carries carbon dioxide. These two functions are essential for the efficient working of muscles.

The packed cell volume (PCV or haematocrit) refers to the percentage of whole blood constituted by red blood cells.

Analysis
A blood sample will indicate the horse's state of health. For example, if the red blood cell count or haemoglobin level is low, the horse is anaemic and must be treated accordingly. A high percentage of lymphocytes and monocytes may indicate some chronic disease. An excess of eosinophils suggests that there is a high percentage of invaders, such as worm larvae, in the blood.

The study of the horse's blood as a guide to performance and treatment is complicated by the ability of the horse to mobilise reserves very quickly; the spleen of the horse acts as a reservoir of blood cells. Thus, a different picture in some aspects (particularly the haematocrit) can be given by the same horse at different times on the same day, depending on alterations in activity and environment, particularly a stimulating change such as a journey, or even a vet who is a stranger.

A blood sample can still provide useful clues which, considered as part of the overall picture, give important pointers to health improvement. Anaemia, larval infestation, virus attack and azoturia are all examples of cases in which the blood can supply necessary information to aid diagnosis and treatment. Table 5.1 sets out the normal range of blood test values.

The heart

The heart is a hollow and cone-shaped organ consisting of muscle contained in a protective cover (the pericardium). It is sited in the centre of the chest, slightly left of the mid-line. The heart is divided into four internal compartments. The upper chambers are called atria (formerly auricles) and the lower are known as ventricles. The function of the heart is to keep up the circulation of blood.

The vena cava brings deoxygenated blood back to the right side of

Table 5.1   Normal range of blood test values.

Haematology	
Red cell count	6.5–12.3 × 10^{12} litre
Haemoglobin concentration	11.2–16.2 g/100 ml
Packed cell volume	32–43%
Mean corpuscular volume	38–46 femtolitres
White blood cells	5000–10500/mm^3
Neutrophils	2000–8000/mm^3
Lymphocytes	1500–4000/mm^3
Eosinophils	100–600/mm^3
Monocytes	100–600/mm^3
Basophils	20–50/mm^3
Biochemistry	
Serum proteins	
total	55–75 g/litre
albumin	25–41 g/litre
globulins	25–41 g/litre (1:1 ratio)

the heart. The blood is collected in the top chamber (atrium), and goes through a non-return valve into the lower chamber, which squeezes the blood up the pulmonary artery to the lungs.

The pulmonary vein brings oxygenated blood back from the lungs into the left atrium; it then goes down through a non-return valve into the left ventricle, which squeezes and forces the blood along the main artery of the body (the aorta) under pressure.

Both sides of the heart operate in parallel, and so both atria fill and then contract, sending the blood into the ventricles. In turn, both ventricles contract and send the blood up the pulmonary artery and the aorta. When a heart chamber contracts, the entry valves close to stop the blood going back the way it came, and as that chamber relaxes these valves reopen. The sound of the contractions and the operation of the valves produces the heartbeat, which can be heard when the horse is stressed or, with the aid of a stethoscope, behind the left elbow. The sound is written, '*LUBB*-dup – *LUBB*-dup – etc.'.

The normal heartbeat at rest is around 35 to 45 beats a minute but at top speed it can rise to about 200. If the rate rises and stays up when the horse is at rest, this is a sign of distress. A slight irregularity of heartbeat is not unusual in horses and may give no cause for concern: only the vet can say. A 'murmur' is the sound of a heart valve working imperfectly, but again this may not be a cause for concern – though it may constitute legal unsoundness. A dropped heartbeat at rest is acceptable, but not during or just after exercise.

Circulation

The circulatory system is shown diagrammatically in Fig. 5.1. Oxygenated blood from the heart is carried round the body under pressure in muscular thick-walled tubes called arteries, which gradually diminish in calibre as their length increases. The main artery leaving the heart is the aorta and its first branches supply blood to the heart itself. It has further branches off to all parts of the body, supplying every organ and structure. The next major branch (the brachiocephalic) goes to the head and forelegs. The aorta goes through the diaphragm and gives off a large branch called the coeliac artery, which supplies the stomach, liver and spleen. The intestines are supplied with blood by the mesenteric arteries: the large cranial at the front, and the smaller caudal at the rear. The renal artery supplies blood to the kidneys, and the iliac arteries supply the area of the hindquarters (see Fig. 5.2).

Every artery divides into smaller arterioles and these subdivide into the delicate capillaries which permeate throughout the body. Water, oxygen and nutrients filter out from the capillaries to the individual cells and some water returns in the same way, together with waste

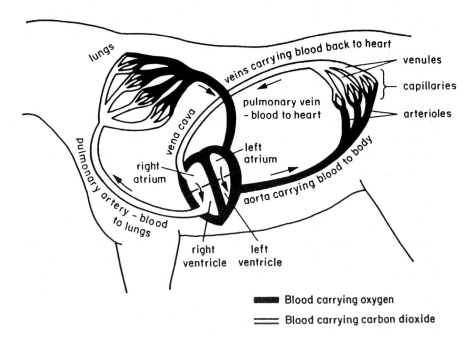

Fig. 5.1 The heart and circulation.

products. Capillaries unite to form venules and these in turn unite to form veins.

Venules are in effect small branches of a vein which receive oxygen-depleted blood from the capillaries and return it to the heart via the venous system. Veins are thin-walled tubular vessels that convey deoxygenated blood on its return journey to the heart. The blood in the veins does not have pressure from the heart to pump it round the body as do arteries; circulation is maintained by the presence of one-way valves within the vein and the massaging effect of the muscles surrounding the veins. Veins are mostly named after their opposing arteries: thus, the vein from the kidneys is called the renal vein. The veins flow into the vena cava which takes the blood back to the heart.

The main exception to this general arrangement is that blood from the intestines needs to be filtered by the liver before going into general circulation. Such blood is collected into the hepatic portal vein, which divides within the liver into a capillary network for filtration purposes before regrouping to form the hepatic vein, which goes into the vena cava.

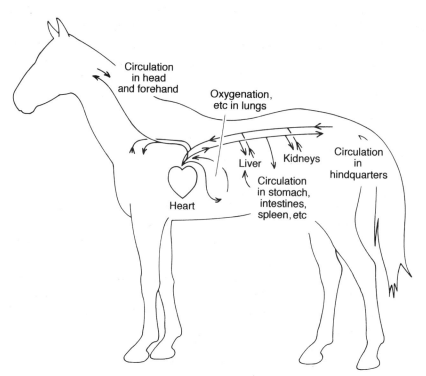

Fig. 5.2 Circulation in the horse.

The whole system is called the systemic circulation system. Pulmonary circulation is the system supplying blood to the lungs. Deoxygenated blood is carried to the lungs by the pulmonary artery, and the pulmonary vein returns it in oxygenated form.

Lymphatic system

Lymph is an almost colourless fluid, chiefly containing white blood cells, which surrounds the tissues of the body. It comes from the blood and has to be returned to it. Some of this fluid is picked up by capillaries, but this collection system is not sufficient. It is paralleled by a second means of collection, the lymphatic system, which is both extensive and important.

Lymphatics are very thin-walled vessels, and their function is to collect the nutrients from digested food and to prevent accumulation of tissue fluid in any part of the body. The lymph capillaries flow into the lymph vessels, which have valves to ensure that the direction of flow is towards the heart. The vessels also have nodes or filters (which are bean-shaped masses of tissue) to check the lymph for infection and if necessary to produce lymphocytes and antibodies to cope with it. If there is infection in an area, the lymph nodes or glands will be enlarged and prominent. This is particularly noticeable under the jaw and inside the thigh.

Disorders of the circulatory system

Anaemia
Symptoms: Pale gums, eyelid linings or other mucous membranes. Heart having to work harder to get oxygen around the body; it beats faster than normal. Lack of best performance and reduction in stamina.
Causes: Shortage of red blood cells or haemoglobin through haemorrhage (bleeding), infection, redworms, bots, or dietary deficiency.
Treatment: The vet must deal with any infection. The horse will need to work less hard during the recovery period. Folic acid, B_{12} or iron supplements may be required in the diet.
Prevention: Control redworms and bots. Grow deep-rooting herbs in the paddock or feed mineral supplement.

Equine rhabdomyolysis syndrome (azoturia, set-fast or tying-up)

Symptoms: Typically, the horse is excited, has done some work, has to wait and is unable to go forward. Examples include after the first draw out hunting, or between Phases A and B in a three-day event, or after warm-up waiting to jump at a show. However, it may occur after the horse is back home from exercise. The horse will sweat up and be unable to walk forward or will do so with difficulty. The muscles behind the saddle and those of the hindquarters feel hard. The horse is distressed by pain. The hind legs may be paralysed. Dark red, strange smelling urine may be passed. Severe cases collapse completely.

Causes: A disease attributed to management but some horses seem to be predisposed towards it. High corn diet and lack of exercise. Glycogen in the muscles is converted during exercise into lactic acid. In cases of azoturia, the lactic acid is not removed quickly enough and accumulates in the muscles, causing them to seize up. It is very like an attack of cramp.

Treatment: Do not move the horse. Rug the horse up and keep it out of draughts. If out, have the horse transported home. Call the vet, who may give drugs for the pain and inflammation. Hot fomentations may ease discomfort.

Prevention: Keep exercise ahead of food – as for lymphangitis (see below). A vitamin E diet supplement may help. The vet may prescribe an antacid or a buffer mixture in the diet.

Dehydration

Symptoms: A fold of skin pinched up will be slow to flatten out. After exercise, the horse is slow to recover its normal pulse and respiration rate. It is dull and lethargic. Prolonged stress such as a long journey or an endurance ride in hot weather can produce an audible diaphragm spasm ('the thumps'). This is a serious condition, the horse being near collapse, and it needs urgent veterinary attention.

Causes: Can be shortage of water, or the horse not drinking enough, or loss of fluid through scouring or excessive sweating from exertion, travel in a confined space, or fever.

Treatment: Ensure that the horse normally has access to water at all times. Check that the water is pleasant for the horse. Salt in feed may encourage it to drink more. The cause of any scouring or looseness in the droppings must be treated.

Performance horses that will be competing in hot weather and sweating heavily should be given electrolytes at the recommended rate immediately before, during and after competition. Electrolytes are sometimes given during endurance rides by syringing concentrated electrolyte solution into the horse's mouth, but this must never be done before the horse has started to drink well, or it will cause fluid to be drawn into the stomach from the tissues and dehydrate the horse even more.

When dehydration is due to lack of available water or after exercise the horse should be allowed to drink small quantities of water (no more than half a bucket), every ten minutes until the thirst is quenched. Once the horse has started to drink, electrolytes can be offered dissolved in water to replace the body salts which have been lost. In severe cases, however, the horse may be given electrolytes intravenously so that the body is rehydrated as quickly as possible.

Endocarditis and pericarditis
Symptoms: Often vague. Loss of interest in work and falling-away in condition.
Causes: The membranes lining the heart or surrounding it are inflamed by bacterial or viral attack.
Treatment: Cure the infection under the vet's direction. Months rather than weeks are required for convalescence, and rest is important.

Grass sickness
Symptoms: Inflamed membranes. Difficulty in swallowing. Depression. No bowel activity. Dribbling. Mucus discharge from nostrils.
Cause: Unknown, but probably viral.
Treatment: None known. The disease is almost always fatal.

Haematoma
Symptoms: Lumps or bulges under the skin.
Causes: Haemorrhage (bleeding), either below the skin or into a muscle to form a lump, generally resulting from a blow. Can be large or small.
Treatment: Small haematomae are absorbed, but large ones require veterinary treatment and a few days' rest.

Lymphangitis (big leg)
Symptoms: Typically, the horse has a swollen hind leg which is warm and tender. The swelling often extends down from the stifle to the foot. The horse shows symptoms of pain and has a raised temperature. Inflamed lymph vessels and nodes can occur in other areas.
Causes: An imbalance between a high corn diet and lack of exercise. It

is often referred to (as is azoturia) as a 'Monday morning disease'. It may also be caused by infection.

Treatment: The vet will prescribe suitable drugs such as pain-killers, sedatives and/or antibiotics. The horse requires a comfortable stable, a laxative diet and hot fomentations applied several times daily to the limb. Lameness will limit exercise, but a little gentle walking in hand will help after the initial swelling has reduced slightly.

Prevention: Keep exercise ahead of food. If the horse is to have a day off, e.g. a Sunday after hunting on Saturday, cut back the food the night before. If possible, put the horse out in the paddock for an hour or more on the rest day. Treat any small wounds quickly to prevent infection.

Overheating

Symptoms: Horse appears exhausted, dull and lethargic, and is sweating. It may be trembling, with a raised pulse and respiration. Temperature may be as high as 42°C (108°F).

Cause: Prolonged or very strenuous exertion in conditions of high heat and humidity.

Treatment: At rectal temperature of 42–43°C (108–109°F) muscle cells within the horse will start to die and it is vital to cool the horse rapidly and effectively by assisting heat loss from the skin's surface. Do not stand the horse still for too long. Reduction of blood to the muscles and skin will lead to lactic acid build-up and the possibility of the horse tying up. In hot weather the horse should have copious amounts of water sponged over the neck, chest, belly, between the hind legs and to the back and quarters as he walks around. This will replace sweating and so aid cooling without further dehydration. Walking the horse in shady areas and the use of large mechanical fans will also assist heat loss.

Ice packs can be used when the weather is very hot but must always be wrapped in a cloth and either applied for a few seconds to one area or kept moving over a large area. Ice should only be used in areas where there are major blood vessels, such as the throat and between the hind legs – the poll is often used so that the melt water runs down the throat.

Cold wet towels are often draped over the neck and quarters: to be effective these must be changed as soon as they become warm – often after only a few seconds – otherwise all they do is prevent heat loss from the area that they cover.

Treat for symptoms of dehydration.

Prevention When high humidity combines with high temperature, take great care to avoid dehydration. Avoid high speed plus long duration and cool the body with cool water as often as possible.

Strangles

Symptoms: Swollen glands under jaw. Nasal discharge. Temperature. Cough. Swallowing is painful.
Cause: Specific contagious bacteria.
Treatment: Isolate. Check spread of disease to other horses. Get the vet quickly as it is highly contagious. Rest. Sloppy food.

Transit tetany

Symptoms: Distress, sweating, fast breathing, stumbling gait, all after a journey (especially of lactating mare in warm weather).
Cause: Lowering of the blood calcium level.
Treatment: Cool, quiet box, water to drink. Call the vet.

Tetanus (lockjaw)

Symptoms: Increasing stiffness of movement. The horse stands in a stretched-out manner. Tapping under the chin will cause the third eyelid to react. Later, the whole of the horse reacts to noise and touch. Muscular spasms. The jaws clamped together.
Cause: A bacterium found in the soil (*Clostridium tetani*). If this gets into an airless situation in a wound, toxins are produced which cause muscle spasm. Entry may be through a puncture wound or even a scratch.
Treatment: Call the vet. Prognosis is not good, but early diagnosis will help. Quiet, dark stable.
Prevention: Vaccinate with tetanus toxoid and give booster injection every other year. Very often this is combined with protection against equine flu. Pregnant mares may get their tetanus booster in the last month of pregnancy to help extend cover to the foal. The foal will need its own protection after about two months.

Thrombosis and embolism

Symptoms: Depends on the site of the problem. The commonest site is the gut and the symptom is colic.
Causes: Obstruction of blood vessels by an attached stationary blood clot (thrombus). The commonest cause of these clots is redworm

larvae in the system. If the blood clot breaks off and flows along the vessel and then jams across a small blood vessel, this is an embolism, and the area served by that vessel will suffer. An embolism may cause part of the body to go out of function for a short while. Sometimes the blood will sort out an alternative route around the system. The larval attack may cause a rupture of the artery wall (an aneurism).

Treatment: Treat the symptom (colic). Call the vet. Control worms, particularly larval stages, migrating through the body.

6 Respiratory System

The main task of this system is to get oxygen into the blood. Without oxygen, all heat production and activity will cease. If the respiratory system falters, the horse will die within a few minutes. Of the horse's three major requirements, food, water and oxygen, the latter is crucial in the shortest time. A horse can go several days without water; it can go weeks without food; but death will occur if it is deprived of oxygen for a matter of minutes.

Tasks of the system

Like several other systems, the respiratory system has a primary function and a number of subsidiary but important ones. The provision of oxygen is the major function of the system. Its other tasks are:

(1) To remove carbon dioxide from the blood.
(2) To help temperature control by breathing out warm air and taking in cool air.
(3) To eliminate water: this is seen readily on a cold day, but happens at all times.
(4) To communicate by sound (voice production).
(5) To act as a sensory input: this is done through both smell and touch (via the nostril hairs).
(6) To act as a filter for air-borne invaders.

Air passages and the lungs

Within the head
Oxygen is taken down into the lungs along a highly specialised route. The extremity of this route consists of the nostrils, which are large,

117

soft, gentle and inquisitive. They change in shape according to the horse's needs. The horse draws air in only through the nostrils and not the mouth. They are easily dilated and form part of the horse's facial expression when it is inquisitive or angry. Facial expressions are backed up by air blown from the nostrils and expelled as a blow or a snort. The hairs between and below the nostrils combine with the animal's sense of smell to investigate strange objects at close range. The airways in the head are shown in Fig. 6.1.

The nasal cavities – one for each nostril – are divided from each other by a piece of cartilage. They are separated from the mouth by the hard palate and, higher, by the soft palate. The cavity is partially filled with wafer-thin, curling bones, called the turbinate bones, which are designed to have a large surface area. This, like the rest of the cavity is covered by mucous membrane which helps to warm incoming air so that it does not strike too cold on the lungs. In warming the air in this way, the body loses heat when the air is expelled. This membrane, in the higher part of the cavity, contains the olfactory nerve endings, which detect smells.

In the skull at the front are air-filled cavities called sinuses, connecting with the nasal cavity. The maxillary sinus is above the molar teeth, and the others are called the frontal, the sphenopalatine and the

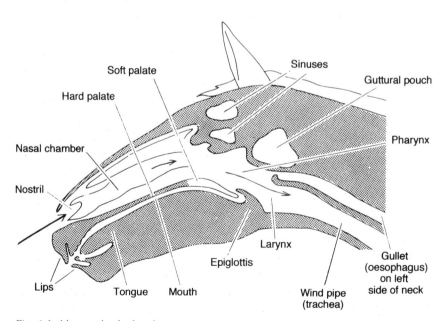

Fig. 6.1 Airways in the head.

ethmoidal sinuses. All exist in pairs, one on each side, and they give the skull strength and form, without excessive weight.

The pharynx or throat is the common passage for food and air, each coming from a different place and going down a different tube, with a crossover mechanism which shoots the food to be swallowed up and over the windpipe and into the gullet. When stomach-tubing a horse, it is necessary to pass the tube up the nostril because of the arrangement of the pharynx. Care must be taken to ensure that the tube goes down the gullet and not down the windpipe.

The Eustachian tubes come into the top of the pharynx. They allow air to pass to the middle ear, and connected to them are the guttural pouches which are sited just above the pharynx.

Within the neck

Air passes from the pharynx through the larynx, which is the organ producing the voice. It is a box of jointed cartilage and the surrounding muscles can alter its calibre. The function of the larynx is to control the air going in and out, monitoring it for foreign objects which must be rejected. It is sited in the throat between the branches of the lower jaw, where it may be readily felt. Food and water pass over its opening (the glottis) on the way down the gullet, and it has a lid (the epiglottis) which closes automatically when the horse swallows. Anything wrong with the glottis or epiglottis causes coughing.

These organs and the vocal cords (which are thick and elastic) produce the horse's sounds of communication or voice. The larynx is thus commonly called the 'voice-box'. The horse can squeal, nicker, whinny and groan. The muscles that retract or draw back these cartilages are controlled by a branch of the vagus nerve which, curiously, is much longer on the left than on the right side. This nerve sometimes malfunctions so as to give wind problems, which are often confined to the left side of the larynx. Despite the larynx's function as a filter, some dust is inhaled by the horse, particularly when eating dry hay or when straw is shaken up when bedding down.

The windpipe (trachea) runs from the larynx to the lungs. It runs along the lower border of the neck and can easily be felt as far down as the entrance to the chest. It is a tube reinforced with rings of cartilage with overlapping ends. The lining of the trachea produces sticky mucus which traps foreign particles which may enter the tube. The particles are wafted up the trachea to the larynx by a carpet of microscopic hairs called cilia. The mucus is then coughed up and swallowed.

Within the chest

The windpipe divides into two bronchi at the entrance to the chest, one branch going to each lung. From this point they divide and subdivide into bronchioles, which end as alveolar sacs. These in turn are subdivided into lots of little alveoli like grapes in a bunch, so as to give maximum surface area (see Fig. 6.2).

The surfaces of the bronchi and bronchioles are protected by mucus and cilia. The bronchioles have fine muscle fibres in their structure enabling the diameter to be changed.

The lungs are two large elastic organs. The horse's right lung has an extra lobe, but the shape of the lungs is not important as they completely fill the cavity of the chest (except for the cavity occupied by the heart) below the backbone and enclosed by the ribs and the diaphragm. The lungs are surrounded by a covering (the pleura), which is a smooth and slippery membrane that prevents friction.

The pulmonary artery brings blood to the lungs from the heart. This blood is described as deoxygenated as it has given up oxygen deep in the tissues of the horse so that normal body processes can take place. In return, the blood carries away a by-product of these processes, carbon dioxide. Both carbon dioxide and oxygen are carried in the red blood cells, chemically attached to a substance called haemoglobin.

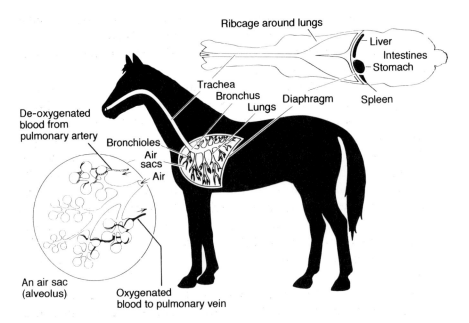

Fig. 6.2 Respiratory system.

Within the lung the pulmonary artery divides and subdivides, resulting eventually in thin-walled capillaries which come into intimate contact with the alveoli. Carbon dioxide and oxygen are able to pass across the fine layers of cells that separate the blood from the air in the lungs in a process called gaseous exchange in which oxygen is exchanged for carbon dioxide. The stale air in the alveoli is exhaled back along the same route from whence it came, while the now oxygenated blood passes into the pulmonary vein to be taken back to the heart.

The diaphragm separates the chest from the belly. It is a strong and thin sheet of muscle attached to the inner sides of the ribs. It begins just in front of the loins, high under the backbone, sloping downwards and forwards to the breast bone. The major blood vessels and gullet go through it as they come from the chest, and like the lungs (which it touches) it is covered with pleura.

Breathing

Breathing is taking the air down into the lungs so that gaseous exchange with the blood is possible. It is one aspect of respiration. The second aspect is the activity in the body tissues where the oxygen is used.

The horse draws in air through its nostrils. The air passes through the larynx, down the windpipe and into the lungs. There, air and blood exchange the required elements and, after a slight pause, the used air is expelled. The process is repeated.

Air is dawn into the lungs by muscular expansion of the thorax or rib cage, and is expelled by elastic recoil of the rib cage. In the horse the rib cage is a single cavity whereas in many animals it is divided into two, with a separate lung in each. It is surrounded by ribs and separated from the abdomen by the diaphragm, which is dome shaped, with the top of the dome nearest the front of the horse. When the diaphragm muscles contract, the dome is pulled flatter and this increases the size of the chest cavity. This diaphragm activity is important for deeper breathing. However, if the stomach and intestines are full, the movement of the diaphragm is impeded. This is why a racehorse has no hay and only a small feed in the morning on a race day.

When the horse is relaxed and at rest, the amount of air taken into the lungs is about one-fifth of the amount taken in when the horse is at full exertion. At rest, the horse usually has a respiratory rate of 8 to 16 breaths per minute, the rate being higher for younger stock. After prolonged rapid exertion this rate may be increased to 120 breaths per minute. Other factors that will cause an increase in the respiration rate include excitement, high altitude, high ambient temperature, high humidity and obesity. The lungs never empty totally, but take in and expel more air when the horse is exerted.

Healthy respiration
In the normal resting horse breathing is a quiet, relaxed process, with breathing in (inhalation) and breathing out (exhalation) taking place in a regular, rhythmical fashion. The nostrils are relaxed and clean, although a slight watery discharge is quite normal. There should be no abnormal sounds such as coughing or wheezing. The rhythm of the breathing is important; normally each breath is followed by a pause and the period of expiration is usually slightly longer than that of inhalation. The length of the pause shortens if the horse is excited, has recently returned from exercise or has a respiratory problem.

Signs of breathing problems
The vet should be consulted if the horse shows any of the following signs:

- Coughing or any other abnormal sound at rest or during exercise.
- Increased respiratory rate or laboured breathing in the resting horse.
- Irregular breathing – for example, a horse may appear to have spells of rapid breathing followed by periods when he does not breathe.
- Reduced exercise tolerance and prolonged recovery rate after exercise.
- Abnormal nasal discharge.

Disorders of the respiratory system

Respiratory disease
Respiratory disease falls into three main categories: infection, inflammation and allergy.

Infection
Many horses travel widely to competitions and mix with other horses, and so they are particularly vulnerable to viral infection. A horse will

recover from a simple, uncomplicated viral infection in about a week, but the virus will have damaged the cells lining the airways so that they are much more susceptible to a secondary bacterial infection, which may take much longer to clear up and cause more damage to the lining of the airways. These infections are often described as chills or cold and the vet will refer to them as upper respiratory tract diseases (URT).

Inflammation

A condition known as Small Airway Disease is associated with local inflammation, which may follow infection, irritation or allergy. Inflammation leads to swelling of the lining of the airways so that the internal diameter is reduced, making breathing less efficient.

Allergy

Blood cells attracted by the inflammation may meet fungal spores which have been inhaled by horses being fed mouldy hay. This causes the muscle of the airways to go into spasm, thus reducing the diameter even further. Dead cells and mucus from the inflammatory reaction accumulate, physically blocking the air flow. Once the mucous linings of the small airways of the lungs have been damaged they may become 'sensitised' to environmental influences, to which they develop an allergy. This is called *Chronic Obstructive Pulmonary Disease (COPD)*. Horses can become allergic to the fungal spores found in hay, while some horses may be allergic to pollens, causing a hay fever type condition.

Respiratory disease is usually progressive; horses rarely develop COPD overnight; there is a build-up of stress on the respiratory system, infection, poor environment and exercise all contributing to inflammation and damage until the lung becomes hypersensitive and COPD results.

Signs of respiratory disease

Increased respiration rate, the effort made breathing out or on expiration becomes more noticeable, and in severe cases the horse will develop a 'heaves line' – the muscles of the abdomen involved with breathing out become enlarged and the horse can be seen making an extra exhalatory effort. There may be an abnormal discharge from the nose and/or eyes; in the early stages of a viral infection this will be watery, but becomes thick and purulent, indicating a secondary bacterial infection. The early stages of a viral infection usually cause a sharp rise in body temperature (normally 38°C or 100.5°F), but this is often very short-lived and is easily missed. Where high performance is vital, temperature should be routinely taken morning and evening. The horse may go off its feed for a few days and this usually coincides with the fever. A cough will develop – this may be an occasional cough in the stable which becomes more severe during and after exercise. All of these factors will combine to stop the horse working as efficiently: indeed, the first thing the rider or trainer notices may be the fact that the horse seems 'not himself'. Temperature taking may indicate a problem before the horse shows any clinical signs.

Treatment of respiratory disease

There is no one cure for respiratory disease but all of the following have an important role to play:

- *Rest.* In the acute stages it is important to allow the horse complete rest. Fresh air is necessary but draughts, cold winds and rain should be avoided.
- *Antibiotics.* The bacterial infection that moves into the cells damaged by the viral infection can be readily and effectively treated with antibiotics.
- *Getting rid of the mucus.* In respiratory disease the cilia that waft away the mucus are reduced in number, and more mucus is produced which is more viscous than usual. If a cough suppressant is used the horse stops coughing and large particles of debris will be left in the airways to cause damage. In the early stages it is better to give the horse a mucolytic agent which helps move the mucus by making it more liquid. Consequently coughing is reduced because the horse can clear the mucus far more easily.
- *Relieving the bronchospasm.* Horses with respiratory problems may suffer bronchospasm: the small airways contain smooth muscle, which in response to irritant substances present in the airway, contract causing narrowing of the passages. This can cause quite severe distress in the horse which will have real difficulty in taking in enough air to breathe – this is equivalent to an asthma attack in humans. The veterinary surgeon can prescribe a spasmolytic drug which acts by causing the smooth muscle to relax, opening the airways and allowing more air to pass into the lungs.
- *Stable management.* Respiratory disease must not be allowed to progress into COPD, the environment should be as dust and fungal spore-free as possible. In severe cases change to a fungal

spore-free alternative such as haylage, good silage, barn-dried hay, alfalfa, grass nuts, hydroponic grass or high-fibre cubes. If this is not a viable alternative the hay will have to be soaked; the idea is that the fungal spores swell and are swallowed, not inhaled. In order to accomplish this hay must be soaked for several hours.

Dust-free bedding should be used; wood shavings, although often dusty, contain few spores – let the dust settle after putting in new shavings before returning the horse to its box. Bedding should be kept scrupulously clean. Bad drainage means a damp bed – paper and peat are very prone to dampness. A damp bed produces ammonia, which irritates the lungs and paralyses the hair-like cilia which waft the mucus away from the alveoli and up the bronchial tree.

Fresh air is essential. The stable should be draught-free with air vents in the roof apex which are large enough to carry away stale air. The air inlets – half door and window – should be on more than one side, so that air movement outside will always get into the stable. Air movement around the stable should be free – buildings, hedges and trees can all obstruct air flow.

The stable should be kept as clean as possible: the dust from floor to ceiling should be vacuumed or washed away – dust, cobwebs, ledges and cracks all harbour spores. The hay fed to the rest of the horses in the yard should also be soaked – spores can be blown on the wind and the position of the muck heap and where hay and straw are stored must all be away from the stabling.

The horse should be turned out as much as possible especially in acute cases of COPD, regardless of the weather and time of year – you will just have to invest in a sturdy New Zealand rug!

If exposure to the allergens responsible for a horse's 'asthma attack' is unavoidable a spasmolytic drug can be given as a liquid that can be inhaled using a mask and a nebuliser. Treatment by inhalation on three or four successive days will protect a horse for up to three weeks and can be given in anticipation of exposure to fungal spores if, for example, being stabled away from home.

Chill or cold (upper respiratory tract diseases, URT)
Symptoms: A clear, thick discharge from the nostrils which later may become whitish; swollen throat glands; a gentle or wheezy cough;

possibly some difficulty in swallowing and a slight rise in temperature.
Cause: A virus causes the primary infection. The horse standing in an
area which is poorly ventilated, such as a stable or lorry, or when first
stabled after being out at grass, is more susceptible to the virus.
Treatment: Isolate the horse, keep it warm but allow plenty of fresh
air, use paper bedding or arrange for the horse to be out of the stable
when the bedding is shaken up or fresh bedding is laid. Hay, if fed,
should be soaked and fed on the ground; give soft food and green
food. An antiseptic electuary may be given. An ointment designed for
human nasal congestion and 'chestiness' can also be rubbed not on the
chest and throat but into the outer nostril, twice a day. Inhalations of
friar's balsam may also be used. The condition will generally clear up
in a week and will respond well to antibiotics, which control secondary
infections. Keep the horse on walking exercise until the condition is
completely cleared.
Prevention: Avoid stuffy conditions for horses and take particular care
when getting them up from the grass. Do not let horses drink from
public troughs at shows. Avoid allowing the horse to stand in a
draught, especially when it is cooling.

Influenza or 'the cough'
Symptoms: Generally similar to a cold. The horse may first appear
shivery or off its food. Raised temperature.
Cause: A virulent virus which has different strains.
Treatment: Call the vet without delay. Antibiotics help. Proceed as for
a cold or chill. Generally, avoid hard or fast work for one week for
each day of raised temperature.
Prevention: Once the virus is in the yard it is nearly impossible to stop
it going from one horse to another. When 'the cough' is known to be in
the area, it is, therefore, safest to avoid contact with other horses.
There is a vaccine which gives protection against many but not all of
the flu strains. Vaccination is compulsory before attending many
competitions.

Laryngitis, tracheitis, bronchitis
Symptoms: Coughing. A drop in temperature. Discharge from the
nostrils. Difficulty in breathing. All three diseases are similar.
Cause: Infection of the upper respiratory tract.
Treatment: Keep the horse warm and give plenty of fresh air. Damp
the food before feeding. Electuaries, antibiotics and steaming may
help.

Lungworm

Symptoms: A dry cough. Laboratory examination of droppings is necessary to confirm an attack.
Cause: Worm larvae.
Treatment: Call the vet. Fit animals are most resistant to infestation.
Prevention: Keep the pasture clean.
   Note: Some horses and most donkeys can carry the disease without showing symptoms.

Nose bleed (epistaxis)

Symptoms: Blood appearing at the nostrils. The bleeding may occur from the lungs following fast work. It may come from the guttural pouch, the top of the throat, or from the nose following stomach tubing.
Cause: May be associated with viral infection.
Treatment: Keep the horse quiet; often the bleeding will stop of its own accord. The vet may be able to offer a line of treatment.

Pneumonia

Symptoms: Rise in temperature up to 41°C (107°F). After 12 hours, quickened pulse and respiration; cold extremities. The animal is 'tucked up'. Coughing.
Causes: Inflammation of the lungs caused by a virus, bacteria, a fungus or a parasite.
Treatment: Call the vet. Keep the horse quiet and warm, with plenty of fresh air. Steam inhalation may help. Long convalescence.

Sinusitis

Symptoms: Grey nasal discharge, generally from only one nostril. The area below the eye on the affected side may be swollen and tender.
Causes: Infection, often following a cold or strangles. A diseased tooth.
Treatment: Call the vet who may drain the sinus. Antibiotics and sulphonamides will help.

'Wrong in the wind' (whistling, roaring, 'makes a noise')

Symptoms: Abnormal noise as horse inhales at canter or gallop.
Diagnosis: Some cases are clear cut and easily identified; others are a matter of opinion and the experts may agree to differ as to whether the horse is unsound in the wind, or has a temporary infection which affects respiratory function, or is merely unfit and rather 'thick in its

wind', which will come right with improved fitness. Viewing with a laryngoscope may show if there is some lack of vocal cord movement.
Cause: Usually, it is the nerve to the left side of the larynx which malfunctions; thus that vocal cord and its neighbouring cartilages are not drawn back during inspiration and the noise is created by air rushing past this obstruction.

Treatment: This problem used to be treated by 'tubing' (tracheotomy), which allows air directly into the windpipe and by-passes the obstruction. Commonly now the horse is 'hobdayed', which is a simple operation to clear the obstruction. The wound after the operation should drain freely and heal well, during which time the horse is kept stabled and quiet. A modification of the Hobday operation includes a prosthesis, which is a man-made spare part.

Prevention: As big horses seem more susceptible to this trouble, the very greatest care must be taken when getting them fit. The British Ministry of Agriculture lists the disease as hereditary but not everyone would agree. Horses that have been hobdayed are not eligible for show hunter classes.

7 The Skin

The skin is many things. It is the body's outer protective (integumentary) layer or covering and the largest organ of the body. It is a very tough and complex packaging system. Horse hide, for example, is used to make leather suits to protect motorcycle speedway riders, who frequently crash at high speed on an abrasive surface.

This envelope to contain the horse is also a protective covering for the underlying tissue, but has several other functions. It stabilises body heat, eliminates waste products in solution with the sweat and provides camouflage for the horse in the wild. The skin also has specialised nerve endings through which the animal receives the sensations of touch, pressure, cold, heat and pain, as explained in Chapter 4.

The thickness of the skin varies with both breed and area of the body. Thus, the skin of the Thoroughbred and similar types such as the Arab is thinner than in the less aristocratic breeds, and the skin across the back, for example, is thicker than that of the face.

The skin is also an indicator of health. Movement of the skin over the ribs shows the presence of subcutaneous fat even in a fit horse. Similarly, a pinched-up fold of skin may give an indication of dehydration if the fold is slow to disappear.

Structure

Skin

Skin (see Fig. 7.1) is the tissue forming the outer covering of the horse's body. It consists of two layers: the inner layer, known as the dermis, and the outer layer or epidermis.

The epidermis is covered with hairs, which form the coat, and it is modified at the extremities of the horse's limbs to form the hooves. It is a superficial layer which is being shed constantly in the form of scurf because, like most cells within the body, its cells are continually dying

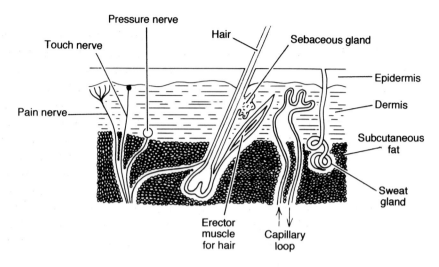

Fig. 7.1 Skin.

and being replaced. The scurf needs to be groomed from the body so that it does not litter the surface and impede some of the skin's other functions.

Horses in the wild do not need grooming. It is not in their nature to dash around working up a sweat. In the wild, the dead cells mix with grease, mud and so on, and the accumulation falls off gradually. In contrast, the ridden horse is being asked for sustained activity and high performance. Regular grooming increases the power of the skin to work at high pressure as well as being an aid to cleanliness and a preventive of disease.

The dermis or inner layer of the skin is deep and sensitive. It contains blood vessels, nerve fibres, glands producing sweat and oil, and hair roots. The hairs and the tubes of the oil and sweat glands pass through the epidermis to the surface, where their openings are known as pores.

The skin is very elastic, varying in thickness according to the amount of protection required. It moves freely over the horse's flesh and should feel loose when handled. The inner layer is seated on a thin layer of subcutaneous fat.

The sweat glands lie deep in the skin, and are little coiled tubes continuing to the surface by a thin duct through which the sweat is discharged. They are in action constantly although this will not be visible when the horse is at rest.

Hair

Almost the whole of the horse's body is covered by hairs. They grow from the hair bulbs, set deep in the skin, and come out at an acute angle with the surface so that the coat lies flat and smooth. The skin carries several kinds of hair: permanent hair such as the long hair of the mane, tail and heel 'feathers', tactile hairs of the lips, nostrils and eyes and the temporary hair of the coat which is shed and changed for a new growth in spring and autumn, the length of the new growth depending on the season. Hair is also shed, a little at a time, constantly throughout the year, being replaced by new growth. Each hair is lubricated by oil which exudes from a small gland at the base, and has a tiny muscle which can pull it into an upright position. The hair is part of the mechanism for stabilising body heat. Some hairs, such as the whiskers on the muzzle, are modified so as to act in a sensory capacity, rather like antennae.

The colour of the hair is due only to a single pigment which, by its variation in quality and grouping, gives the colour range we know. This ranges from grey, through chestnut to black, or almost any combination of these colours. There is no pigment in white hairs. A roan-coloured horse has a mixture of white and coloured hairs, grouped to one side of the hair. In an albino there is no pigment in either the hair or the skin: the pinkness comes from the blood below.

Protection

The colour of the skin and the coat gives protection from sunlight. The skin is not necessarily the same colour as the coat, as in the case of a grey. The albino, being devoid of pigment, is more vulnerable to exposure to sunlight and often has a lower resistance to infection. The coat also gives protection from thorns, brambles and the like. The skin is tough in its outer layer, is attached loosely and is free-moving so as to minimise the risk of its tearing. It keeps water out, and yet is able to expel excess moisture as required. This is done through the sweat glands. The subcutaneous fat under the skin acts as a padding to protect the horse's body from minor bumps.

Stabilising body heat

The muscular activity of the body generates heat, which is then lost from the body by radiation and the evaporation of sweat. If the weather is hot or there is intense muscular activity (as in galloping), the blood vessels in the skin expand to radiate more heat and to stimulate the sweat glands to greater activity. This is then noticeable as 'lathering up', particularly in Thoroughbred horses.

The skin is cooled by the action of the sweat evaporating off the skin. The hairs of the coat lie flat against the skin, so trapping the minimum amount of air and allowing the sweat to evaporate as quickly as possible. Sweat evaporates more slowly in very humid conditions and so the cooling effect is then less. Horses that have sweat dripping off them are creating sweat faster than it can evaporate; it is likely that they are not losing heat effectively as evaporation may be slow. To work a horse hard and long in hot and humid conditions creates for the body the serious problems of overheating and dehydration, which cause unacceptable distress to the horse. In extreme circumstances this can result in death.

The horse needs to conserve its body heat in cold weather and therefore the blood vessels in the skin contract. Less heat is then lost by radiation. When the horse is ill, there is often a battle between the invading germs or bacteria and the body's defences, and this leads to sweating.

The horse's coat keeps the body warm, and the oil produced by the glands under the skin's surface greases the hairs and renders the surface waterproof. In cold weather the hairs stand on end, so increasing the air trapped in the coat which also grows longer, thus providing yet more protection. In hot weather the hair lies flat and is much shorter, replacing the long coat that has been shed in spring. Horses of Eastern origin, such as the Arab and the Thoroughbred, have a shorter and finer coat than British native stock.

When the horse is debilitated, the subcutaneous fat is reduced so the horse gets cold and to cope he tends to make the hairs of the coat stand up or 'stare'. Want of condition, neglect or ill health will also cause the coat to look dull and feel harsh. In good health, the coat lies flat, feels quite smooth and has a good gloss.

Where a horse is clipped out, as is the hunter during the winter, the balance must be put right by the provision of rugs, blankets, and food. Clothing on horses stops the hair growing so quickly by reducing the need for a warm coat.

Waste disposal

The function of eliminating waste products in solution with the sweat is particularly important for the horse under stress. Where horses sweat a lot from other reasons, it is evident that they will get rid of more salts from the body than are surplus to requirements. In such circumstances, therefore, greater care must be taken with nutrition to make good the deficit. Extreme cases of such losses of essential salts (electrolytes) may occur in three-day eventing or long-distance riding in hot weather. On completing their activity such horses may need a solution of these salts that are required by the body.

For this aspect of the system to work efficiently, it is important that the pores in the skin be kept open. They have a tendency to become clogged with dirt, and debris such as dead skin cells. The horse in work therefore requires efficient use of the body brush. This is most effective when the horse is still rather warm after exercise, as the pores are then open.

Camouflage

The horse's coat colour is a means of camouflage in its wild stage, enabling it to escape the notice of its enemies by allowing it to blend into the background. This can be seen in the wild ponies on both Exmoor and Dartmoor, where the coat colour tends to blend in with the bracken and other background foliage. The striped coat of the zebra, which is a member of the horse family, is another example of camouflage.

Formation of vitamin D

Vitamin D, known as the 'sunshine vitamin', occurs as two provitamins which need the ultraviolet component of sunlight acting on the skin to be converted to the vitamin. The main function of vitamin D is concerned with the body's ability to utilise calcium and phosphorus. Horses rarely exposed to the sun may run short of vitamin D.

Disorders of the skin

Skin diseases and disorders are a common occurrence in horses.

Cracked heels
Symptoms: An inflamed area with hard skin and red raw cracks, causing pain and lameness.

Cause: Allowing the heels to get wet, scratched, or muddy, and not attending to them properly at the end of the day. This complaint especially affects clipped-out horses.

Treatment: Acriflavine cream rubbed in gently each day. The scabs must be removed.

Prevention: When washing the feet, put the thumb in the deep groove in the heel to ensure that it is cleansed. Grease heels with udder cream or similar protection before going hunting in wet conditions. Dry heels gently when wet and do not brush out mud with a stiff brush.

Girth gall

Symptoms: A sore area under the girth.

Causes: Sensitive skin. Girth causing rubbing, especially a dirty girth.

Treatment: As for a cut. By placing a cotton wool pad over the area, the horse can normally be ridden again after a few days. Exercise in hand in the meantime.

Prevention: Surgical spirit can be used to harden the area once healed.

Mange

Symptoms: Intense skin irritation. Small lumps on the withers, back, neck and shoulders.

Cause: Parasites (mange mites).

Treatment: The vet must be informed as some forms are notifiable to the authorities. An affected horse should be isolated. (*Note:* this is a very rare disease in Britain.)

Mud fever and rain scald

Symptoms: Inflammation of the skin often leading to swelling with serum oozing through the skin so that the skin eventually cracks and a secondary infection may then occur. It is frequently found in the heels and lower legs of horses in wet weather, the belly, back and quarters can also be affected. Mud fever often goes with cracked heels. The horse may be lame and the hair looks matted and tufted. The tufts will lift off exposing grey-green pus on the bottom of the scabs.

Cause: A bacterium called *Dermotophilus congolensis* enters skin which has been saturated by rain or mud. Horses with clipped legs have little protection and are more susceptible to infection as are horses with feathery legs as these take a long time to dry. There would appear to be a higher incidence in some areas and some years. Poor hygiene will also contribute to horses becoming affected.

Treatment: House affected horses. Remove excess feather and clean and dry the area. A dilute iodine solution can be used. Antibiotic cream should then be applied.

Prevention: Do not brush belly and legs of a tired muddy horse; either apply stable bandages and clean next day or wash clean, towel-dry and apply stable bandages. Remove excess feather but do not clip legs. Use barrier creams to waterproof the skin.

Lice

Symptoms: Skin irritation in the mane, neck and side of the chest, especially in spring and early summer.

Cause: Lice.

Treatment: Dust with louse powder. Check general condition and improve diet if necessary. Clean coat thoroughly.

Ringworm

Symptoms: Young horses are particularly at risk but ringworm can affect horses of all ages. Early signs are circular tufted areas of hair, about 1–2 cm in diameter, the hair falling out to reveal scaly skin which may become infected, accompanied by the formation of pus.

Cause: Fungal infection. Ringworm fungi are able to survive for at least a year in stables, in horse transport and on wooden fences from which horses can pick up infected hairs by rubbing themselves. Horses can also be infected by other animals, grooming kit, tack or clothing.

Treatment: The horse should be isolated, the affected area clipped with scissors to remove the hair and then treated with a fungicidal dressing. An antifungal drug may also be given in the feed. Contaminated woodwork should be pressure-hosed and the horse's tack and clothing disinfected. It is advisable to take hygiene precautions such as wearing rubber gloves as ringworm may occasionally be contracted by the horse's handlers.

Sit-fast

Symptoms: A dying lump of flesh under the saddle patch.

Cause: Severe pressure from a saddle.

Treatment: Poultice until the dead area comes away, then bathe clean daily and apply antibiotic ointment. The vet's help may be needed.

Prevention: Use a properly fitted saddle.

Sore back

Symptoms: Tender back. Sometimes there are sores.

Cause: Loose girth. Poorly stuffed or dirty saddle. Bad rider.

Treatment: As for girth gall (above).

Sweet itch
Symptoms: The mane, back, quarters and tail look inflamed and rubbed. Sores.
Cause: Allergic dermatitis. Midge bites make certain horses allergic to some proteins in their diet. It is found particularly in ponies, generally in spring and summer, on animals at grass.
Treatment: Stable at dawn and dusk. Keep the affected area clean. Apply the parasiticide benzyl benzoate every other day. At first occurrence, get the vet to check for mange.

Urticaria (nettle rash)
Symptoms: Raised areas or swellings on the skin, caused by accumulation of fluid under the skin.
Cause: There are several possible causes. It may be an allergic reaction to plants, bites or stings, but it sometimes indicates an excess of protein in the diet.
Treatment: A day's laxative diet, such as a bran mash with a little Glauber's or Epsom salts, then use calamine lotion or 2 tablespoons of bicarbonate of soda in half a litre of water, applied externally. Antihistamines may be helpful.

Warbles
Symptoms: Firm nodules or swellings on the back. After a fortnight or so the swellings are bigger and may have a hole in the top.
Cause: Warble-fly larvae. The fly lays its eggs on the coat, and the larvae eventually make their way to the skin, usually in spring and early summer.
Treatment: It can be dangerous to try and squeeze out the larvae. If they are squashed under the skin, for example by the saddle, a massive allergic reaction can occur. The condition is therefore best left alone. Poultices should not be used except when a grub has been squashed and an acute reaction has occurred.

8   Digestive System

The function of the digestive system is to process and extract most of the nutrients from whatever foodstuffs are put into it. The system consists of the teeth, the accessory organs, and the alimentary canal, which runs the length of the horse's body.

The digestive tract starts at the mouth and ends at the anus. Food and other materials passing along it are not part of the horse's body, but are merely travelling through it. Nutrients are extracted and waste matter is voided. The digestive tract is both lengthy and complex, and if the horse is fed contrary to its natural requirements, problems will arise. The tract tends to be prone to invasion by parasites and relies on the horse and its keeper to be selective over what is put into it.

Teeth

The teeth provide a cutting and grinding system which is both simple and yet highly specialised. The horse's teeth (Fig. 8.1) are divided into the cutting teeth at the front (the incisors), and the grinding teeth at the back (the molars). All male horses and some mares have four tushes or canine teeth situated between the incisors and the molar teeth. Horses, like human beings, have two sets of teeth: in infancy they have milk or deciduous teeth and later these are replaced by a second or permanent set of teeth.

The molars are unique in their adaptation for grinding coarse hard herbage. The horse's tooth is made up of layers of three substances:

- Dentine in the centre;
- Then a layer of enamel which is the hardest substance in the body; and
- Finally a layer of cement which cushions the tooth to stop it being brittle. Human teeth do not contain cement.

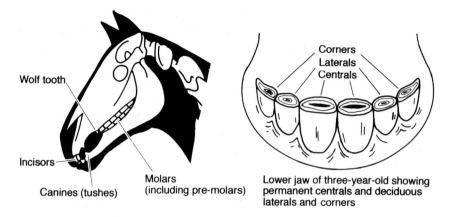

Wolf tooth

Incisors

Canines (tushes)

Molars
(including pre-molars)

Corners
Laterals
Centrals

Lower jaw of three-year-old showing
permanent centrals and deciduous
laterals and corners

Fig. 8.1 Teeth.

The molars have big surfaces or 'tables' and the enamel is folded to
make funnel-like depressions in the tooth which become filled with
food to look black. Inspection of the black infundibulum or 'cup' on
the incisors is used to help age horses.

As the horse chews by moving its jaws from side to side, the molars
grind the food; they also wear against each other. New permanent
teeth have a large crown, much of which is below the level of the gum,
so that in a five-year-old horse most of the jaw is filled with teeth. The
tooth wears down as it is used but that is compensated for as the
growth of the tooth root forces the crown upwards. However, because
the lower jaw is narrower than the upper, the wear on the tables is
sometimes uneven. Small areas at the sides of the tables do not get
worn down and they stick up as sharp edges. This may cause sores on
the cheeks or the tongue. Potential areas of trouble are the inside edges
on the lower jaw and the outside edges on the upper jaw. Rasping (see
Chapter 2) will deal with this problem.

Ageing the horse

As the biting surface of the incisor teeth wears away the pattern on the
surface of the tooth changes so that, with experience, the age of the
horse can be estimated by examining its teeth. The first essential is to
be able to distinguish the milk teeth from the permanent teeth; milk
incisor teeth are small and white and appear to be pointed at the gum
while the adult teeth are larger and yellower. The incisor teeth are

called centrals (the pair top and bottom in the centre), laterals (the teeth next to the centrals) and the corners (see Fig. 8.1). After a permanent tooth has erupted it takes six months to become 'in wear'.

Once the horse has a full mouth of permanent teeth the age is estimated by the changing pattern on the tooth table, the angulation of the teeth which protrude more as the horse ages, and the shape of the tooth which changes from oval to triangular with age. As the horse gets older the 'cup' becomes shallower until it is known as the 'mark'. As the tooth wears down, the pulp cavity which carries nerves and blood vessels is exposed and, to avoid pain, secondary dentine is laid down to protect the pulp cavity. This gives rise to a raised 'dental star' on the tooth table. For a short time both the dental star and the mark are seen on the tooth table but as the horse ages only the dental star is visible and it becomes increasingly central on the tooth table (see Fig. 8.2).

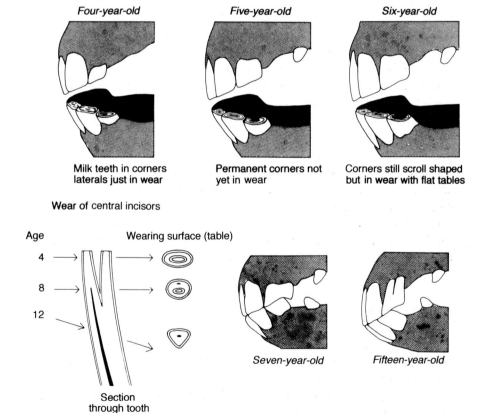

Fig. 8.2 Ageing.

Table 8.1 The eruption of the horse's teeth.

Age of eruption	Incisors				Premolars	Molars
	Centrals	Laterals	Corners	Tushes		
0–1 month	★					
1–3 months	★	★			★ ★ ★	
9 months	★	★	★		★ ★ ★	●
18 months	★	★	★		★ ★ ★	● ●
2.5 years	●	★	★		● ● ★	● ●
3.5 years	●	●	★		● ● ●	● ●
4.5 years	●	●	●	◇	● ● ●	● ● ●

★ milk teeth
● permanent teeth
◇ tushes

The age of foals can be judged by looking at the growth of their tail and the stage of development but generally the milk central incisors erupt by the time the foal is four weeks old and the laterals erupt between one and three months. By the time the foal is a year old it will have a full mouth of neat, white, temporary incisors but the edges of the corners will not meet.

The two-year-old will have a full mouth of temporary incisors which are all in wear. At about two and a half the temporary centrals will be replaced by permanent teeth so that the three-year-old will have permanent centrals which are in wear. At about three and a half the lateral incisors are replaced so that the four-year-old has four permanent teeth in wear. At about four and a half the corners are replaced so that the five-year-old has a full mouth of permanent teeth with the corners just in wear at the front edge. The tushes will have erupted by then in most geldings and some mares.

The six-year-old will have a well-formed mouth with all the incisors in wear with level tables and obvious dark 'cups'. In the seven-year-old the 'cup' in the centrals will have worn out, leaving the 'mark' which is not as dark. The top teeth may overlap the bottom ones so that there may be a little 'hook' on the back of the corner incisors.

By eight years the cup will have worn out of the laterals, leaving a mark, and the centrals will have a dark line called the 'dental star' near the front of the tooth. The hook will have disappeared.

By nine the cup will have worn out of the corners, leaving a mark and the dental star will be apparent on the laterals. There may be a small hook and the centrals will have rounded off, giving a triangular shape. Galvayne's groove appears as a dark groove on the upper corner teeth at between nine and ten.

The ten-year-old will have stars and marks in all teeth but the marks will be more indistinct and the stars will be more clear. The laterals will have rounded off to be more triangular. Galvayne's groove gradually grows down the tooth.

The 12-year-old will only have dental stars in the centrals and the teeth are more triangular. The 15-year-old will only have dental stars on the tooth tables and the teeth will have increased slope, while Galvayne's groove extends about halfway down the corner incisor.

Once the horse has a full mouth of permanent teeth, ageing can only be approximate as the type and level of nutrition of the horse can affect the changes outlined above.

Accessory organs

Liver

The liver is the largest gland in the horse's body and lies up against the diaphragm. It is said to have over a hundred different functions. It supplies a fluid called bile to aid digestion, and also stores energy in the form of glycogen. The liver also converts amino acids into proteins. It regulates the blood and controls the nutrients carried in it. Because it monitors all that the blood carries, its functions may be impaired as a result of damage caused by infections, toxins and other poisons. In some cases this damage is cumulative, for example through eating ragwort. Inflammation of the liver is called hepatitis, and jaundice is a symptom of various forms of liver malfunction as a result of damage or disease. The liver can repair considerable damage to itself.

Pancreas

This large gland produces digestive juices. It also produces the hormones insulin and glucagon to control blood sugar levels.

Digestive tract

The digestive tract of the horse is shown diagrammatically in Fig. 8.3. The horse's lips are specially mobile and adapted for grasping. Its incisor teeth are used for biting off herbage, in contrast to the teeth of

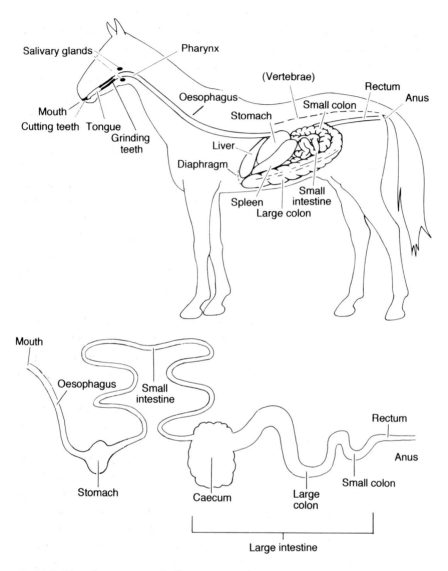

Fig. 8.3 Digestive system and alimentary canal.

cows where the tongue is used in conjunction with the teeth meeting a hard pad. In the mouth, the food is moved by the tongue which transfers it from the front towards the back and sides so that the molar teeth can grind it. During this process the salivary glands (the parotid, the mandibular and sublingual glands, arranged in pairs), produce saliva, which wets and warms the food. Finally, the tongue forms a portion of food into a bolus, which is rolled off the back of the tongue. This triggers the pharynx to operate the epiglottis so that the bolus passes through the pharynx, entering on the lower channel and leaving on the upper to go along the oesophagus or gullet. This is a tube 4 to 5 ft (up to 1.5 m) long, which goes from the back of the throat down the neck. Food being swallowed can be seen on the left side of the neck passing down just behind the windpipe or trachea. The oesophagus goes through the chest, passing between the lungs, and on through the diaphragm into the abdominal cavity where it enters the stomach. The abdominal cavity is lined with a smooth membrane (the peritoneum), which also covers the intestines and helps them slide easily against each other like a tub full of writhing snakes. Food is moved along the gut by waves of muscular contraction called peristalsis. Movement down the oesophagus is aided by the lubrication provided by the saliva.

The empty stomach is only about the size of a rugby football but fills to contain 9–18 litres (2–4 gal). The ring muscle controlling the inlet into the stomach is called the cardiac sphincter; the muscle at the outlet is the pyloric sphincter.

The stomach is followed by the small intestine, which has three parts. The first metre (3 ft) is called the duodenum, into which flow the ducts from the liver and pancreas. The main part of the small intestine is the jejunum. This is nearly 20 m long and its final part (about 2 m long) is called the ileum. These three parts hold about 50 litres (12 gal). The diameter of this long tube is greater than that of a garden hose but smaller than that of a fireman's canvas hose. The small intestine is held up in loose coils by the mesentery that is formed by the peritoneum being folded or looped around the gut and attached to the roof of the cavity. It carries blood vessels and nerves for the gut.

The small intestine empties into the first portion of the large intestine, the caecum. The caecum is a muscular, blind-ended sac with a capacity of about 35 litres (8 gallons) and runs from the point of the hip to the girth on the left side of the horse. Close to the point where the small intestine connects with the caecum is the exit from the caecum into the large colon. The large colon is three to four metres long and can hold about 80 litres (16–20 gallons); it has muscular walls and runs from the hip along the base of the abdomen to the sternum and diaphragm. The large colon leads to the small colon which is about the same length but has a much smaller diameter and hence only holds about 16 litres (3 gallons). The final 30 centimetres of the alimentary canal is the rectum which stores the faeces prior to defaecation and the rectum ends in a sphincter muscle called the anus.

The horse's gut is designed to glean maximal nutritive value from grass and poor quality herbage; readily available nutrients are extracted in the stomach and small intestine while fibre is broken down slowly in the large intestine. Domestication and the resulting change in the horse's diet to fit in with our requirements has led to the horse being highly susceptible to digestive disorders such as colic and azoturia.

Digestion

The complex foods that the horse eats consist of water, vitamins, minerals, carbohydrates, lipids and proteins. These last three form the bulk of the digestible food. The carbohydrates have to be broken down into simple sugars, which are the source of usable energy. Lipids, which are fats and oils, are broken down to fatty acids and glycerol, which may be used or stored. Proteins are broken down into amino acids which are the building blocks from which much of the body is made.

Little digestion occurs in the mouth because horse saliva, although copious in quantity, is low in enzymes, the chemicals that create changes of state in foods. The food is mixed with gastric juice in the stomach. This is secreted by glands in the wall, and acidifies the food by means of hydrochloric acid. It also contains three enzymes: pepsin, which starts breaking down proteins; renin, which coagulates milk in foals; and lipase, which starts work on lipids.

Although the horse's stomach is rarely empty, food stays there only for a short period of time, between 30 minutes and 3 hours depending on the type of food. The food leaves with the most liquid portions first: water, carbohydrates, proteins and fats, in that order. Five hours after eating a full meal, a horse will usually feel hungry again. Provided the duodenum is empty and the food in the stomach is sufficiently acid, the food is passed on from the stomach to the small intestine.

Secretions from the liver and the pancreas flow into the duodenum. The liver produces bile, which flows down the bile duct into the duodenum and emulsifies lipids, thus aiding their digestion and absorption. Bile turns the acid contents of the stomach into an alkaline mixture to go down the intestine. The horse has no gall bladder; it is meant to be a continuous feeder. Feeding little and often is therefore better for good digestion and the efficient use of food.

The pancreatic juice is alkaline and contains sodium bicarbonate to counter the acidity of the stomach. It also contains enzymes, including trypsin (which breaks down proteins into peptides and then into amino acids) and amylase (which breaks down starch into maltose which, in turn, is broken down into glucose by the enzyme maltase).

Digestion continues along the main length of the small intestine (the jejunum). At this stage the food of most animals is a creamy smooth mixture. In the horse, however, this mixture still contains the coarse fibre which is an essential part of the horse's diet. Peristalsis, the process of muscular contraction that moves the food along, also mixes it with the digestive juices and forces it against the intestinal walls where it can be absorbed. The intestinal wall has little protuberances (villi) all along it, which are like the pile on a carpet and thus give a greater surface area. Here the amino acids, glucose, minerals and vitamins pass into the blood stream and some of the fatty acids and glycerol pass into the lymphatic system. Between the villi are little crypts which produce further juices to aid digestion. There is no clear division from the jejunum into the ileum, but there is a valve to control flow into the caecum.

The caecum acts as a holding chamber to keep the large colon topped up. The breakdown of food in the large colon may take several days which is why it is so bulky, and why the grass-fed horse has a big belly. To enable it to carry this considerable weight, the horse has a strong back. Because the large colon is so large, at one point it turns sharply back on itself at the pelvic flexure; this sharp turn is sometimes a site of blockage. Bacteria live in the caecum and the colon, and break down cellulose to release volatile fatty acids which can be used as a source of energy by the horse. These bacteria are of many types and have very short lives. They are fairly specific to different foods so it is important to change food sources gradually so that the population of bacteria can also change to adapt to the new diet. Besides breaking down foods, the bacteria can also build them up into essential vitamins.

Food passes from the large colon into the small colon, where nutrients and water are still being extracted. It reaches the rectum where further water is removed. The waste material is formed into balls of dung or faeces, which are evacuated at intervals through the anus. On average, the food takes three to four days to pass through the horse. Examination of faeces after feeding whole grain will show that some foods pass through more quickly than this, and indeed some grains remain intact.

Parasites of the digestive tract

Flatworms

Flatworms are rarely important. The *liver fluke* (which is a form of flatworm) is found in wet conditions. To complete its life cycle it has an intermediate host, the mud snail. Control of an area includes draining land and killing the snails. The liver fluke normally attacks cattle and sheep, but where a horse is invaded it will cause unthriftiness, and will stunt growth and lead to anaemia.

The other flatworm to note is the *tapeworm*. Tapeworms can grow to 80 cm (2½ ft) long, but are usually 5 to 8 cm (2 to 3 in) long. They live in the large and small intestine. Their intermediate host is a mite. They rarely produce symptoms but may cause unthriftiness. Tapeworm are controlled by a double dose of a specific wormer.

Roundworms

The three important roundworms that affect the horse are the seat- or whipworm, the large round whiteworm and the red bloodworm.

The *seatworm* (*Oxyuris*) female lays eggs at the horse's anus. Larvae develop in the eggs, drop to the ground and get eaten with food. The small (up to 15 cm (6 in) long) adult worms live in the caecum and colon. The worm causes the horse to have an itchy anus and may lead to tail rubbing. The yellow eggs may be seen round the anus. Routine worming controls this pest.

Whiteworms (*Ascarids*): these large round worms are up to 1 ft long (15–30 cm) and as thick as a pencil. They live in the small intestine. The female lays eggs (at a laying rate of 8000 per hour per worm), which are passed out in the droppings. In favourable conditions on pasture, eggs hatch to form larvae which remain inside the eggshell for protection. The eggs are infective for a period of from 30 days to up to 3 years. When eaten the larvae go through the gut wall and migrate via the liver and heart to the lungs where they get coughed up and reswallowed. They then become adults.

Whiteworms cause some loss of condition for horses under three years old. Principally they are a foal problem. Adult horses that have whiteworms must be treated if foals have access to their pasture.

Redworms (*Strongylus*) are tiny worms, as thin as cotton and as long as a fingernail. They live in the intestines, where the female lays eggs that pass out with the droppings. Redworms can be extracted from the droppings after 'worming', and their eggs can be identified with a microscope. The eggs hatch when conditions are suitably warm and moist. The third-stage infective larvae crawl up blades of grass and get eaten. They then burrow into the gut linings, and although some complete their development there in three or four months, others travel further. Some invade the liver after an eight-month journey. The larvae of one species (*Strongylus vulgaris*, the large redworm) get into the arteries supplying the intestines and travel against the blood flow until reaching the anterior (cranial) mesenteric artery (see Fig. 8.4). This is the main blood vessel supplying the intestines. They develop there for several months before returning down the blood vessel and back into the intestine. These expeditions lead to damaged artery walls and blood clots where the worms settle. These clots (thrombi) may break off and block blood vessels, thus stopping blood supply to the part of the intestine served by that vessel. The symptoms of this worm damage may include loss of condition, anaemia, distended stomach, staring coat, diarrhoea and colic. Control includes removing droppings from the paddock, grazing with cattle and sheep, and rotating grazing. Drugs used against worms are known as anthelminthics and some can now kill the wandering larvae as well as

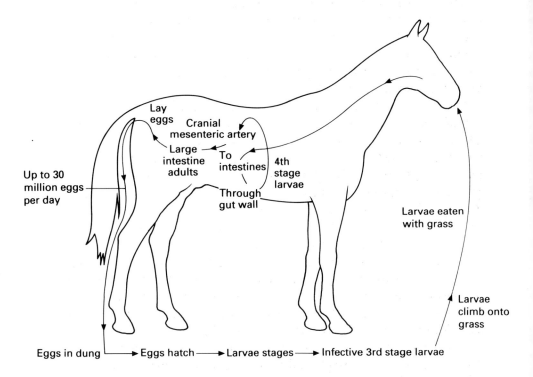

Fig. 8.4 Life cycle of large redworm (*Strongylus vulgaris*): 200 days.

the adult worms. Thus, when dosing the horse, there can be a more complete cleansing of the system from these parasites. This possibility has changed the pattern of worm control. Generally speaking, horses should be wormed every four to six weeks and there should be a change to a chemically unrelated wormer every 12 months to prevent the worms building up a resistance to one product.

Bots

Bots (*Gastrophilus*) are a non-worm parasite, the larval stage of the gadfly. The adult female lays its eggs on the coat of the forelegs from June to September. The eggs hatch to larvae, which the horse licks off. These burrow into the tongue or cheek, where they remain for 2 to 3 weeks; they then migrate to the stomach and attach themselves to the stomach wall. In spring they let go and pass out with the droppings, maturing into flies. They cause unthriftiness. The eggs should be wiped off with a paraffin rag or scraped off with a knife. Anti-fly aromatic protection (such as a daily dab of oil of citronella) on the forelegs is beneficial. Horses should be treated with a wormer such as ivermectin that is effective against bot larvae in early winter after the flies have been killed by the first frost of the autumn. A further dose in February will kill any remaining larvae before they pass out in the horse's droppings.

Disorders of the digestive system

Choking

Symptoms: Dribbling, attempts to swallow, head repeatedly down to chest with tensed neck.
Cause: Potato, apple, carrot or lump of dry feed.
Treatment: Keep the horse calm. As long as it can inhale air it will not die. *Do not drench or give water.* Proceed as described in First-aid Procedure (Chapter 2).
Prevention: Do not give concentrates to a very hungry horse. Give a small drink and a little hay first. Horses cannot vomit, though they can pass liquids back through the nose. Sugar beet nuts should be soaked thoroughly before feeding.

Colic

Colic is a name used to describe abdominal pain caused by a wide variety of disorders. Whatever the cause, the horse tends to display the same symptoms.

There are several types of colic as follows:

(1) *Spasmodic colic* is a condition of an irritated gut wall becoming overactive leading to spasm of the muscular wall of the intestine.
Symptoms: The horse is moderately distressed, sweating, constantly going down and getting up, looking at and kicking at flanks, and may roll often getting cast. The pulse rate may rise to 68–92 beats per minute and be over 100 in severe cases. The temperature and respiration rate will be up and the horse will pass few droppings. Spasmodic colic may come and go quite quickly.
Causes: Damage to intestinal wall by migrating worm larvae, feeding and drinking too soon after fast work.
Treatment: Relaxant drugs usually relieve the condition rapidly.

(2) *Impactive colic* – this accounts for about 30% of all colics and is due to impaction or blockage of food material in the gut, usually the large intestine.
Symptoms: The horse looks dull and off-colour and gets up and down in an uncomfortable manner. It may roll more than usual.
Causes: Eating bedding, the change from an all grass diet to a hay ration. Not usually in great pain.
Treatment: The vet will perform a rectal examination to try to feel where the blockage is. The horse may be given pain killers and liquid paraffin via a stomach tube.

(3) *Distension or tympanitic colic*
Symptoms: Usually very painful; the horse will sweat and roll violently.
Cause: Build-up of gas in gut which may occur in front of an impaction, be due to a twist in the gut or fermentation of food in the stomach or small intestine.
Treatment: Dependent on the cause.

(4) *Intestinal catastrophe*
Symptoms: The horse is in extreme pain and may be uncontrollably violent.
Causes: The gut has become twisted, telescoped into itself or rotated about its mesentery, all of which obstruct the blood supply and will eventually lead to death of the affected part of the gut.
Treatment: Immediate veterinary attention is vital as abdominal surgery is necessary.

Predisposing factors: Faulty teeth causing poorly chewed food. Too much or unsuitable or badly prepared food. Bolting food. Irregularity of meal times or too long between meals. Poor quality food. Accidental access to food, or to food in the wrong form, e.g. short grass cuttings. A sudden change of diet. Excess of cold water to drink when horse is hot. Over- or under-work. Working immediately after feeding. Watering after feeding. Crib-biting or windsucking. Kidney- or bladder-stones. Taking sand up when drinking from a stream. Parasites – probably the most common cause.

Care of the horse: The horse should be brought into the stable if outside. It should be encouraged to stale. The bedding should be topped up and banked round the walls, and any obstruction should be removed. Call the vet. Temperature, pulse and respiration should be taken, and the horse should be kept warm with light clothing. Do not feed but offer water. An occasional walk in hand round the yard may help. The vet may use drugs to relieve pain, relax the horse and ease spasms. He may also administer saline solution and lubricant. Immediate surgery is required in the case of a twisted gut.

Prevention: Feed each horse as an individual, feed concentrates little and often, keep to regular feeding times, make changes to the diet gradually, feed good quality feed and store it away from vermin, keep to your routine, even when away from home, cool the horse thoroughly after strenuous work before allowing it to drink and eat large amounts, have the teeth checked and rasped regularly, stop horses bolting their feed by adding chaff or putting a salt lick or large stones in the manger, keep to a regular effective worming programme.

Constipation
Symptoms: Small, hard or no droppings.
Cause: Poor diet.
Treatment: Soft laxative diet of green food and bran mashes. Purgatives should not be used except on the vet's advice.

Diarrhoea
Symptoms: Obvious.
Causes: Nerves. Sudden change of diet or too much green food. Too much rich food. Faulty teeth. Inflammation of the gut from irritant food or worms. Infection.
Treatment: Remove the cause where possible. Diet of hay and a little dry bran. Check temperature: if it is high, an infection is the cause. Treat for dehydration.

Parrot mouth

Symptoms: Horse in poor condition.

Cause: Malformation with short lower jaw (mandible).

Treatment: In severe cases, feed with complete cubes so that the horse does not have to bite.

Poisoning

Symptoms: Diarrhoea, colic, convulsions, coma, dilation or constriction of pupils, distressed breathing, muscular inco-ordination, sensitisation, blood in urine, etc.

Cause: Ingestion of a substance that harms the body internally by interfering with function.

Treatment: Call the vet at once.

Sharp teeth

Symptoms: Quidding, i.e. chewing food without swallowing. Cautious eating, sometimes with head on one side. Lacerations of tongue and cheek.

Cause: Uneven tooth wear leaving sharp edges.

Treatment: Rasping, as described under Tooth care (Chapter 2). Sloppy food for a few days if there are lacerations. Sponging the inside of the horse's mouth with salt water will ease the lacerations and aid healing.

Sore throat

Symptoms: Poor appetite, cough, running nose.

Cause: Bacterial activity, often as a secondary infection.

Treatment: The horse should be isolated, kept warm and allowed ample fresh air. Inhalations may help. Dusty bedding and food should be avoided. Sloppy food fed from a bowl on the ground. The vet may prescribe antibiotics.

Wolf teeth

Symptoms: Horse tosses its head when it has a bit in its mouth.

Cause: Natural formation – not always present.

Treatment: Ask the vet about removal.

9 Reproductive, Urinary and Mammary Systems

The reproductive, urinary and mammary systems are interrelated. The reproductive system's task is to ensure the continuance of the species. Like most animals, the female horse is subject both to cycles and to seasons of the year in her sexual behaviour. For reasons of safety, performance and convenience, the male horse is commonly neutered or gelded. Although horses in the wild appear to breed with a high degree of efficiency, in the domesticated horse the number of foals reared compares unfavourably with the number of mares going to stallions each year, particularly in the Thoroughbred. A major reason for this is that the stallion is allowed to cover the mare only when man dictates and man is not as good at detecting the optimum time as the stallion when left to his own devices. Also, an artificial breeding season has been imposed on the Thoroughbred so that foals are born early in the year to give the two-year-old racehorse an advantage. This means that mares and stallions are expected to breed successfully out of their natural breeding season, when fertility is low.

The mammary system provides nourishment for the young, and although the udder is more discreetly placed than in cattle, the mare will provide large quantities of milk. Indeed, in some parts of the world she provides milk for human consumption.

The urinary system filters impurities from the blood, temporarily stores them, and then disposes of them.

The male reproductive system

The reproductive organs of the stallion (see Fig. 9.1) are designed to create a sperm and place it in such a position within the mare that it can unite with an egg. Sperm is created in the testes, which function best at a slightly cooler temperature than the rest of the body. They are therefore slung in a thin skin 'purse' (the scrotum), which is located

Male

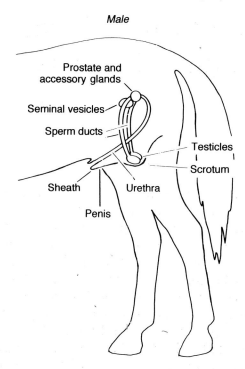

Fig. 9.1 Male reproductive system.

between the hind legs for protection. The testes start life in the abdominal cavity but usually have descended down the inguinal canal into the scrotum by birth. Although the testes may reascend, they are dropped permanently by 12 months. Where one or both testes are retained in the canal or abdomen, the horse is called a 'rig' or cryptorchid. A 'rig' may be purchased in mistake for a gelding. Although the retained testis will not produce fertile sperm, it will create the male sex hormone testosterone, which is responsible for male behaviour. Accordingly, a rig must be treated like a stallion. Rigs may be used as 'teasers' to ascertain whether a mare is in season.

In the mature horse, the testes are round, long, and of a size that would fill a cupped hand. Each testis weighs about 300 g (10 oz). The sperm created by the testes are stored in small coiled tubes, joining into one, the epididymis. This is attached to the upper edge of each testis. The epididymis has a tube (the vas deferens) which leads up into the body. The two tubes, one from each testis, run side by side as the route for sperm during the sexual act. In the abdominal cavity they lead past the two seminal vesicles which lie either side of the bladder and which, with neighbouring accessory glands, produce seminal fluid. The sperm and seminal fluid together form semen. A stallion will release 40–120 ml (2–5 fl oz) of semen at a time, and this will contain about 4000 million sperm. A common duct (the urethra), which carries both semen and urine, runs from the bladder, down to and through the penis, which, at rest, is enclosed in the sheath (prepuce).

When the stallion is sexually aroused, blood flows into the erectile tissue of the penis, which becomes thicker and longer – up to about 50 cm (20 in). When the penis is erect, the stallion can, with practice, insert it into the vagina of a receptive mare. This is called intromission. The head of the penis (the glans) is further enlarged inside the mare, thus securing a tight fit. After some thrusting, semen is ejaculated into the mare and this is accompanied by flagging of the stallion's tail. The penis then starts to reduce in size and the stallion withdraws from the mare's vagina. From mounting to dismounting, the whole operation commonly takes less than a minute. The penis quickly shrinks back into the sheath, which consists of double folds of skin lubricated by smegma. The sheaths of both stallions and geldings need to be kept clean inside and out.

Castration is the operation of removing the testes, and the operation is usually carried out in spring or autumn. A castrated stallion is called a gelding, and it sounds, looks and behaves like a mare out of season.

In general, the male genitalia function well. The vet can take a sample of semen and check it for quality. Occasionally, germs may affect the stallion's penis. They may be picked up from a mare during service. An example is a venereal disease caused by a herpes virus, which causes spots or 'coital exanthema'. This takes the form of blisters on the penis, and necessitates two or three weeks of rest for the stallion. A stallion may also be damaged in use by being kicked by a mare, so causing a swelling filled with blood (a haematoma) on the penis, or one filled with mixed fluids (oedema) on the scrotum.

The female reproductive system

The mare's reproductive system (Fig. 9.2) is designed to produce an egg (ovum), which will unite with a sperm to form an embryo. The system also provides nutrition for the embryo and a good environment in which it can develop.

Ova are produced by the ovaries. At birth, these contain all the egg

Female

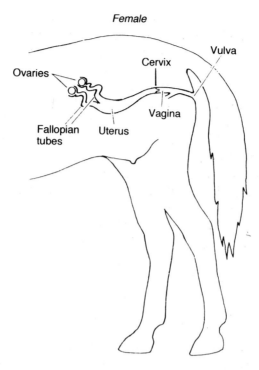

Fig. 9.2 Female reproductive system.

cells needed, and eggs are released at intervals during the mare's fertile life. The two ovaries are attached high in the abdominal cavity, just behind the kidneys. An expert can feel them through the wall of the rectum. They are bean-shaped and each is about the size of a chicken's egg. An ovum is passed down from an ovary through one of the oviducts (also known as the fallopian tubes), where it may be fertilised. Each fallopian tube runs into a horn of the uterus or womb. This is Y-shaped, with two horns and a main body; it is suspended in the abdominal cavity. At its rear end there is the sphincter muscle (cervix), which closes it for most of the time. A short passage (the vagina) leads from the cervix to the outside. The vagina ends in the vulva, which has two lips or labia on the outside and a small penis-like organ (the clitoris) on the inside.

When the mare is in season, she can flash open the lips of the vulva in an action called 'winking'. This is quite often done after she urinates in the distinctive and slightly squatting position of the in-season mare. Instead of being tightly closed, when the mare is in season the cervix relaxes and opens slightly. When she is covered by the stallion at mating, the mare's vagina takes the stallion's penis. Some of the semen will be lost in the vagina, although most should be ejaculated directly into the uterus, sperm then swim across the uterus and up the fallopian tubes in search of an egg. On finding it, the sperm swim round it trying to gain entry. Only one sperm will succeed and unite with the egg.

Generally, the female genitals function well. However, germs may invade the genital tract and cause problems. They may gain entry during mating (coitus) or because the mare has a poorly shaped vulva which allows air to enter and take in germs. This defect is corrected by stitching using 'Caslick's operation'.

Two diseases which cause – or have caused – great problems are the equine herpes virus and contagious equine metritis. The former results in abortion and also causes 'snotty nose' (rhinopneumonitis) in yearlings. The latter (CEM) is a highly contagious venereal disease causing infertility.

Oestrous cycle

A mare will reach puberty between 12 and 24 months after birth and is then ready to 'come into season'. Normally a mare comes into season (oestrus) at regular intervals through the summer months, the breeding season. Improved food, lengthening days and warmer sun-shine during spring trigger off the process.

The mare's pituitary gland produces FSH (follicle stimulating hormone), which activates her ovaries. One of the ovaries forms a follicle which appears like a hard cyst on the surface. The ovaries also give out the hormone oestrogen (in Greek this means 'to produce mad desire'!). It is this hormone which brings the mare into season (oes-trus). The pituitary gland then starts to produce LH (luteinising hormone), which stimulates the egg to reach maturity and then its release (ovulation) into the fallopian tube. This happens when the mare has been in season for about four days. The crater on the ovary where the egg was sited now fills up like a soft cyst as the yellow body (corpus luteum). This produces the hormone progesterone. Oestrus then ends and the mare 'goes off', having been in season for about five to six days. Ideally the mare is covered during the 24 hours before she goes out of season. The oestrous cycle is summarised in Fig. 9.3.

For the next two weeks the mare has no interest in the stallion. The mare's cycle is now under the control of the hormone progesterone which is being produced by the corpus luteum. Progesterone is known

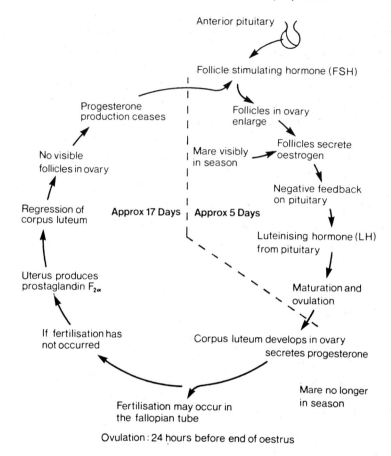

Fig. 9.3 Oestrous cycle of the mare.

as the hormone of pregnancy; under its influence the uterus is prepared to receive the fertilised egg and the mare will reject the stallion and will not come back into season. If the egg has not been fertilised to form an embryo the uterus produces a hormone called prostaglandin which kills off the corpus luteum. Progesterone production ceases and the cycle starts all over again.

Dioestrus is the period between one oestrus and the next; anoestrus is the period over the winter when the cycle stops. The normal cycle lasts about three weeks and in general is consistent for each mare. By observing a mare's normal cycle it will be easier to predict the time of ovulation.

Pregnancy

The mare is pregnant when the ovum and sperm have united to form an embryo. The embryo grows rapidly by division of cells. Initially, this takes place within the egg capsule which is descending the fallopian tube. After two weeks, the embryo is a rapidly growing mass and is lying in one of the horns of the uterus. After three weeks it has taken on body form, utilising the yolk from the egg. By the sixth week the embryo is well developed and is called a fetus, which is nourished by uterine milk. (See Fig. 9.4.) The fetus floats in amniotic fluid, which is parcelled within a membrane (the amnion). This parcel lies within the allantoic fluid ('the waters') and a second membrane (the placenta). The placenta bonds with the lining of the uterus and is a means of nutrient, oxygen and waste product exchange. It is connected to the foetus by the umbilical cord. Except for the lungs and the liver all the systems are working within the fetus. Liquid excreta is passed into the allantoic fluid where some of it solidifies to form a flattish brown piece of matter, the hippomane, which is found among the afterbirth.

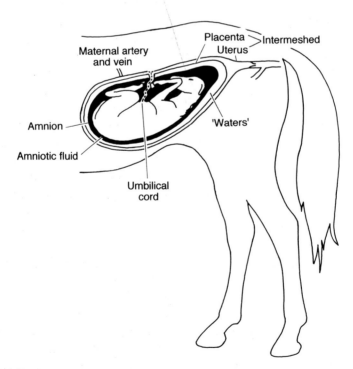

Fig. 9.4 Pregnancy.

Physical movement is noticeable in the later stages of pregnancy when the fetus is growing rapidly.

Inheritance

Genetics is the study of the mechanisms by which the characteristics of the parents are passed on to their offspring. Equine genetics is rather complicated and the genetics outlined here has been simplified to provide a suitable introduction to the subject.

There is coded information on the exact make and shape of the parents in an ovum or sperm. This information is contained in chromosomes. Each chromosome is like a string of beads, each bead being called a gene and having a special function to perform, e.g. coat colour. The adult horse has 32 pairs of chromosomes. Each sperm or ovum (sex cells) produced by an adult horse contains 32 single chromosomes so that when the sperm fertilises the ovum (or egg) the resulting embryo has 32 pairs of chromosomes, half donated by each parent.

Pairs of genes can be described as either homozygous or heterozygous; homozygous means that the genes on the chromosome for a particular characteristic are the same, thus homozygous genes always breed true. Heterozygous means that the genes are different, but in order for the characteristic to be expressed one gene must be 'dominant' while the other is 'recessive'. Thus, the gene for black coat colour (B) is dominant to the gene for chestnut (b), chestnut is recessive to black. The use of capital letters for dominant genes and lower-case for recessive genes is standard practice, the presence of B stops b from expressing itself. This means that horses containing heterozygous genes will not always breed true; if a heterozygous black horse with the genetic make up (Bb), breeds with another heterozygous black horse there is a 25% chance that the foal will have the genetic make-up (bb). This foal will be chestnut as there are no dominant genes to repress the chestnut colour.

In genetics, the gene that results in horses with pricked ears dominates that giving lop ears; similarly the gene for a dished face dominates that for a Roman nose. The genes also determine the sex of the foal, and the sperm always carries the deciding factor.

Recessive genes may show up if *inbreeding* (breeding close relations) is practised. Inbreeding can strengthen the genetic make-up provided there is no history of undesirable characteristics. Close inbreeding

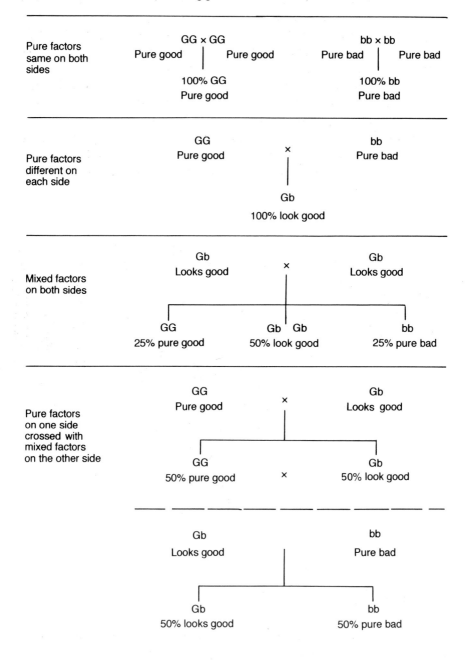

Fig. 9.5 Inheritance of a single trait or character.

includes sire to daughter, dam to son, and brother to sister. Animals born with undesirable characteristics should not be used as breeding stock. *Line-breeding* includes grandfather to granddaughter, grand-mother to grandson, and cousin to cousin. Line-breeding has less risks but takes longer to establish purity. *Outbreeding* is where there is no relation within the previous five generations.

Mating outside the breed is known as crossing. A true hybrid results from mating with another species, e.g. a donkey with a pony. Usually, such hybrids are vigorous but infertile, as is the case with mules. Crossing between different breeds can produce some hybrid vigour. Such vigour was found when horses from the south and east Mediterranean were crossed with English native improved stock to form the Thoroughbred (see Figs 9.5 and 9.6).

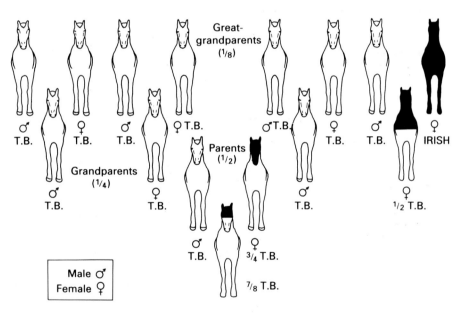

Fig. 9.6 Inheritance.

Mammary system

The mare's udder develops to suckle the foal. The udder consists of the mammary glands in two separate compartments, each leading to a teat. The udder and two teats are located between the hind legs for protection. A big mare can produce up to 23 litres (5 gal) of milk per day.

The mammary glands are well supplied with blood and lymph vessels. The tissues concerned with production are grouped around little sacks called alveoli (similar to those in the lungs), from which run ducts, like the branches of a tree, all joining to go to the trunk. In this case the trunk is the gland cistern. Below this is another gland within the body of the teat (the teat cistern). The teat ends in two small holes, guarded by sphincter muscles, through which the milk is released.

Germs can enter the udder and produce an inflamed condition known as mastitis. The udder then becomes hard and tender to the touch, and swollen lymph ducts will show along the belly. This condition needs veterinary attention.

Urinary system

The urinary system (see Fig. 9.7) is concerned with regulating the water content of the body and removing unwanted substances from the blood by filtering all blood through the kidneys. It supplements the work of the lungs, skin and bowels.

The kidneys maintain constancy in the horse's internal environment, a process known as homeostasis. They regulate water balance, acidity and alkalinity (pH), osmotic pressure, electrolyte levels, etc. The kidneys are affected by the composition of the blood, blood pressure, hormones, stress and drugs. There are two kidneys, each weighing about 700 g (23 oz), located high in the abdominal cavity. Each consists of an outer cortex, in which waste products pass from the blood into collecting tubes. These form an inner medulla and empty into a central pelvis. Inflammation of the kidney is called nephritis or, if only the central pelvis is involved, pyelitis. Urinary calculi or stones may occur as a result of salts crystallising in the urine, but this condition is rare. Urine flows from each kidney down the ureters into the bladder. Cystitis is inflammation of the bladder. The exit to the bladder is controlled by a sphincter muscle which, when released, allows the urine to pass down the urethra to be discharged via the penis or vulva. A horse may pass up to 10 litres (18 pints) of urine per day.

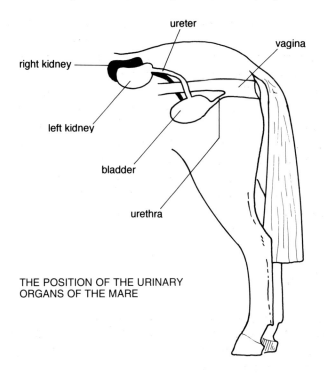

ureter

right kidney

vagina

left kidney

bladder

urethra

THE POSITION OF THE URINARY
ORGANS OF THE MARE

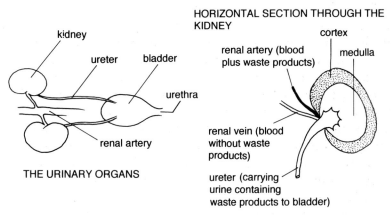

HORIZONTAL SECTION THROUGH THE
KIDNEY

kidney

ureter   bladder

urethra

renal artery

THE URINARY ORGANS

cortex

medulla

renal artery (blood
plus waste products)

renal vein (blood
without waste
products)

ureter (carrying
urine containing
waste products to bladder)

Fig. 9.7 Urinary system.

Part III
Work in the Stable Yard

10 Handling Horses

Basic handling of horses

Horses are large and potentially dangerous creatures; their natural instincts tell them to flee when danger threatens and if their handler is not aware of this the horse can easily become out of control. As with any other animal, young horses, especially colts, are playful. If not disciplined this 'playing' can get out of hand and the horse becomes wilful and difficult to handle. If not handled with consistent competence and taught good stable manners horses will learn their own strength and use it against their handler, a frightening and dangerous situation. It is essential that, no matter how quiet the horse, the handler always works in a safe manner so that it becomes second nature to do so.

Whenever you are handling horses it is important to try and develop a rapport; use your voice. Horses have very acute hearing so never shout at them. They are also highly sensitive to the tone of voice and can be soothed or reprimanded by the use of subtle changes in the way you speak to them. Fear communicates very rapidly from handler to horse; try to anticipate dangerous situations and always be prepared by having the right equipment and by keeping your wits about you. If a potentially hazardous situation arises try to keep calm, talk quietly to the horse and perhaps stroke or pat him, this will keep your nerves under control as well as his. If you are in doubt about your ability to handle a certain horse or situation always seek help or advice.

Approaching the horse in the stable

Horses have good hearing and are very responsive to the handler's tone of voice. Always speak to the horse when opening the stable door; a horse that is taken by surprise may react violently. If the horse is standing by the door he should stand back as the handler enters. If the horse is standing away from the door the handler should enter the stable, close the door and go up to the horse's shoulder, pat him on the neck and put on a headcollar. If the horse is standing with his head in the corner, making it difficult to approach without passing close to the hindquarters, it may be wise to encourage the horse to come to you.

Putting on a headcollar or halter

Before entering the stable the handler should unfasten the headcollar and uncoil the rope, slipping both safely over one arm. Once the horse has been approached the lead rope should be placed round the horse's neck just below the poll; this is to help control the horse should it try to move away. The cheekpieces of the headcollar should be held in either hand and the noseband slipped round the horse's nose. Then the headpiece should be lifted with the right hand and gently flipped over the horse's poll, catching the end with the left hand which also holds the buckle of the headcollar. Care must be taken not to startle the horse or to let the free end hit the horse in the eye. The buckle should then be secured so that the noseband is two fingers' width below the projecting cheekbone or facial crest and any excess length of headpiece

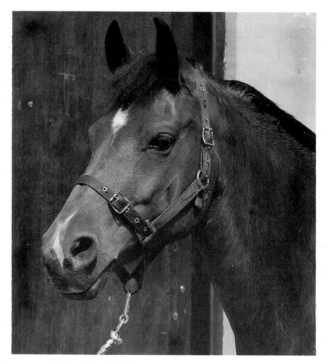

Fig. 10.1 A correctly fitted headcollar.

should be tucked through the headcollar ring out of the way (Fig. 10.1).

Some headcollars are fitted with a browband to prevent the head-piece slipping down the neck. Others have a throatlash secured with a clip and the headcollar is merely slipped over the horse's nose, over the ears and the throatlash is clipped up. The throatlash should be quite loose, allowing a fist between it and the cheekbones. The lead rope should be clipped onto the headcollar under the horse's chin with the open side of the clip under the jaw not the chin and pointing away from it; thus if the horse pulls back he will not catch the fleshy part of the chin in the clip (Fig. 10.2).

Halters consist of rope and incorporate a lead rope. They can be adjusted to fit most horses. However the lead rope must be knotted at the noseband to avoid it tightening on the horse's jaw (Fig. 10.3).

As with all tack, headcollars, halters and lead ropes should be checked regularly and repaired if they are showing signs of wear. Nylon headcollars are not suitable for leaving on horses that are turned out in the field as they do not break should they catch on anything; leather headcollars are safer.

Securing the horse

It is safe practice to tie the horse up when the handler is working in the stable. The horse should be tied with a quick-release knot to a string loop on the tie-up ring (Fig. 10.4). The string loop is designed to break if the horse panics and pulls back. Baling twine is practically unbreakable and should not be used. Horses should never be tied to objects that may move, for example, the stable door or a gate. Mares with foals and untrained young horses should not be tied up.

Horses kept in stalls are tied to a rope which passes through a ring and is then fastened to a sliding log by means of a knot at the end of the rope. As the horse moves in the stall the heavy log takes up the slack of the rope so that there is no danger of the horse putting a leg over a loose rope (Fig. 10.5). Horses may also be cross-tied using two ropes, one from each side of the headcollar, passing to tie-up rings on two posts or two sides of a stall. This is a useful way of keeping the horse still and secure while handling the horse as it limits the range of movement.

The handler must speak when approaching a horse that is tied up to ensure that the horse knows that the handler is there. Do not walk straight up to the horse's bottom and pat him; let him see you and reassure him before touching him.

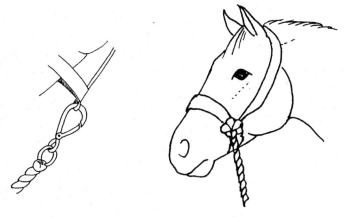

Fig. 10.2 A correctly fitted lead rope clip.

Fig. 10.3 Halter.

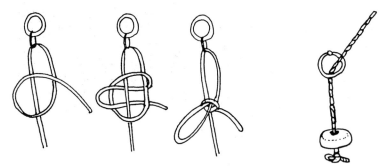

Fig. 10.4 Tying a quick-release knot.

Fig. 10.5 A sliding log and rope arrangement for securing a horse.

Leading a horse in hand off-road

Before taking any horse out of the stable the handler must be sure that they are in control; a quiet, reliable horse can be led in a correctly-fitting, sound headcollar with a lead rope (Fig. 10.6). The handler should be wearing suitable shoes and gloves – nothing hurts like a rope burn – and should never wrap the lead rope around the hand. An overhand knot should be tied in the end of the lead rope. Even so, a naughty horse can quickly learn to pull a short lead rope out of the handler's hands and if there is any doubt about how the horse is going to behave, for example, a young horse or a horse that has been in the stable for a while, the handler should wear a hard hat and lead the horse in a bridle or headcollar with a lunge line attached.

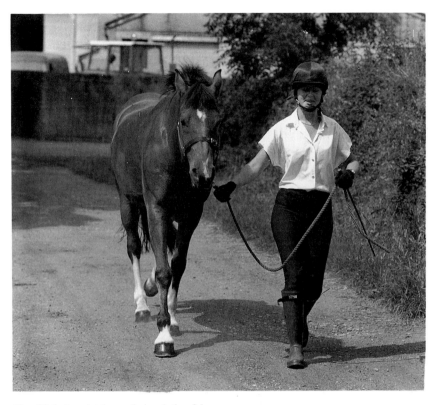

Fig. 10.6 A quiet horse being led safely.

Care must be taken when leading the horse through openings such as stable doors or gateways; do not hurry or take short cuts – the stable door should be open wide and the horse led straight and slowly so that he does not catch his hip. If there is a danger of the gate or door swinging closed on the horse, it should be fastened back or held by a helper; a horse that has had a door or gate swing shut on him may rush, increasing the risk of banging himself or slipping. Once the horse is in the stable, carefully turn him to face the door making sure that he does not slip and then close the door, release the horse and leave the stable.

The horse should be led from the near (left) side with the right hand holding the rope close to the headcollar and the remaining rope coiled in the left hand. The horse should walk freely forwards with the handler at the horse's shoulder. Do not pull on the rope or look back at the horse, if he hangs back either get a helper to encourage him or carry a long whip in the left hand which can be used to tap the hindquarters. (See also Chapter 12, 'The Equine Road Users Code'.)

Presenting a horse for inspection

At some time in his life the horse will have to trot up in hand – it may be for the vet to check soundness or to show the horse off to a potential purchaser – and it is important for both horse and handler to know what they are doing. Ideally there will be a level, straight stretch of hard surface about 40 m long so that there is enough room for the horse to trot forward freely, pull up and turn.

First the horse should be made to stand up straight, square and with his weight equally balanced on all four feet, with the handler standing in front. If the horse is wearing a bridle the reins should be taken over his head and each rein held a little below the bit either side of the head to keep the horse straight and still. When asked, the handler should move to the horse's near side and walk the horse in a straight line away from the examiner until asked to turn. The horse should then be turned to the right, away from the handler, and walked back straight towards the examiner. This is then repeated in trot allowing the horse a few walk strides to balance himself and get straight after turning, before asking him to trot. The horse should not be pulled, held too tight or have his head turned towards the handler as this will prevent the head 'nodding' – the sign of lameness the vet will be looking for.

Turning out into a field

Horses can become quite excited in anticipation of being turned out into a field and the handler must be suitably equipped with gloves, stout shoes and, possibly, a hard hat. The horse should also be suitably restrained. If a normally quiet horse becomes excited and is only wearing a headcollar it can give more control if the rope is placed over the horse's nose from the off side and secured through the noseband of the headcollar. The field gate should be opened wide enough to avoid any risk of the horse banging itself. If there are other horses barging at the gate, help should be sought rather than struggling to squeeze the led horse through and risking injury to horse and handler.

Once the horse is in the field, turn him, close the gate and release him. Horses should never be chased once released. If several horses are being turned out at the same time they should all be led well into the field, turned to face the fence, well apart from each other and released at the same time. The last person in the field closes the gate and tells everybody else when ready to let their horse go. Horses often have a buck and a kick, so turning them to the fence means that they have to turn round to gallop off, giving the handlers a chance to step back out of the way.

Every time a horse is turned out in the field a quick check should be made for hazards such as litter, broken fencing and poisonous plants and action taken as necessary – either clearing up the problem or reporting it to the person in charge.

Catching a horse in the field

Depending on the horse's temperament, catching one horse in a field containing several horses can either be easy or a very frustrating, not to say dangerous, exercise. Go prepared with a suitable headcollar and rope and a few nuts in a bucket if necessary – if there are several horses a bucket can be a liability as they all crowd around to get a mouthful. In this situation the reward may be better hidden in your pocket and just offered to the horse you are trying to catch; this is one situation where giving a horse a titbit is justified.

Having shut the gate, approach the horse's shoulder slowly and quietly with the headcollar discreetly held over your arm or shoulder; do not march straight up to the horse, almost pretend it is not him you are after. Avoid staring at the horse. When you are close, speak to him and offer the food, give him a couple of nuts, a pat and place the rope around his neck before fitting the headcollar. This way you can discourage the horse from moving before you have got the headcollar on.

Quietly lead the horse to the gate, avoiding the other horses, open the gate, lead him through, turn him and close the gate. Assistance may be needed at this point if all the horses decide they want to come with you. Squeezing your horse past may result in him getting caught in the gate or the other horses escaping. If you are on your own scatter some feed on the ground away from the gate to distract the other horses while you lead the caught horse out of the field.

Catching a difficult horse

Some horses are always difficult to catch, while others may become upset by other horses galloping about or by wild, windy weather. Some may let you catch them and then pull away from you; again be prepared and use a headcollar and lunge line or bridle to lead the naughty horse. If possible get help and quietly aim to confine the horse in the corner of the field, with one person either side. Each should carry a headcollar and have some feed for the horse. Never try to herd or chase the horse as it will only make him worse and be very careful that the cornered horse does not spin round and kick out or gallop over the top of you.

Occasionally, leaving the horse, giving him time to settle down and coming back later will work; horses do not like to be ignored. Talking to other horses in the field or catching another horse may excite his curiosity and make him more amenable to being caught because he thinks he is missing out on something! Always assume that youngsters are going to be difficult to catch; this way they are unlikely to get into bad habits.

Simple methods of restraint
It is always safer to have an assistant when treating a horse, trimming or clipping and it is important that the helper is not nervous and is

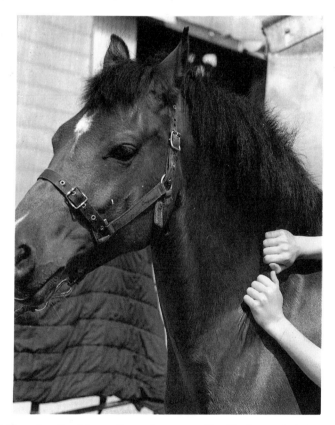

Fig. 10.7 Grasping the skin on the neck can provide effective restraint.

alert, aware and knows what to do. Always start off quietly; a small feed may be enough to distract a horse, or he may respond to being held in a bridle. Do not just put a twitch on the horse with no regard for the horse's temperament.

A simple and gentle restraint is to hold up a horse's front leg; the helper should always be on the same side as the person treating the horse as the horse is more likely to jump away from the treatment than towards it. The horse should be untied and the foot picked up as if the helper is about to pick out the foot and then held by the toe so that the helper can stand upright. Care should be taken that the horse does not snatch the foot away and get a leg over the rope that the helper is holding. If the helper feels about to let go of the foot the other person must be warned so that they can stop what they are doing; remember the other person is relying on the helper for safety.

Grasping a large fold of skin in the middle of the horse's neck is frequently enough to make the horse lower his head and be submissive and is a useful emergency restraint (Fig. 10.7).

Some horses will need more severe restraint and here a twitch is used. A twitch can be made from a piece of broom handle 75–150 cm (2.5–5 ft) long with a piece of stout cord or plaited baling twine looped

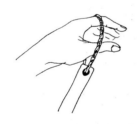

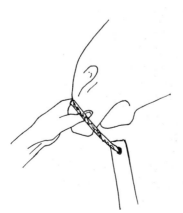

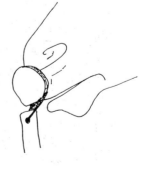

Fig. 10.8 Applying a twitch.

through a hole drilled near the end of the stick. The loop of the twitch is passed over the hand and put on the horse by grasping the upper lip, sliding the loop onto the lip and twisting it tight, adjusting the tension according to the horse's response (Fig. 10.8). The twitch must be put on and taken off quickly or horses will learn to fight it. Most horses react well to the twitch, becoming quiet and amenable. However, a few may try to avoid it, becoming quite dangerous. A sedative or tranquilliser prescribed by the vet may be used for these horses. The horse's ears or tongue should never be twitched and the twitch must not be left on for prolonged periods of time.

Another humane twitch is shaped like a large nutcracker which is passed round the horse's upper lip and then fastened at the open end by a piece of cord. This twitch can be used without an assistant, but this is not recommended because if the horse panics it may be difficult to catch the horse and take the twitch off.

11 The Daily Routine

Yard routine

Routine is as important to those working in the yard as it is to the equine inhabitants; an efficient, yet flexible, routine ensures that all the necessary tasks are completed and gives horses peace of mind. The routine to be followed will vary from yard to yard depending on the type of horse and the priorities of the yard manager. The following routine is rather old-fashioned and would be suitable for hunters or competition horses. Many livery yards would not start until 8 AM while racing yards tend to start earlier.

7.00 AM	*Morning stables*
	Check the horses and refill water buckets
	Tie up, adjust rugs and give haynets
	Muck out
	Quarter
8.00 AM	Feed horses, sweep yard and have breakfast
9.00 AM	Skip out stables
	Tack up and exercise (may be ride and lead)
	On return allow to drink and stale
11.30 AM	Groom and replace rugs. (If there is a second group of horses to exercise, grooming may be done at evening stables)
12.30 PM	Water, hay and give lunch-time feed
	Set fair stable and yard
1.00 PM	Break for lunch
2.00 PM	Carry out daily or weekly chores
	Clean and put away tack

4.00 PM	*Evening stables*
	Tie up, skip out, pick out feet, water and rug up
	Set fair stable, give hay and sweep yard
4.30 PM	Give tea-time feed
7.00 PM	*Late night check*
	Give last feed, water and hay if necessary
	Adjust rugs
	Skip out stables

This routine ensures that the horse's health is checked before he is fed and leaves the horse in peace and quiet to eat his breakfast. However, in many yards the first job of the day is feeding; this is often carried out by a senior member of staff 30 minutes before the rest of the staff arrive. It is important to note and report back whether the horse has eaten all the last night's feed and if there are any signs of ill-health (the signs of health that should be monitored in an early morning inspection are detailed later in this chapter). Mucking out, tidying the muck heap and sweeping the yard are normally done before breakfast, helping to work up a healthy appetite!

Over breakfast it will be decided which person is to ride which horse and how much exercise the horse needs. Once the horse returns from exercise he is cared for promptly and rugged up again. Many yards try to get all horses ridden in the morning. The horses are then given hay and fed and staff have their lunch break.

The afternoon may be needed for tasks such as clipping and trimming. After the weekly chores any horses not yet fully groomed are attended to and all of the horses are 'done up' for the night. Droppings are picked up from the stables (skipping or skepping out), the banks and the bed are tidied up (setting fair), rugs are changed or straightened, the horses given hay and water and the yard swept. Finally the horses are fed and the yard is locked up for the night. Where possible the horses are given a late night check, water buckets are topped up, rugs straightened, and hay and a late feed given if it is in the ration.

On top of the routine outlined above there are other jobs that need to be done. Every day the water buckets and feed mangers must be scrubbed out and automatic drinkers cleaned. Once a week the horses' shoes must be checked so that a shoeing list can be drawn up, the grooming kits should be washed and each horse's rugs shaken out. Yard maintenance routines are described in Chapter 12.

Housing

Although horses are hardy creatures and may be kept at grass all year round, it is often desirable that they should be housed in stables. Stabling provides protection for the horse and convenience for its owner. A horse that is fit has lost its protective fat; a groomed horse no longer has the natural protective oils in its coat. Such horses need protection from the elements. Where the horse is clipped out, as is the case with many working horses, it has lost its coat. Stables protect the horse from the cold, wet and wind during the winter months, and from heat, flies and sun during the summer.

From the owner's point of view, having a stabled horse is a convenience. The horse is at hand, is clean and dry, and is easier to feed and water. Even where adequate pasture is available, stabling the horse saves the grass. Indeed, it is possible to keep a horse without pasture at all, provided it is adequately housed. This is done at some racing stables by choice, and of necessity by some horse-owners in towns. Stabling also provides security and safety. This is especially so where the stables are near the house.

There are many other advantages of stabling. Obviously, it is easier to monitor and control the horse's food and water intake when it is inside. The stabled horse is easier to control, both as regards exercise and, where necessary, restraint. Stabling is, indeed, essential in cases of ill-health or sickness when isolation is desirable.

Requirements of a stable

Sound stabling is a good investment from every point of view. Stabling need not necessarily be grand but ideally it should be purpose built. Although this represents a substantial capital investment, in most cases a stable block adds to the value of the property. Brick- or block-built stables are the best, but are very expensive, and most private owners today are content with stabling of the sectional wooden type. This is available from a number of manufacturers and varies considerably in both quality and price.

Whatever type of stabling is used, there are certain essentials to be borne in mind. Stables should:

- Be warm and dry.
- Have dry foundations.
- Have free drainage.
- Have good ventilation with adequate fresh air yet free from draughts.

- Have good light, both natural and artificial.
- Have a water and electricity supply.
- Be accessible.
- Be arranged to minimise on labour.
- Be *safe* – no projections, and with all electric wiring and lighting protected.
- Be able to be thoroughly disinfected.
- Have adequate fire precautions.

Wood, brick and blocks create a better environment than galvanised iron sheets or asbestos. Galvanised iron in particular has no insulation value and buildings constructed wholly or partly of this material are prone to condensation and overheating. This can be overcome to some extent by providing adequate insulation and boarding over the interior of the stable.

Siting the stables

The ideal site probably does not exist. However, the site should be level and well drained and, if starting from scratch, a concrete base should be installed with a good drainage system. The best ground to build on has a sub-soil of gravel or deep sand which gives a firm base and is dry and free-draining. Rocky soil such as limestone, chalk and granite is next best while clay, peat or marshy soils are the worst and need extensive drainage surrounding the stable yard. Buildings require proper foundations, and in the case of new buildings, planning permission is needed. Approval by the local authority under the Building Regulations is always necessary. The stables should be protected from the prevailing wind, particularly from the north and east. Too many surrounding trees and buildings can prevent the free circulation of air, which is essential to health. If the stabling is to be erected near a dwelling house, the stable block should be sited downwind of the house. Consideration must also be given to ease of access, not only for people but also for routine and emergency vehicles.

The stable block

Today, most private owners prefer loose boxes (see Fig. 11.1) as opposed to stalls where the horse is tied up. However, if converting an existing range of outbuildings not designed as stabling, the arrangement may dictate that the buildings are better converted to stalls.

The stable block itself, large or small, consists not only of loose boxes or stalls, but also of ancillary accommodation. Provision must

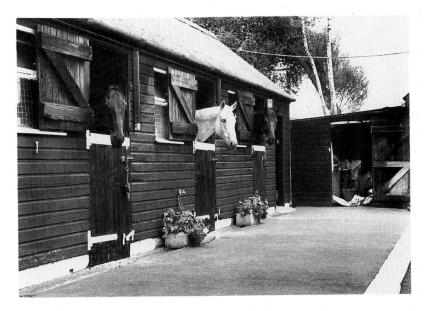

Fig. 11.1 Individual loose boxes.

be made for the storage of feed in the form of concentrates, and of hay and straw or alternative litter. A secure tack room is needed, and there must be somewhere to dry rugs and so on.

In a commercial stable there are additional requirements, e.g. an office and possibly a staff restroom or lounge. In every case, various items need to be stored: tools, wheelbarrows, horse-box or trailer, etc., and there must always be somewhere to dispose of manure.

A variety of housing systems, modern (see Fig. 11.2) and traditional, are in use. Stalls are traditional, but still have their place; however, in modern practice, loose boxes with ancillary accommodation are generally the answer.

Choosing a loose box

Size
The first requirement for a loose box is that there should be adequate head room with a minimum of 3 m (10 ft). The recommended dimensions for loose boxes are:

Large hunter: 3.7 m × 4.3 m (12 ft × 14 ft)
Pony: 3.7 m × 3.0 m (12 ft × 10 ft)
Foaling box: 4.6 m × 4.6 m (15 ft × 15 ft)

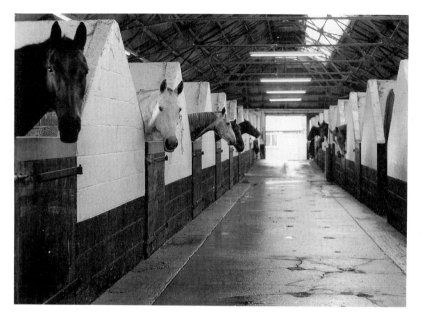

Fig. 11.2 Stabling in an 'American barn' system.

The single box should give not less than 42 m³ (1500 ft³) space per horse.

Stalls should be 1.8 m (6 ft) wide by 2.7 m (9 ft) long, with a passage behind with a minimum width of 1.8 m (6 ft). Dividing partitions should be 2 m (6 ft 6 in) high at the front and 1.5 m (5 ft) high at the rear.

The aim is to provide a minimum of 28 m³ (1000 ft³) of air for each horse housed in the building.

Roof

The stable and its roof should be designed to keep the temperature below 15°C (60°F), even in the hottest weather. Horses tolerate cold, but high temperatures cause them distress. A sloping roof provides a large air space with light and good ventilation. Flat roofs are used if there are lofts or living quarters overhead, but this may reduce ventilation. The roofing material used should be durable, quiet, non-flammable and insulating. The ceiling inside the box should be non-conductive or moisture in the warm air coming off the horse will condense as it hits the cold surface and drip onto the horse. There must be an adequate air outlet at the highest point of each stable.

Floor

Floors should be laid on a solid foundation and raised above the outside ground. They should be non-slip, smooth, durable and insulating so that it does not strike cold to the horse. Concrete is the most commonly used material today but possible alternatives are brick, tarmac, slats or chalk. Floors should be level from side to side but slope front to rear or vice versa to allow for drainage; slopes are usually 1 in 60 in the loose box and 1 in 40 in any gutters. There should not be an open drain in the stable; instead, there should be a trapped drain at the front or back. The drain should be free of sharp angles and closed; underground drains must be checked regularly.

Stable doors

The stable door should be 2.4 m (8 ft) high for horses and a minimum of 1.2 m (4 ft) wide. It should open outwards or sideways. The door should be divided in two, the top part being hinged outwards and left fastened against the wall so that the horse can look out. The bottom half of the door should be about 1.4 m (4 ft 6 in) high for horses with a metal covering along the top edge to prevent the horse chewing the wood. Weaving grids or grilles can be attached to the bottom door if necessary. Weaving grids usefully limit horses chewing the door and its surrounds so are fitted as standard in some yards. Door latches should be horse-proof, strong and easy to use and should not project on the edge of the door when it is open. Proper stable bolts are best, with a kick bolt at the bottom.

Windows

Each loose box should have an opening window protected by a grille or mesh. The best is the hopper type 'Sheringham window' which directs cold air upwards so that it mixes with the warm air in the stable. Windows on the wall opposite the door greatly improve light in the stable; they also enable a pleasant breeze to be available in summer.

Kicking boards

The walls of the boxes should have strong kicking boards up to 1.2 m (4 ft) high. These give the horse protection and can have ridges along them to help prevent the horse getting cast.

Stable fittings

Generally speaking, the fewer stable fittings the better – considerable care is needed to make them accident-proof.

There should be securely fitted tie rings – one at chest height and one at eye level. Feed mangers should be placed in the corner 1.1 m (3 ft 6 in) from the ground. The manger should be large, with a rim too broad for crib-biting, smooth and with rounded corners. Some boxes are designed so that there is access to the manger without going in to the stable, thus saving time and increasing efficiency and safety.

Hay may be fed from a rack at horse's eye level but this is an unnatural position for the horse and hay seeds can fall into the eyes; they are, however, more labour-saving than hay nets. An alternative is a large deep hay manger but there must be suitable provision for removing debris which would otherwise accumulate below it. Many people prefer to feed hay on the floor. Again, labour economy needs hay to be fed without having to open stable doors.

Automatic drinkers are efficient and labour-saving although costly to install – they must each have a cut-off tap and the whole system must cope with frost. The amount the horse is drinking cannot usually be monitored with drinkers. They should be placed away from the manger and hayrack. Strong plastic buckets are an adequate alternative where labour is cheap: they should have the handle removed and be placed in the corner near the door. Alternatively the bucket handle can be clipped to a ring. Empty bucket-holding brackets are potentially dangerous.

Lighting

Artificial lighting in each box is important as there must be adequate light to work both early and late during the winter months. Electric light fittings should be protected by a wire grille or be of the self-contained type. All fittings should be tamper-proof, and switches and power points are better outside the box protected from rain.

Stalls

Stalls are individually partitioned areas in which the horse is tied up with hay, feed and water placed in front of him. Stalls are also useful as day standings for horses brought in from the field, such as in riding schools. Stalls allow more horses to be housed in a smaller space and are warm, labour-saving, inexpensive and require less bedding material. Mares are particularly easy to muck out in stalls.

Yards

Young horses or riding school ponies may be yarded, in other words several are housed together in a large pen inside a barn. Yards are

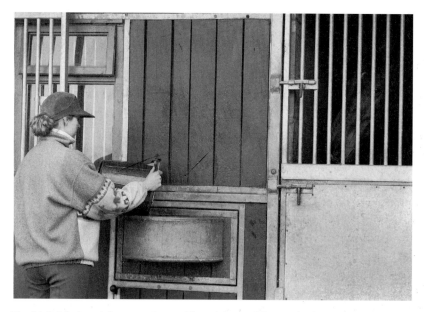

Fig. 11.3 Modern labour-saving stables with provision to feed concentrates from the outside.

usually deep littered with straw. Providing that they are watched for bullying at feeding time and no one horse is being 'picked on' this is a natural way to keep horses inside as they are herd animals. In some yards the horses are tethered apart at feeding times.

The stable environment

The horse's respiratory system must be kept healthy if the horse is to perform at its best. All stabled horses face a constant challenge to their lungs due to dust, mould spores, mites, viruses, bacteria, humidity and noxious gases (including ammonia) present in the stable environment. This challenge can be reduced using 'dust-extracted' bedding, paper, and shavings and by feeding soaked hay and semi-wilted forages.

Arguably the single most important factor in reducing this respiratory challenge is to ensure that the stable is adequately ventilated. Many stables are poorly ventilated due to the widely held misconception that good ventilation leads to cold and draughty boxes where horses 'don't do well'. With the correct positioning and size of air inlets and outlets and the use of air baffling techniques, there is no reason why a well ventilated box cannot provide a 'comfortable' environment. Cold, fresh stables are better than warm, stuffy ones – the horse can always wear an extra rug. The only temperature change likely to be harmful results in chills caused by hot, tired horses standing in a draught. Essential for a good stable environment are:

● Generous air movement, free from draughts.
● A dry atmosphere with no condensation.
● A reasonably uniform temperature.
● Dry flooring with good drainage.

Ventilation

Good ventilation provides a constant supply of fresh air, removing air-borne micro-organisms, noxious gases and excess moisture. Natural ventilation relies on three forces to provide air movement:

● The stack effect – warm air rises and is replaced by cool air.
● Aspiration – as wind passes over the roof air is sucked out.
● Perflation – air movement from side to side and end to end of a building.

The stack effect is the key to natural ventilation – air warmed by the horse's body rises creating a flow of air through the stable.

Air inlets should be designed so that fresh air is evenly distributed to all parts of the stable without creating low level draughts, with a generous air change rate above the horse and gentle currents at horse level. Inlets may be the top half of the stable door, hopper and louvre vents and windows. Hopper windows should open inwards with side cheeks to reduce down-draughts. The aim is to direct incoming air above the horse, with secondary currents providing ventilation at horse level.

Air outlets should be at the highest point of the stable roof – in a pitched roof building the air outlet should be a ridge vent. A pitch of 15° or more is recommended; a lower roof pitch will inhibit air movement and may limit the available air capacity.

There has been much debate about correct ventilation rates for stables, often quoted as the number of air changes per hour or as cubic metres per hour per kilogram body weight. The aim is to avoid stagnant air or draughts. The optimum ventilation rate is determined by the percentage of dust and mould spores in the air. As a general rule, a stable with a high air volume per horse will have a lower requirement for air changes and vice versa. Where horses occupy a shared air space in American barn-type stabling, a higher air change rate is needed. If the natural ventilation is not adequate electric fans may have to be installed; such a system must meet minimum ventilation rates, avoid creating draughts and be easily controlled manually.

Beds and bedding

One important aspect of stable management is to provide a clean and safe environment for the horse. This involves 'mucking out', the one job that all grooms are determined not to spend the rest of their lives doing. Mucking out is much like doing the housework – a boring, menial task that is repeated every day while being taken completely for granted by the inhabitants of the house! Yet providing and maintaining suitable bedding is essential to the horse's health and fitness.

A bed is necessary to:

- Prevent injury and encourage the horse to lie down.
- Prevent draughts and keep the horse's lower legs warm.
- Encourage staling and absorb or drain fluid.
- Cushion the feet.
- Keep the horse clean.

Types of bedding material
Ideally the bed should be economical, dry, soft, absorbent of fluid and gases, clean to use, easily obtainable, good quality, not harmful if eaten, light in colour and readily disposable. Few materials can satisfy all these criteria.

Straw
There are three common types of straw which can be used for bedding horses: wheat, barley and oat straw. Generally wheat straw is considered to be the best as it is less palatable to horses and they are less likely to eat it. It is also said to be harder and shorter than the other straws making it easier to handle. However, the horse owner is not always in a position to choose which sort of straw to buy and it is more important that the straw is free from dust and mould. Straw is less absorbent than some other beddings and is best suited to a stable that drains well. Wastage also tends to be greater as it is more diffi-

cult to separate clean and dirty straw than, say, clean and dirty shavings.

Straw will rot down and can be spread onto fields as a fertiliser. However, disposal of straw muck heaps is becoming more difficult and European regulations look set to escalate the problems. Although cheap and easily available, straw is not a suitable bedding for horses with a respiratory problem and an alternative should be sought. Dust-extracted chopped straw packed into plastic bags is available; this is more expensive than ordinary straw and may still be eaten by the horse. Hemp straw can also be used; it is highly absorbent.

Wood shavings
Increasing numbers of horses appear to be suffering from respiratory disorders and in an attempt to make the horse's environment as dust-free as possible shavings have become a very popular bedding material. Shavings are compressed and packed into plastic bales and can be bought singly or stored outside, an advantage for the one-horse owner who does not have much storage space. Alternatively the shavings can be bought loose. Shavings are highly absorbent, suiting a poorly drained stable or a deep litter system. Horses are also unlikely to eat shavings making it a very popular bedding for competition horses. One minor disadvantage is that it does tend to get everywhere; rugs need to be shaken out thoroughly and shavings are not a suitable bed for a foaling box. Shavings take a long time to rot down so disposal can be a problem.

Paper
Shredded paper is another dust-free bedding which is highly absorbent. Its use is not so widespread for several reasons: it is expensive, unappealing to the eye and difficult to get rid of. The shreds of paper are very light and tend to blow in the wind so it is useful to put a muck sack over the barrow on the way to the muck heap.

Peat moss
Shavings have largely replaced peat moss which is a dark, dusty and highly absorbent bedding. The dark colour gives the stable a dull look and makes mucking out more of a chore as the droppings and wet patches soon become lost in the bed and regular skipping out is essential. It is very expensive and is sold in plastic-wrapped bales which can be stored outside. It is inedible.

Other materials
The search for economical dust-free bedding continues, with one of the least conventional alternatives being rubber matting covering the stable floor; the matting allows urine to drain away and appears to be comfortable and warm for the horse to lie on as well as being non-slip. As muck disposal becomes more difficult it may be that rubber stable floorings become more popular.

Mucking out equipment
Forks, rakes, shovels and barrows are all potential hazards in a busy stable yard. Observe these guidelines for safety's sake:

- Never leave tools where a horse can reach them and do not put barrows in the stable doorway if the horse is not tied up.
- Store tools out of the way of passing people and animals.
- Do not use tools in need of repair and make sure repairs are safe – string holding something together is not safe.
- During mucking out, prop up outside the stable those tools not in use.
- Move the horse out of the way so that you never have to use the fork close to him.
- Stout footwear is essential as it is only too easy to stab one's foot with the sharp prongs of the fork. Many people wear gloves for protection and hygiene.
- String or plastic from forage or bedding must be disposed of safely in a special bin and not left lying round the yard to cause a hazard.
- Wheelbarrows should be rinsed daily and the remaining tools washed weekly to prevent the muck and urine causing them to rot prematurely.

A three- or four-pronged fork is needed to muck out straw while a special many-pronged fork is used for shavings. Straw beds can be laid with a two-pronged fork. A brush and shovel are needed to tidy up, while all waste is put into a wheelbarrow or muck sack. A skip or skep is a small container used for removing droppings during the day; plastic laundry baskets make an inexpensive skip.

Caring for a straw bed
Ideally the horse should be placed in a separate box while mucking out takes place; this is better for his wind, avoiding the dust that is shaken up during mucking out, and allows more efficient and safe mucking

out. If this is not possible, put a headcollar on the horse, tie him to a loop of string on the tie ring and move the horse to one side of the box so that all obvious piles of droppings can be picked up. Remove water buckets and then, starting at the door, use a fork to throw clean straw to the back or one side of the stable. As the straw is shaken the heavier, soiled material falls through the prongs and can be collected on a muck sack or in a wheelbarrow.

Once a week clear and sweep the floor, disinfect it and allow it to dry. The horse should never be asked to stand on bare floor as this is slippery. If the horse has to stay in the box put a thin layer of straw down to stop slipping and yet allow the floor to dry. Regularly turn the banks of straw at the sides of the stable to prevent mould forming; thus throw the bedding to a different side every day.

Then replace the bedding, shaking it well. First build the banks. Banks are useful in preventing draughts and helping to prevent the horse getting cast. Throw the straw up against the wall and then pack it firmly using the back of the fork so that the bank stands above the bed a minimum of 30 cm (12 in) high. Lay the bed so deep that the fork does not strike through to the floor; straw is easily displaced as the horse moves round the box so the bed must be deep enough to ensure that the floor is not exposed – 23–30 cm (9–12 in) should be adequate. Depending on the horse – some are much cleaner than others – allow half a bale of straw per day to keep the bed deep and clean. Large horses in small boxes or brood mares with foals at foot may use as much as a bale a day.

Place the soiled straw on a muck heap, which should be close-packed and neatly squared off. The saying goes that if you want to know if a yard is well run go and look at the muck heap!

Scrub out the water buckets, refill and put back in the stable; do not place them in the doorway or under the haynet or manger, but in a corner where they are visible from the door. If the stable has a fitted manger or drinker check this to make sure that no straw has fallen into it and if necessary clean it out. Both mangers and drinkers should be cleaned daily.

Caring for a shavings bed

The initial cost of laying a shavings bed can be quite high with a 3.7 m^2 (12 ft^2) loose box needing five or six shaving bales to start it off. As before when mucking out, the horse should be taken out of the box or tied up and moved to one side of the box. The piles of droppings can then be picked by hand (wearing rubber gloves) into a skip and then transferred to the barrow. A shavings fork can be used, but, although quicker, this tends to be more wasteful as some clean shavings will be removed. Working from the door the bed can then be thrown up. As the forkful of shavings is thrown against the wall droppings will fall to the bottom of the bank to lie on the floor and can be forked up. As shavings are highly absorbent the wet patches tend to be consolidated like cat litter, not spreading to the rest of the bed. Clean shavings can be scraped off to uncover the wet patches which should then be forked into the barrow.

Once the floor is uncovered it can be swept and, as with straw, either left to dry or have the shavings replaced and new shavings scattered on top. Many shavings are very dusty when fresh and if possible it is better to wait until the horse is out of the box before mucking out. Some people like to put down some clean shavings every day while others put them down a bale at a time when needed. On average two bales of shavings a week should keep the bed topped up adequately, providing that the bed was thick enough in the first place; a foundation of 15 cm (6 in) is the minimum to encourage the horse to lie down and prevent injury.

Deep litter system
Both straw and shavings can be used on a deep litter system. The bed is laid as normal but no droppings or wet patches are taken out. Clean bedding is added whenever necessary. This system is particularly useful when young horses or ponies are yarded together or the stable floor is very uneven or poorly drained. The advantages of the system are that it tends to be economical, less bedding is used on a day-to-day basis, it is labour-saving and provides a solid bed which does not move when the horse rolls.

The system does have some disadvantages: at the end of the winter the bed must be completely removed, often a job for a tractor as it is very heavy work to do by hand; the horse's feet must be regularly picked out; and if the bed is not cared for properly it will become unhygienic and unsightly with the horses covered in muck like cattle. Some yards use a similar system in loose boxes, just taking out the droppings but leaving the wet patches, as outlined in the next section.

Semi-deep litter system
The semi-deep litter system is a useful compromise between a thorough daily mucking out and leaving all the waste in. The way in

which yards manage a semi-deep litter system varies from leaving in all the wet material and removing only the droppings daily to removing the wet material and droppings daily but not moving the banks. The latter is a useful way of managing a shavings bed which has very high banks. The banks are left untouched to become quite solid while the middle of the bed is mucked out and the floor swept as normal.

Skipping out

Skipping out involves removing droppings without taking out any bedding. A heavy-duty pair of rubber gloves can be used, particularly in shavings beds. Alternatively a fork can be inserted beneath the dropping and, with the skip tipped towards the dropping, it can be flipped into the skip. The stable should be skipped out every time you go in; this is hygienic and saves bedding from becoming soiled. In any case the stable should be skipped out at lunch-time and evening stables. As long as the stable door is secured and the horse is placid enough it is not necessary to tie the horse up in order to skip out the stable.

Disinfecting boxes

Any stable that has been occupied by a horse suffering from an infectious disease should be thoroughly disinfected before being used by another horse.

- All bedding and left-over hay should be removed and burnt.
- Any salt lick should be thrown away.
- The walls, door, manger and other fittings should first be thoroughly cleaned, possibly with a pressure washer, and then scrubbed with a suitable disinfectant.
- The stable can later be rinsed and left to dry.
- If necessary the walls can then be repainted and the woodwork creosoted.
- Any equipment used on the infected horse or in its stable should also be treated; this includes haynets, grooming kit, buckets, rugs, blankets and tack.

The early morning and late night check

Two important yard routines are the early morning check made before feeding the horses and the late night check made in the evening. The checks are made to ensure that the horse has eaten up its food and looks healthy. In addition the late night check must include a check on the security – everything should be locked and the stable doors secured.

Prompt recognition of the subtle signs of ill-health allows rapid treatment and, consequently, speedy recovery. In order to identify the sick horse the horsemaster must be able to recognise the everyday signs that indicate that the horse is healthy. This should be second nature, a subconscious routine, every time the horse is handled.

The signs of health

- The horse should be alert.
- The horse's stance – it is normal to rest a hind leg, but resting a front leg may indicate problems.
- The horse's mucous membranes (eyelids, gums, etc.) should be a salmon–pink colour.
- The coat should be smooth and glossy, with the skin moving freely over the underlying tissues.
- The frequency, consistency and smell of the droppings and urine should be correct for that horse.
- Disturbed bedding and dried sweat marks may indicate that the horse has been distressed.
- There should be no abnormal heat, pain or swelling on any areas of the horse's body, especially the lower limbs.

If any of these signs are abnormal the first thing to do is to check the horse's vital signs: temperature, pulse rate and respiration rate (TPR). To obtain 'normal' values each of these measurements should be taken while the horse is calm and at rest, for example between feeding and the daily exercise.

Temperature

The horse's normal resting temperature is 38°C (100.5°F). Any deviation from normal may indicate stress of some sort, most commonly illness. A clean veterinary thermometer, lightly greased with petroleum jelly, is used to take a horse's rectal temperature (Fig 11.4). Standing to one side of the horse's hindquarters, lift the tail and gently insert the thermometer into the rectum with a twisting action. Place the thermometer full-length into the rectum, pressing it gently against the wall of the rectum for one to two minutes. Then slowly remove the

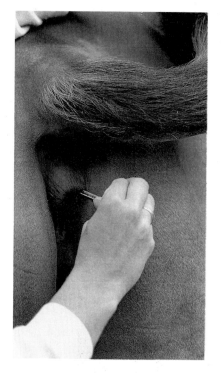
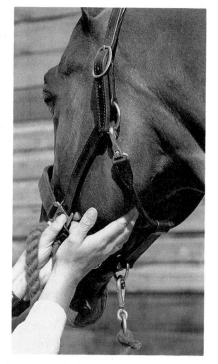

11.4 Taking the temperature.   *Fig. 11.5* Taking the pulse.

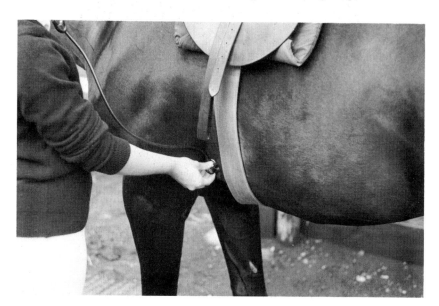

Fig. 11.6 Using a stethoscope.

thermometer with a rotating movement and read it. Digital read-out thermometers, although more expensive, are easy to read and are a useful addition to the first-aid kit.

Pulse

The horse's normal resting pulse rate is 36–42 beats per minute and this corresponds to the heart rate. The easiest place to take the horse's pulse is where the facial artery runs over the cheekbone (Fig. 11.5). Run the fingers down the inside of the horse's left cheekbone until you feel a moveable lump, about the diameter of a pencil, running across the bone. Gently press your first two fingers along this lump, cupping the cheekbone, and count the pulse for 10 seconds. Multiply by six to give the pulse rate per minute.

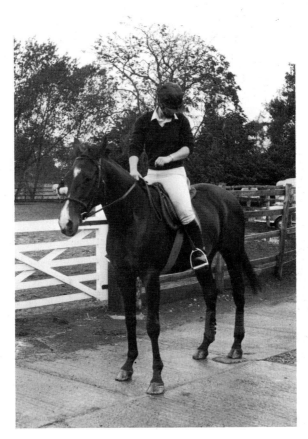

Fig. 11.7 Recording the respiration rate.

A stethoscope can also be used on the left side of the horse, just behind the elbow and in front of the girth (Fig. 11.6). Also, the mounted rider can lean down and press the back of their ungloved hand against the horse in front of the girth. Once the horse has had a canter the heart can be clearly felt hammering against the ribs!

Respiration

The horse's normal resting breathing rate – how often the horse breathes in and out – is 8–16 breaths per minute. To take the respiration rate, the in and out motion of the ribs or rise and fall of the flanks is observed (Fig. 11.7). Each combination of in and out is counted as one. The rider can also put a hand close to the horse's nostrils and count as the horse breathes out – beware the horse does not sniff your hand looking for titbits! In cold weather the horse's breath can be seen as he breathes out.

12 Yard Work and Riding Out

Yard maintenance

Safety is paramount; horses are large creatures which evolved to take flight or lash out when threatened and it is essential that anybody involved with horses realises the potential danger. The yard routine and layout should be organised in such a way as to minimise any risk to the health and safety of both horse and handler. One of the most simple and yet important things is to keep the yard tidy during and after daily chores are carried out. For example, during mucking out tools and barrows should be placed where they will not interfere with the movement of horses and humans, and after use should be stored in a convenient place which is out of the way (Fig. 12.1).

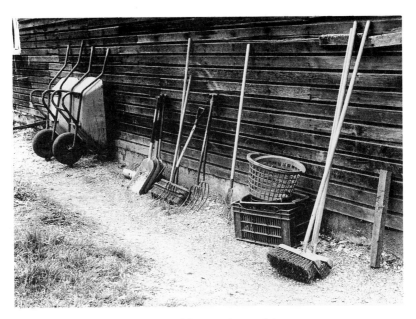

Fig. 12.1 Yard tools and barrows safely stored out of the way.

Disposal of manure

Siting the muck heap
The muck heap should be sited within easy reach of the yard to save
too much time spent wheeling barrows back and forth, yet it should be
out of sight of the car park and yard entrance. The road or track
leading to the muck heap should allow access for the tractor and
trailer or lorry that will remove the manure. The base of the area that
is going to contain the muck should be concreted and surrounded on
three sides by railway sleepers set in steel joists up to a height of 1.8 m
(6 ft). An alternative and time-saving method of muck disposed is to
have a trailer parked below a ramp and to empty the wheelbarrows at
the top of the ramp directly into the trailer which is emptied when full.

Building the muck heap
The muck heap needs daily attention if it is to be kept under control.
The heap should be built in steps with a flat top and vertical sides
which should be raked down to prevent loose pieces of straw blowing
around the yard (Fig. 12.2). The surrounding area must be swept and
kept clean. The secret of success is to pack the soiled straw down as

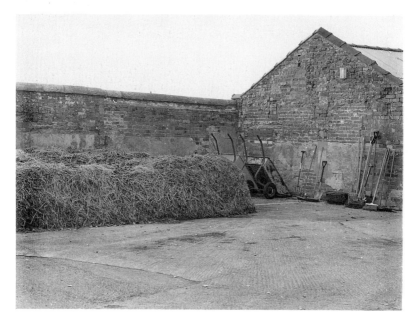

Fig. 12.2 The muck heap.

firmly as possible by stamping it into place; any straw that falls to the floor is thrown up onto the heap and trampled down again. A muck heap built in this way can store more muck in the same area and rots down better because it heats up throughout.

Removing the muck heap

Disposal of manure is a problem for many yards. Straw muck may be regularly collected by firms supplying market gardens and mushroom growers or local farmers may be prepared to spread either shavings or straw muck on their fields. Providing the horses have been regularly and effectively wormed and that the manure is well rotted then the muck may be spread on fields belonging to the yard once or twice a year.

A limited amount of shavings manure may be added to the floor of an indoor school. A muck heap can be burned, but the fire may smoulder for days and sometimes weeks. It can be a fire hazard and may cause considerable nuisance to neighbours.

Weekly chores

As well as keeping the yard and stable area neat and tidy on a day-to-day basis (Fig. 12.3) there are yard maintenance jobs which need to be done on a weekly or seasonal basis. These include:

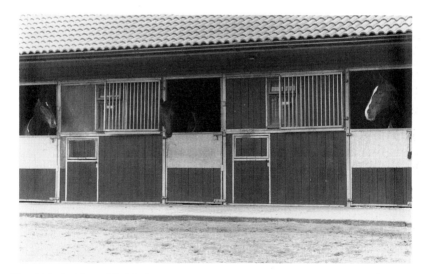

Fig. 12.3 A tidy stable block.

- Cleaning stable windows and removing cobwebs.
- Clearing out drains.
- Checking first-aid kits and fire-fighting equipment.
- Replacing light bulbs.
- Cleaning stored tack.
- Brushing out rugs.
- Cleaning out the feed room, hay and straw shed.
- Scrubbing out feed and water containers.
- Checking feed stocks.
- Ordering and collecting feed.
- Disinfecting stable floors.

Unfortunately many of these jobs are often neglected with staff having more than enough to do caring for the horses. This is short-sighted as maintenance is important for appearance, safety and long life of equipment and fittings.

Clearing drains
Once a week drains and sinks should be flushed with cold water to ensure that they are working properly and then disinfected. Occasionally drains will become blocked and have to be cleared; this unpleasant job should be done with care as there is a health risk involved. Heavy-duty rubber gloves are vital and drainage rods should be used where possible to loosen the material clogging the drain. To prevent some drains blocking they can be fitted with a removable grid or trap which catches solid material and can be cleared regularly. In cold weather drains may freeze over and should be melted with liberal applications of salt.

Disinfecting stable floors
Although desirable, it is unlikely to be feasible to take up the bed once a week, scrub the floor with disinfectant and allow it to dry before putting the bed back down. Thus many yards only do this twice a year and in the meantime sprinkle powdered disinfectant on the swept stable floor once a week. This is a useful compromise which keeps the stable sweet-smelling and is not time consuming.

Personal hygiene

There is little point in maintaining a high standard of stable management if this is not reflected by the staff. Working with horses is a grubby job and yet every effort should be made to maintain personal hygiene: clothing should be clean, hair tied back, fingernails kept short and easy to scrub and no dangling scarfs or jewellery worn which may be unsafe.

Lifting heavy objects

Back pain is the major reason for people being off work, yet lifting heavy and often awkward objects is unavoidable in stable work. Safe procedure will help avoid accidents which often result from careless short cuts (Fig. 12.4). Whenever possible bales and sacks should be moved on a wheelbarrow but they still have to be lifted onto the barrow. To minimise the risk of back injury, any weight should be picked up from the ground by standing in front of it and bending the knees. Avoid lifting a bale or muck sack, swinging it onto your shoulder and turning at the same time; lift it straight up to rest on something and turn before taking hold of it again and carrying it on your shoulder.

Load a barrow with the weight towards the front, over the wheels. Although the temptation is great, avoid overloading barrows, trying to carry too much or moving things single-handed. Full water buckets are easier to carry if the weight is equally distributed so carry one in each hand.

Bales and muck sacks are not the only heavy objects that need to be moved; bags of feed have to moved and stored. Small bags which can be lifted high and held against the chest can generally be carried comfortably, but if you need to lean back to support the weight, the bag is too heavy and should be put on a barrow.

The feed room

The feed room should be conveniently sited to avoid wasting too much time going back and forth to it. It is best constructed of brick or concrete blocks to discourage vermin. It should also be secure so that there is no possibility that a loose horse could stray into the feed room. Large yards may have a feed room and a separate feed shed to allow storage of large quantities of fodder. If this is not the case the feed room should be accessible for door-to-door delivery of feed.

Ideally the room will have a tap, sink and draining board,

- *Assess the situation:*
  Dress – boots, gloves, etc.
  Equipment – pitch fork, bale hook, pulley, trolley, jack, lever, etc.
  Assistance – machine, team, mate, etc.
  Reconnoitre – safe object, safe route, safe landing zone, safe weight.

- *Stance:*
  Feet apart – balanced; one foot forward.
  As close as possible to the object.
  Back straight, chin in.
  Legs bent.

- *Grip (lifting from floor):*
  Hand close and under weight or object clutched close to body.

- *Vision:*
  Do not block your view.

- *Lift:*
  Up and forwards – use leg muscles (calves, thighs, buttocks) but *not* back muscles.
  Do *not* twist or bend your spine.
  Keep weight close to body.

- *Carry:*
  Do not hurry, easy breathing, short steps.

- *Deposit:*
  Reverse of lift.

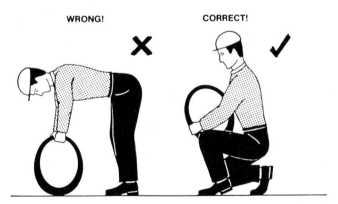

WRONG!   CORRECT!

Fig. 12.4 Safe lifting technique.

encouraging regular washing of feed bowls and utensils. An electric socket for boiling a kettle should be well away from the wet area.

All types of feed will deteriorate if kept in poor conditions; ideally the feed room should be built and designed so that it is always cool with little variation in temperature. It should be well ventilated, dry and light but protected from direct sunlight and free from vermin such as rats, mice, birds, insects and mites.

It is almost impossible to make a feed room vermin proof and so open bags of feed should be stored in galvanised feed bins, raised off the floor on small wooden blocks, or in plastic dustbins with well-fitting lids. These should be cleaned out regularly and always emptied before a new bag of feed is emptied on top. Unopened bags of feed should be stored on pallets to raise them off the ground and prevent dampness. Damp food soon becomes stale, mouldy and unappetising to horses.

The feed room floor should be swept daily; a commercial type of vacuum cleaner with a long tube will help to keep awkward areas clean. There should be room around the bins for a terrier or cat to patrol and discourage vermin. Empty feed sacks and other rubbish must be collected in a dustbin which should be emptied once a week and any left-over feed should be buried in the muck heap. Simple housekeeping measures like this may not be enough to keep rats and mice away in which case a pest control programme will be needed; rats are a constant health hazard, eating food, making it unpalatable to horses and possibly passing on the disease leptospirosis to horses, dogs and sometimes humans. Rats are not the only problem; mice and birds can also rip bags and leave droppings on the floor and in food.

The feed room may also be fitted with a shelf for supplements, a lockable cupboard for medicines and a feed board.

The hay barn and plastic-packed forage

Hay may be stored for daily use in a store in the yard, but large stocks are usually kept in a barn, sited away from the stable because of the fire risk, yet easily accessible to staff. The barn should also be accessible to a tractor for the delivery of hay and straw and there should be no overhead wires which could be damaged by high loads. Even well-made hay loses quality with age, but good storage conditions will help keep it palatable for longer. Hay must be protected from the weather and from damp rising up from the ground. Also air should be able to circulate through the stack so the stack should be raised on pallets or bales of straw and there should be small gaps between the bales. Storing hay in a barn is better than covering it with plastic sheeting as that allows damp and mould to grow – ventilation is very important.

The safety regulations apply to the hay barn as well as the stable yard. String should be knotted and put in a waste bin or bag, any loose hay should be used or cleared up immediately and the bales should not just be taken from the front but removed layer by layer from the top.

Plastic-packed forage will only stay palatable if the bags are not punctured. The bags must be protected from rats and mice which chew the bags and from sharp edges which may rip the bags. Careful handling is also very important. Protecting the bags from direct sunlight will prolong their life.

Monitoring feed stocks

Every week feed stocks should be checked and if necessary ordered or bought. Small yards may visit the local supplier and collect what they require; larger yards may have a weekly or fortnightly delivery. Delivered goods should be checked off against the delivery slip as they are unloaded. This slip should then be checked against the subsequent invoice before paying the bill. It is wise to have an agreement with the feed merchant that if any bags are not up to standard they will be replaced free of charge.

Riding out

When riding out, responsible people know and follow two codes: the Country Code and the Equine Road Users Code (Fig. 12.5).

The Country Code

- Enjoy the countryside and respect its life and work.
- Guard against all risk of fire.
- Fasten all gates.
- Keep dogs under close control.
- Keep to public paths across farm land.
- Use gates to cross fences, hedges and walls.
- Take litter home.
- Help to keep all water clean.
- Protect wildlife, plants and trees.
- Make no unnecessary noise.

Remember that you have a responsibility to yourself, your horse, the

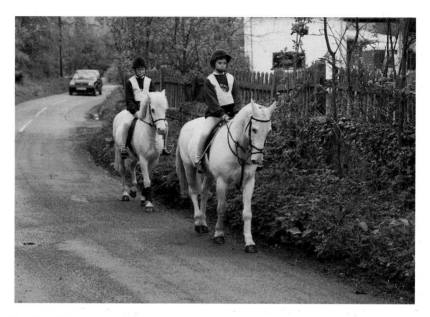

Fig. 12.5 Riding out safely dressed and equipped.

land, farmers and other path users. Behaviour which spoils other people's pleasure, causes accidents, damages crops or stock or inconveniences landowners leads to barred gates and a 'horses not welcome' attitude.

The Equine Road Users Code

- Untrained horses or inexperienced riders may not go on the road alone, nor may they go on busy highways until the rider is experienced and the horse well behaved on quieter roads.
- Riders and drivers must be familiar with the Highway Code and the British Horse Society publication *Riding Safely on the Roads*.
- Horses must stay on the left. Led horses should be on the left of their leader.
- Horses may not go on pavements.
- Riders must wear fitted, properly secured hats to current BSI specifications.
- Footwear must have heels, soles should not have heavy cleats and stirrups must be wide enough.
- Tack must be in good order and properly fitted.
- Bright wear is advisable and in poor light it is essential on both

horse and rider. After sunset a lamp (white – front, red – rear) is required.
● Respect other road users and adjacent pedestrians.

13 People in the Stable Yard

There has been a natural tendency for people involved in working with horses and yard management to concentrate on the horses. They are concerned about the stables, the bedding, the feed, the exercise and so on, but they rarely ask 'Are the staff all right?'. This chapter is about people. If the people are not right then the horses will be unhappy, poorly cared for and unsuccessful.

There was a time when 'girl grooms were two a penny', or so some people seemed to think. There seemed to be enough stable staff so devoted to the needs of the horses in their care that they would work all hours for very little money, living in terrible conditions and getting rare appreciation and few thanks. Mercifully, times have changed and there is now an awareness that staff deserve a square deal and good staff are a sound investment. Furthermore, it makes sense for a horse business to invest in people. Yards that offer fair conditions of service plus staff training tend to keep their staff and have successful results.

Yard staff

Work with horses seems attractive from a distance – cuddling those noble creatures and galloping about with one's hair blowing in the breeze! In reality it is tough, dirty and repetitive. It sometimes calls for courage and a cool approach to tense situations. It requires great pride in one's work, good attention to detail and resourcefulness. Also the person must have that quality of empathy with horses, which in a non-sentimental way creates a good working relationship with them.

What makes a really good worker? The following qualities give some useful pointers:

● *Responsibility* – taking responsibility means that the horse, other people in the yard and all concerned can be quietly confident that each job will be done properly. A person can only work to the best of their ability, but that does include taking pride and interest in the work. Nowadays people rarely have to do a job just because someone says so. They like to understand why the job is necessary and why they do it in a particular way; then personal pride ensures that not only will the job be well done but that everybody can rely on the person to do it.

- *Reliability* – being reliable means that not only can someone rely on the person to do the job but also that it will be done in the agreed manner and at the agreed time. If it is not possible to achieve the plan then the reliable worker will always let the appropriate person know so that a contingency arrangement can be made.

- *Efficiency* – using time efficiently does not mean dashing about, puffing and blowing, driving everyone else to despair and turning the horses into nervous wrecks. It means being well prepared, thinking first and making a plan. Someone who uses time efficiently is also punctual. This does not mean always being early, but it does mean that if the horses have to be loaded at 8.30 AM then by 8.25 AM they are all ready and that one can enjoy the five minutes in hand to mentally check that everything is in its right place according to plan. Sometimes in the horse world this aspect of leaving on time means an early start. The alternative is tasks done badly, the horses flustered and then having a horrid journey because the driver is going too fast for their comfort.

- *Skill* – being skilled means that one has taken the trouble to study how jobs should be done. Then with the aid of good tuition backed up by careful practice the skill is developed, first to a high standard and then to a fair speed. With horses and ponies there is always the extra dimension that the worker must consider the animal and work accordingly.

- *Realism* – each person has to recognise their own limitations and present skill levels. Perfection is usually an impossible dream. Once a person recognises these things then they can work to improve their knowledge and skills.

- *Resourcefulness* – initiative is a great gift and sadly some people have only a short supply. Working with horses means that nothing is predictable. All animals and much of nature have this factor which makes them so intriguing. One has to cope to the best of one's ability with this unpredictableness. A person must also be willing to say if they do not understand or they need assistance or guidance about how best to proceed. There will also be times when a person finds that their knowledge and skills are not sufficient; in these situations it is generally best to get expert help. It is wrong to feel that one always has to find a solution to every situation independently.

- *Safety* – safe is good. Taking unnecessary risks is bad. Never attempt makeshift repairs – they will let someone down. Try not to skimp jobs by taking short cuts; agreed practice is safe practice. Some people seem accident-prone and disaster seems to follow them around. Watch such people and see why things go wrong. Generally they do not allow enough time; then they fail to engage the brain before starting on the job. It is very important that a person working in the yard does not put others at risk.

  For example, there is a dark corridor and you switch on the light; 'pop' – the light bulb blows. It is essential that the bulb is replaced before someone has an accident wandering along in the dark. You put down a rake the wrong way round and someone steps on it; 'bang' – they get hit in the face. You are carrying a bucket and rush to answer the phone; 'crash' – someone has tripped over the bucket. You park your wheelbarrow in the stable doorway because you are late and to save tying up the horse; 'crash, scrape, clatter' – the horse has tried to hop over the barrow or squeeze past it, has fallen in the process and now needs the vet. You open the door of the indoor school; 'crunch, – someone was riding past. You are lungeing a quiet horse without wearing gloves; 'bang' – the farmer over the hedge shoots at a pigeon, your horse leaps in fright and your hands get a nasty burn from the lunge line. The list is endless. All too often accidents do not happen, they are caused.

- *Care* – equine welfare is a concern of every animal lover. Because they are working with horses routinely, some people occasionally lose sight of the animals' needs, or they fail to recognise that each horse is different with individual needs. One must care for the horses' physical and mental well-being.

  In competition there is a delicate balance: the event rider or long-distance rider knows that their team-mates and maybe their country depends on them but their horse is exhausted. The prize is within sight – should they press on? No. One must realise that it is fine to stress a horse in competition but he must not be over-stressed. The balance calls for fine judgement, but if there is doubt then the balance must tip towards the horse's well-being rather than competition success.

In riding and driving there is a risk for both horse and handler; riding is a risk sport. However, one must never lose sight of the welfare considerations. Furthermore, at any time or place where one sees unacceptable standards of horse care or misuse of horses one must be prepared to act. The animals which give us so much are owed this.

- *Loyalty* – loyalty is an important quality and takes many forms. A person is loyal in support of their horses and workmates. It is also important to be loyal to the yard and the business; this may entail keeping confidences. During World War II there were posters reminding people that 'Careless talk costs lives' – enemy spies were about. Nowadays one would do well to remember that careless talk costs reputations. Sadly some horse people delight in speaking ill of others.

- *Representativeness* – a final quality of a good worker is that of an ambassador. Everyone is an ambassador, firstly representing themselves, their appearance and pleasant manner immediately establishing a good first impression. Remember, 'You never get a second chance to make a first impression'. One also represents one's team of workmates – one scruffy or loudmouthed person in the team stands out and lets the side down. In addition one is an ambassador for the stable and every stable needs a good reputation. It is a great honour to work for an establishment that is held in high regard. Professionals find that having worked at a yard with a good reputation will always stand them in good stead for the rest of their career.

Working relationships

For most stable staff it is important that they have good relationships with others. Single-handed jobs need a special, strongly-motivated person who can take pleasure from working alone. But most stable yards rely on a team approach and that needs some extra qualities to those already listed.

Everyone in a yard needs to 'pull their weight'. If one person is a slacker then everyone else has to work harder or else standards fall. Also each person must contribute positively to a team approach; some people take the attitude that it is always someone else's job to greet a stranger, pick up litter, change a light bulb or do any other task. The other crucial ingredient for a good team worker is that they promote good relationships and have a good effect on the rest of the team. Everyone has 'off' days when workmates find the person grumpy or a bit difficult; there is generally a good reason. On these days the rest of the team will make allowances. Similarly, there will be times when one is relied upon by workmates.

Maintaining good working relationships with others is important and should not be taken for granted. Working as a team is enjoyable and, if well done, aids efficiency. It is important to be able to take orders and deal with requests; some people all too easily take offence when none is intended. If it is something which cannot be done now then it is helpful to clearly and politely say so. If a problem crops up between one person and another it is important to try and talk it through and resolve it; if necessary a senior person may be brought in to help. The great thing is that the team should be strong and harmonious.

There is a golden rule for being a member of a team: it comes from the Bible in the Sermon on the Mount – 'In everything, do unto others as you would have them do unto you.'

Meeting and greeting

One of the first tasks anyone in the yard must master is how to greet callers. The person may be a client, a potential burglar, have got lost or is just being nosey. A stranger wandering around is an accident risk, and every yard should have an agreed procedure for visitors. Usually there will be an area where they can be 'parked' while the person they need to see is located. A conversation with a stranger in the yard may go like this:

'Good morning. May I help you?'
'No thanks. I'm fine.'
'We have a policy in this yard that no visitor may proceed unescorted. Now, how may I help you?'
'I want to see the boss.'
'I am sorry but Mr Jones is not here at present. Would you like to see the Head Girl?'

Politeness and firmness are the best policy. Anyone without a convincing explanation should have their car registration number and a brief description of their appearance noted in the day book. Then if there is a break-in in the vicinity inform the police. However, never lose sight of the possibility that an unexpected stranger may be a journalist about to write-up your yard in the local paper, or they may be a newcomer to the district seeking to place a lot of business with your yard. Remember too that every message is important. There must be a good system for passing on messages accurately, speedily and reliably.

Supervisory skills

The job of the Head Girl, Senior Lad, supervisor, or whatever title is used, is crucial to the atmosphere of the yard, the level of horse care, tidiness and much else besides.

A good supervisor is easily identified by two particular aspects of the yard:

- Good practice – for every yard there must be selected and agreed safe, effective and efficient ways of doing all routine tasks. All staff including trainees must adopt and stick to these practices. The supervisor is the arbiter of good practice.
- High standards – standards of quality, tidiness and, where appropriate, of work rate are consistently high. The supervisor leads from the front with a forthright cheery example.

A good supervisor has two particular attributes:

- Reliability – reliability is not just necessary from the employer's point of view; it is also sought by all team members. A good supervisor will always do their best, both for the employer and for the staff; where their needs conflict the supervisor may seek a compromise but ultimately has to enforce the employer's requirements with tact, loyalty and authority – it is sometimes a tough job.
- Skill – change must be brought in with understanding, clarity and ongoing enforcement. The supervisor should use their authority without giving rise to resentment. Problems should be dealt with clearly but pleasantly, be they problems with jobs, people or horses. The supervisor advises, demonstrates, refers and helps both individuals and teams in order to achieve high performance. Yet after listening to and discussing others' ideas the supervisor

should always be willing to accept improvements. This person should be a good communicator; they should accept that a good relationship with the team is a two-way process and show authority and sensitivity in making it good.

A particularly difficult skill is that of counselling. Staff have problems and may seek help. The skill lies in listening and then helping the person to reflect wisely on possible alternative scenarios. The mistake is to give pat solutions or trite advice for others' problems. Where appropriate it may be best to tactfully encourage staff towards suitable help from specialists.

Staff training

The yard supervisor together with the employer will design the staff training programme, basing it on an assessment of each person's needs and ambitions. As training proceeds each individual will be given the opportunity to report on their own perception of their progress and how this affects their training plan. The supervisor will review the effectiveness of the training methods being used.

Often the supervisor is the trainer, so they will plan and deliver the training. Staff will need encouragement and will want to know how well they are progressing. The employer will also want to know how beneficial the training is proving to be.

In many cases National Vocational Qualifications (NVQs) will be used which means that staff will have plenty of ongoing feedback on their level of skills and on their progress. British Horse Society qualifications, or those of other organisations, may also be used in parallel with NVQs.

The supervisor has to develop as an effective trainer and so will need training themself to be skilled and up-to-date on qualifications, training techniques and resources.

14 Health and Safety

In Britain there is a Health and Safety Executive which gives advice on good practice and which enforces the relevant laws. People working with horses should know what the law has to say, in general terms, about matters which affect them in their work.

The points below are set out in the Health and Safety at Work Act 1972, a shortened copy of which has to be on display or given to each employee. The Management of Health and Safety at Work Regulations 1992 requires employers to assess risks to staff and others so that risks are minimised; this should lead to proper staff training and supervision to ensure that agreed procedures are followed. The law also requires that records are kept, staff are trained, safety equipment is tested, accidents and incidents are recorded, safety clothing is used where appropriate and dangerous substances are properly stored and used.

Duties of employers

The employer must make reasonably sure that the workplace, all machinery and systems of work are safe. All the kit and anything used must be safe and handled, stored and moved about safely. The employer must make sure that all staff are taught how to do jobs safely and that they are supervised so that they adhere to safe practices. There must also be provision for welfare, such as a first-aid kit, lavatories, hand-washing facilities and somewhere to get warm after working outside in winter.

Duties of staff

Staff, including trainees, must cooperate on safety and health matters. Staff must also take reasonable care for themselves, their workmates and anyone else who may be affected by what they do or fail to do. Those who are self-employed are both employer and staff all rolled into one and so must take on the responsibilities of both.

Safety policy and records

If there are five or more staff the employer has to write a safety policy which staff must be familiar with and obey.

Reporting incidents

Staff should always report incidents when things go wrong. The person in charge can then decide if the matter should be entered in the accident or incident book. Such a book is compulsory for BHS and ABRS approved riding schools; it is also required by the 1981 First Aid Regulations. The entry must show the time, date and place of the incident; it must include the names and addresses of witnesses; it must give a clear account of what happened; it must include the names of the horses and people involved and state who was in charge and who was hurt, with added details of any injury sustained and treatment given; it should include a plan or diagram of the accident, plus informative notes, clearly written, and be signed by both the person in charge and, if possible, the person who suffered the incident. If a loose leaf form is used it should be kept in a file with an index of contents.

Reporting hazards

Any machinery or equipment which is faulty or anything hazardous must be reported to the person in charge as soon as it is noticed. That person has a duty to act straight away. A simple notice stating 'Faulty – do not use' could be the first step, or 'Slippery surface – take care'; then further steps must be taken to put the matter right.

Reporting injuries, diseases and dangerous occurrences

Certain matters have to be reported to the local environmental health department; this is enforced by the Reporting of Injuries, Diseases and Dangerous Occurrences Regulations (RIDDOR) 1985. These matters have to be reported immediately by telephone and then confirmed in writing; the yard has to keep its own record for at least three years.

Examples of injuries which must be reported include:

- Death in an accident at work.

- When a member of staff is off work for more than three days following an accident at work.
- Most broken bones (but not fingers and toes).
- Eye wounds.
- Amputations.
- Injury or unconsciousness from electric shock or lack of oxygen or due to absorption of a substance through breathing, eating or drinking it or from having it spilt on the skin.
- Acute illness from bacteria or fungi or other infected material.
- Any injury which results in the person being admitted to hospital for more than 24 hours; this includes clients at riding establishments.

'Dangerous occurrences' which have to be reported are more likely to occur in factories or on building sites.

Reportable diseases include:

- Asthma caused by working in consistently dusty conditions.
- 'Farmers Lung' which is a breathing difficulty caused by regularly handling mouldy hay or straw.
- Leptospirosis (Weils disease) which can be contracted when working in places infested by rats.

First aid

Under the Health and Safety (First Aid) Regulations 1981 the yard must have first-aid provision. This means that someone must always be in charge and take responsibility for calling an ambulance if it is needed. Ideally this person should have first-aid training. First-aid boxes and kits should be kept at the stables, in vehicles and taken on expeditions.

Accident procedures (when a person is badly hurt)

Accidents can and will occur; frequently they involve a rider falling from a horse on the road, in the school or in a field. Whatever the cause the procedure to follow is much the same. Most importantly remember to *keep calm* and use your *common sense*. The telephone number of your local doctor and vet should be beside the telephone or carried with you on a hack. Remember that a telephone is no good locked in the house; yard staff must always have access to one. A small emergency first-aid pack must be taken with you on a hack, along with money, a phone card or a mobile phone.

Immediately after the accident has happened, secure the scene in order to minimise the risk to yourself and any others in the vicinity. Do this by standing guard over the hurt person while sending others to catch the loose horse and to summon the police and/or ambulance if appropriate. The first priority is the casualty who should be reassured and examined. Be sure to take no unnecessary risks. The next thing is to remember the accident ABC:

- A is for approach and airway. Approach the hurt person being careful not to get hurt yourself, and once you have reached them ensure that their mouth and windpipe are free of obstruction.
- B is for breathing; mouth-to-mouth resuscitation may be necessary.
- C is for circulation; if the person is bleeding, pressure must be applied to the area to stop the bleeding as rapidly as possible.

Check for consciousness
Speak loudly and clearly to the casualty, watching the eyes to see if they flicker or open. If the person is conscious they should be asked if they have any pain in the back or neck and if the answer is 'yes' they must not be moved and you should stay with them until help arrives.

Open the airway
The unconscious casualty's airway may be blocked making breathing difficult or impossible. It is vital to, firstly, remove any obvious obstruction from the mouth and, secondly, to open the airway. This is done by placing two fingers under the chin to lift the jaw. At the same time the head should be tilted well back. If a head or neck injury is suspected the head should only be tilted just enough to open the airway.

Check for breathing and a pulse
Look for chest movements, listen for the sound of breathing and feel for breath on your cheek. The pulse can be felt on the neck, between the Adam's apple and the strap muscle that runs across the neck to the breastbone.

The recovery position and mouth-to-mouth resuscitation
If skilled help is not going to arrive quickly the casualty can be put in the recovery position. This prevents the tongue from blocking the throat and allows the unconscious casualty to be left if necessary. It involves turning the casualty with minimum movement of the head, neck and spine. In order to turn an injured person without help:

(1) Open the airway.
(2) Straighten the legs.
(3) Kneeling at the person's side, bring the arm nearest you out at right-angles to their body, with the elbow bent and the hand palm uppermost.
(4) Bring the other arm across the chest and hold the hand, palm outwards, against the casualty's cheek.
(5) With the other hand grasp the thigh furthest away and pull the knee up, keeping the foot flat on the ground.
(6) Keeping the hand pressed against the cheek, pull at the thigh to roll the person gently towards you, supporting the head all the time.
(7) Once the person is turned, tilt the head to make sure the airway is open and adjust the hand under the cheek to ensure that it stays open.
(8) Bend and bring forward the upper knee to prevent further movement.

In serious cases the casualty may be unconscious and not breathing. Immediate action must be taken:

● Undo the chin strap of the hat, but leave it on.
● Press back on the person's forehead and lift the jaw up and forwards to open the air passage to the lungs.
● If this does not start their breathing support the jaw, pinch the nose and blow a normal breath into their mouth, repeating every five seconds.
● Watch to see if the chest begins to rise and fall; if not check that the airway is not still obstructed.
● A Laerdal pocket mask is available to avoid the risk of transmission of disease from mouth-to-mouth resuscitation.

Even if the fallen rider appears to be unhurt, if there is any doubt call for medical assistance or send the person to hospital for a check-up and remember to fill in an accident report no matter how minor the incident. Anyone who has, or might have been, concussed must not ride or drive again that day.

Control of Substances Hazardous to Health (COSHH) Regulations 1988

The COSHH Regulations require the employer to make sure that exposure to hazardous substances is prevented or adequately controlled. Such substances include those that are toxic, harmful, irritant or corrosive. They include disinfectants, detergents, insecticides, mouse and rat poison, creosote and veterinary products. The Regulations also cover exposure to harmful micro-organisms such as those which cause tetanus and to quantities of dust from feed, bedding or arenas, or exposure to any material at work which can harm health.

Precautions
The employer must list the hazards, assess the risks, introduce appropriate controls, ensure that these control measures are adhered to and monitor, train and supervise staff concerning risks and precautions. Some matters call for education and training; for example, staff should know that toilet cleaner and bleach are hazardous when mixed; weedkillers should not be decanted into smaller containers as only the original container will be labelled safely.

Sometimes a change of practice is called for, for example, the sump oil used for horses' feet can give grooms acne. Other matters may call for expensive equipment, for example, riding arenas should not be excessively dusty and need to be kept damp, perhaps requiring an irrigation system. Inexpensive equipment may be needed such as simple dust masks for those grooming muddy horses or stacking old straw. Precautions may involve providing equipment and giving training, such as in the use of rubber gloves, aprons and boots when handling horses with ringworm.

Some of the simple precautions call for an absolute insistence on basic hygiene. Waterproof plasters should cover cuts and hands should be washed before eating (or smoking!). These simple measures reduce the risk of leptospirosis following handling of straw which has had contact with rats. Everyone working with horses should be vaccinated against tetanus.

Safe storage

All pesticides must be stored in a safe lock-up away from staff and feeds. Agricultural pesticides may only be used by staff who have been trained and certified as competent. Veterinary products should be kept in a locked cabinet; only those with adequate training should use these products. If a syringe and needle are used then the needle must be disposed of into a 'sharps bin' – generally found in the back of the vet's car.

Accident prevention

Good housekeeping reduces trips and falls. Pot holes, broken steps, defective gates, projecting nails, items left in passages, tools lying about and any obstruction can cause an accident. Children should not roam unsupervised around work areas.

Those riding or leading horses on the road should keep to the left and the horse should be on the handler's left. Both horse and handler should be properly trained and equipped; inexperienced or overfresh horses should be escorted by a car.

Approved hard hats must be properly fitted and fastened before mounting and remain so until dismounting. Footwear for riding must have a sharp-edged heel (trainers or Wellington boots must never be worn). Footwear for stable work should be robust and, when handling young horses, toe protection is advisable. Gloves should be worn for lungeing and leading young and fresh horses. Bridles give greater restraint than a headcollar.

All electrical appliances and extension cables should be connected using a safety cut-out (residual current device or RCD). Tractors, and even lawn mowers, must only be used by trained staff, as should chaff cutters and oat rollers which must be guarded. Horse walkers should be in a fenced-off area and staff trained before using them. Pressure washers combine water and electricity so need special care. The use of ladders requires caution: the base must not slip so it may need securing on a shiny floor; the top must be at least 1.05 m (3 ft 6 in) above the landing place. If a ladder is left in place, a board must be tied to it so children cannot climb up. Agreed procedures must be implemented when entering riding schools. Finally it is best to keep visitors and traffic away from horses. Wandering visitors should always be greeted and escorted to a safe place. Safety is everyone's responsibility.

Part IV
Horse Care Skills

15 Care of Tack and Horse Clothing

Apart from the tack in which the horse is ridden, the domesticated horse wears rugs, blankets and sheets, bandages and boots.

Care of tack

The majority of a horse's tack is made of leather and both leather and stitching will rot if exposed to sweat, water, heat and then neglected. Thus it is important for appearance, safety and durability that it is kept clean and supple. It is also an ideal time to check the stitching and leather for signs of wear and damage. Unsafe tack should be put to one side and not used again until it is mended, otherwise it may break and cause an accident. The stitching on stirrup leathers tends to wear relatively quickly. To check it, grasp the sewn-down end and pull firmly; if the stitching is weak it will be possible to tear the end away. Remember, tack that has broken and been repaired, for example reins, are weakened and should not be used for competition or other strong work.

Many yards only clean the bit and wipe the tack over on a daily basis, just removing straps from their keepers to clean and soap underneath. If this is the case the tack should be taken apart and cleaned thoroughly once a week. If the tack is exposed to much mud and rain then it should be treated with a leather dressing such as neat's-foot oil on a monthly basis. Over-oiling will make reins difficult to hold and may rot the stitching. The stirrup leathers and surface of the saddle should be treated with care or the leather dressing will come off onto the rider's clothing. Similarly, if a saddle is used without a numnah, leather dressing used on the lining of the saddle may stain the horse's back or cause a reaction on a sensitive horse.

Leatherwork should be rubbed clean with a damp cloth or sponge which is regularly rinsed in warm water. Saddle soap should then be rubbed well into the leather, particularly the fleshy or rough side, using a slightly damp sponge. Saddle soap comes in many forms: glycerine, tins, tubes and liquid. Read the instructions and remember not to use too much or to make the sponge too damp.

Only if the tack is caked with mud is it necessary to use more water and get the tack really wet. Wet leather should be dried with a chamois leather or dry cloth. If the leather has been soaked with rain it should be wiped clean and left to dry naturally. A suitable leather dressing or oil should be used before the leather is soaped to replace the oils lost and to prevent the leather drying out and becoming brittle.

Leather may become mouldy or dry during storage. This can be prevented by dismantling the piece of tack, treating it with a leather dressing, wrapping it in newspaper and then putting it in a plastic bag.

Cleaning saddles

The saddle should be placed on a saddle horse and the girth, leathers, irons and numnah removed. If the irons and stirrup treads are very dirty they can be taken off the leathers, separated and dunked in warm water in a bucket. First the underneath of the saddle should be wiped with a damp cloth or sponge, a clean stable rubber put on the saddle horse and the saddle replaced.

The rest of the saddle should be cleaned, removing any lumps of accumulated grease (jockeys) with a pad of horsehair. The seat of the saddle may not need wiping if it is clean. The leathers, girth, irons and treads should be washed, paying particular attention to any folded areas. All the leather should then be soaped, taking care to do both sides of buckle guards and girth straps. The seat and saddle flaps should be wiped with a dry cloth to remove excess soap which may stain the rider's breeches. Irons and treads should be dried with a towel and polished if necessary. Any suede, serge or linen surfaces should not be soaped but brushed clean. After cleaning the leathers, the irons should be replaced, run up and the leathers put through and under the irons. The girth can be laid on top of the saddle and the saddle covered with a cloth or cover before being returned to its rack.

Cleaning girths

Leather girths should be carefully cleaned after use or they will become hard and rub the horse. The inner felt lining of three-fold girths should be removed, oiled and replaced regularly.

Nylon, string, lampwick and webbing girths should be brushed off every time they are used. If they are muddy or stained they should be soaked in a non-biological detergent, scrubbed and thoroughly rinsed. Care must be taken not to soak any leather parts and if they are hung up by both buckle ends to dry this will prevent the buckles rusting. Finally, any leather parts should be soaped or oiled.

Cleaning numnahs

Quilted cotton, linen-covered foam and synthetic sheepskin numnahs should be shaken or brushed after every use and washed by hand or machine when necessary. Some horses have sensitive skin in which case soap flakes or a suitable washing powder should be used. Sheepskin numnahs must be washed by hand in soap flakes, rinsed and have oil applied to the skin side to prevent it hardening.

Cleaning bridles

Hang the bridle up and remove the bit or bits which should be soaked in warm water, hang the reins up and take the rest of the bridle apart, remembering which holes the pieces were done up on. All the leather should be cleaned and soaped as described above and the bit washed, dried and the rings polished. If oiling is necessary this is the time to do it and to check stitching and the condition of the leather where it is folded or bent. The bridle should then be put back together again in the following order (Fig. 15.1):

- The headpiece should be threaded through the browband, ensuring that the throatlash is to the rear.
- The headpiece should be hung on a hook – for a double bridle the bridoon headpiece (sliphead) should be threaded through the near side of the browband, first under the main headpiece and buckled on the off side.
- The noseband headpiece should be threaded through the browband from the off side to buckle on the near side. It should lie under the headpiece.
- The two cheekpieces should now be attached. A double bridle will have two buckles on each side.
- The bit or bits should be attached the right way up and the lip strap if fitted put on. The lip strap should be pushed through the 'D's on the bit from the inner side to the outer side and buckled on the near side.
- All straps should be placed in their runners and keepers and the noseband placed around the bridle and secured by a runner and keeper.

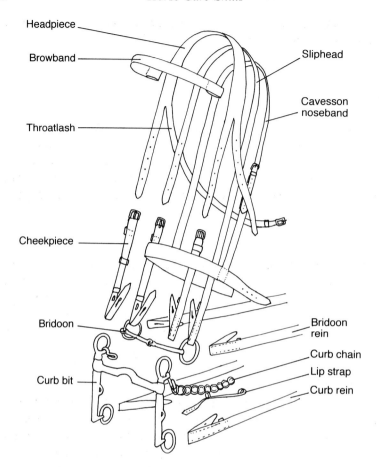

Headpiece

Browband

Throatlash

Cheekpiece

Bridoon

Curb bit

Sliphead

Cavesson noseband

Bridoon rein

Curb chain

Lip strap

Curb rein

Fig. 15.1 Assembling a double bridle.

- The reins should be replaced; on a double bridle the wider rein attaches to the bridoon while the narrower rein goes on the curb bit.
- The curb chain should be hooked on with the lip strap ring hanging down and the lip strap then fastened through the ring to prevent the chain being lost.
- The bridle can then be 'put up' by passing the throatlash around the bridle in a figure of eight, through the reins and securing by a keeper and runner.

Remember, buckle fastening always goes to the outside while billets (fixed hooks) go on the inside. The rough or flesh side of the leather goes against the horse's skin.

Rugs

Rugs are worn in winter to keep the horse warm and dry and in summer to protect him from flies and to keep him clean and improve the appearance of the coat. Rugs are generally fastened at the front and then secured by a roller or surcingle round the horse's girth; more recently cross-over surcingles and leg straps have become a popular way to secure a rug effectively.

Types of rug
The many different types of rug on the market are enough to confuse any new horse owner. It is important to buy the right rug and one that will last. The clipped horse will need a minimum of a stable rug and one or more blankets, a sweat sheet or cooler and a summer sheet. If turned out during the day in winter the horse will also need a New Zealand rug.

Night or stable rug
The night rug or stable rug is a heavy-duty rug for use on cool summer nights and all day and night in winter. Traditionally they were made of jute or canvas lined with blanket and fastened with a roller. A number of blankets can be worn under the rug to suit the weather conditions; heavy striped woollen blankets, although expensive, are warm, but layers of thinner blankets may be used.

Man-made fibre and quilted rugs are now commonly used; while expensive they are light, warm, easily washed and tend to stay in place better as they come with cross-over surcingles or similar fastenings (Fig. 15.2). There is also less pressure on the horse's back than when using a roller.

Day rug
The day rug is woollen with a contrasting binding and most stables only use them for special occasions. They are fastened at the front and may have a matching surcingle (Fig. 15.3).

Sweat rug or cooler
A sweat rug or cooler is used to cool off and dry horses after exercise.

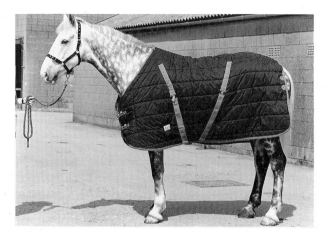

Fig. 15.2 Quilted stable rug with cross-over surcingles.

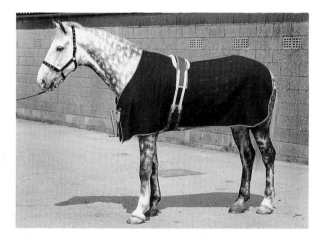

Fig. 15.3 Day rug.

The open mesh type works on the same principle as a string vest, trapping pockets of air to insulate and dry the horse. To work effectively a top rug or sheet must be put over a sweat rug. Coolers are rugs made of material with special properties; the moisture from the horse's body is not soaked up by the rug but taken from the skin/hair through the rug to condense on top of the rug, leaving the horse warm and dry underneath. These make useful travelling rugs.

Summer sheet

The summer sheet is a light-weight rug designed to protect the horse from flies and to keep the dust off the coat in summer. In hot weather it can be used on travelling horses and over the top of a sweat rug (Fig. 15.4). Additionally they can be used as an under-sheet in winter to protect a thin-skinned horse from possible irritation from wool. Washed once a week they help keep the horse's skin and coat clean.

Exercise or quarter sheet

Exercise sheets or quarter sheets can be used under the saddle on cold days or on horses that have been tacked up prior to ridden exercise, for example, race horses in the paddock. The sheet runs from the withers to the top of the dock, reaching down to just below the saddle. It is kept in place by a fillet string and a matching surcingle on the unsaddled horse; if used under the saddle the corners of the sheet are folded back under the saddle flap and girth straps or held in place by loops through which the girth runs.

Hood

A cloth hood can be used in the stable or during exercise to keep the horse warm and thus to prevent the coat on the head and neck growing too rapidly. Stretch or waterproof hoods can be used with a New Zealand rug to keep the horse clean and dry in the field. Hoods can be worn all the time or just when out riding.

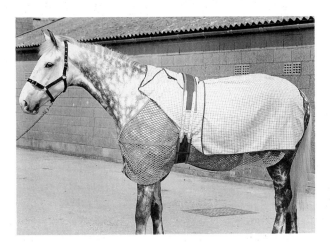

Fig. 15.4 Sweat rug with a summer sheet on top; the front corners of the summer sheet have been folded back and secured with a roller.

New Zealand rug

The New Zealand rug is used to keep outwintered horses and ponies warm and dry and to protect and keep clean the stabled horse which is turned out for a few hours in the day. The rug is made of lined waterproof canvas or synthetic material and is designed to be self-righting so that it stays in position when the horse rolls in the field (Fig. 15.5). The inexpensive types usually have a surcingle stitched to the rug which passes through the sides of the rug and buckles under the horse's belly and leg straps which pass round the hind legs and buckle back to the rug. This design can put pressure on the horse's spine and tends to slip, rubbing the shoulders. More expensive versions may have cross-over surcingles and/or leg straps.

It is imperative that a New Zealand rug fits correctly; it should fit snugly round the neck so that it cannot slip back and press on the withers and rub the shoulders. Some rugs have an adjustable front fastening allowing for the different shapes of horses. The rug should reach to the top of the tail and be of adequate depth. If fitted with a surcingle this should never be knotted to shorten it; take the time to sew it. The leg straps may be made of nylon or leather, which should

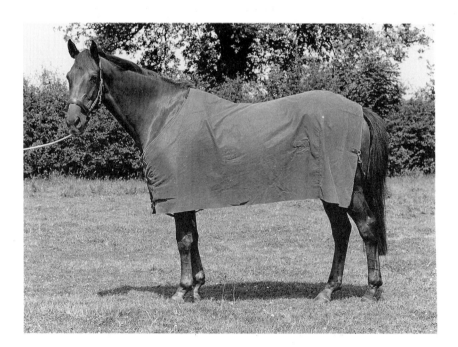

Fig. 15.5 New Zealand rug.

be oiled to keep it soft so that it does not chafe the horse. The strap can be passed round the horse's upper thigh and clipped back to the 'D' on the same side, or crossed to the opposite side; if fastened back to the same side the straps are usually looped through each other. The straps must allow adequate room for movement without dangling by the horse's hocks (Fig. 15.6).

Horses living out in New Zealand rugs should be checked twice a day; a severe rub can develop in a short time if the rug slips. Each horse should have two rugs so that when necessary a dry one can be put on and the other dried. Stitching, leather and buckles must be checked daily for wear, a horse can panic and gallop uncontrollably

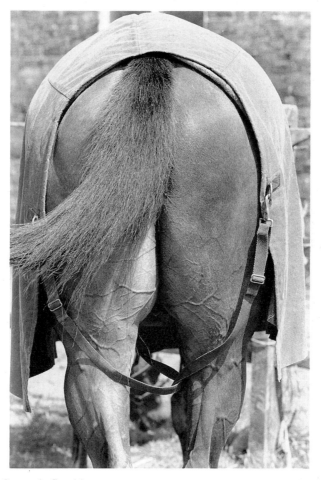

Fig. 15.6 Correctly fitted leg straps.

around the field if the rug slips due to a poor fit or a broken strap. Always catch the horse and get somebody to hold him before trying to adjust a rug in the field; otherwise you may find yourself in a very tricky and potentially dangerous situation.

A young horse can be frightened by a flapping New Zealand rug so initially put it on in the stable to allow the horse to become accustomed to it and then walk and trot him in hand before turning out.

When taking off a New Zealand rug always clip the leg straps back to their 'D's so that they do not hit the horse when you put the rug back on. Clips should always be fastened facing inwards so that they cannot catch on wire fencing.

Keeping rugs in place

Rollers
Rollers are made of leather or webbing and are fastened round the horse's girth to keep rugs in place. Leather rollers are long-lasting but expensive. Webbing or jute rollers are a less expensive alternative, but make sure they are wide enough for the size of horse or they will soon concertina into a narrow band under the horse's girth. A roller has padding either side of the spine, but it may still be advisable to use a thick pad under the roller to minimise pressure on the spine (Figs 15.3 and 15.4).

An anti-cast roller has a metal arch over the withers designed to stop the horse getting cast. Unless this arch is large it is unlikely to work as it merely gets buried in the stable bed (Fig. 15.7). A thick pad is needed under the roller as it tends to concentrate pressure either side

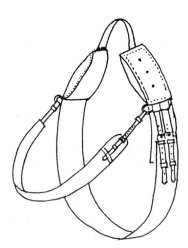

Fig. 15.7 Anti-cast roller with breast girth.

of the horse's withers. There should be buckles on both sides so that it can be undone if the horse does get cast.

Specialist leather rollers can be used for breaking in horses. These have 'D's for side reins, a crupper and a breast girth.

Breast girths

The breast girth is a leather or webbing strap which is fastened to a strap attached to the front 'D's either side of the roller (Fig. 15.7). It is designed to stop the roller sliding back. It should fit closely around the chest just above the point of the horse's shoulder. A similar strap can be used with a saddle, in racing for example.

Surcingles

Surcingles are narrow unpadded straps which hold rugs in place. They are usually stitched into place and care must be taken that pressure is not put on the horse's back.

Cross-over surcingles are stitched at an angle on the off side of the rug, passed under the horse's belly, crossed over and fastened on the near side. These hold the rug in place effectively and with little pressure on the back (Fig. 15.2).

Belly straps

Some quilted rugs have broad bands of matching material which pass from one side of the rug, under the horse's belly and fasten on the other side. Some designs of rug have bands of material which also pass between the front legs in a nappy-type arrangement.

Leg straps

Some night rugs are held in place by leg straps in the same way as a New Zealand rug. Some designs also fasten around the front legs.

Measuring for rugs

Rugs are generally sold with reference to the length of the horse from point of shoulder to point of buttock. For example, a 16hh horse requires a 1.8 m (6 ft) or 6 ft 3 in rug depending on its build. It is worthwhile taking a few more measurements and measuring the rug before buying it. Measure the distance around the horse's neck where the rug should lie; many rugs are far too big around the neck, slip back and sit on the withers. Measure from just in front of the withers to the top of the tail and from the centre of the horse's breastbone to the point of buttock to ensure that the rug will be long enough. A well fitting rug is more comfortable for the horse and lasts longer as it is less likely to get torn.

Putting rugs on (Figs 15.8–15.12)

The horse should be tied up and should stand still while having the rug put on. Always speak to the horse first. If a blanket is worn, collect up the blanket with the left side in the left hand and the right side in the right hand. Fold the blanket in half before throwing it onto the horse's neck. The top half should be drawn back and adjusted so that it is even on both sides and then eased back over the loins to a hand's-breadth from the top of the tail. The front part of the blanket must lie well up the neck and should never be pulled against the lie of the coat; if it is wrong, take it off and start again. It is better to put the blanket on the same way so that soiled areas are always at the quarters.

Unless it is secured the blanket will slip so it is usually turned back over the front of the rug and secured under the roller; both front corners of the blanket should be folded to the top of the withers. The rug should then be either folded and put on like the blanket or gathered up and gently thrown over the neck and withers. The front buckle should be fastened and the rug folded back or eased back over the quarters. The triangle of blanket should then be folded back over the withers, the pad and roller placed on top of the folded blanket and the roller fastened firmly but not tightly.

As long as the horse is placid it is useful to organise the rug and blanket by standing behind the horse to ensure both are even and straight. If attached surcingles are used, they should be checked from the off side so that they are not twisted and then fastened on the near side.

Taking rugs off

Again, no short cuts can be taken; the horse must be tied up and reassured before unfastening the front buckle of the rug. The surcingle or roller should be unfastened, removed and placed over the door, in the manger or, if it is a straw bed, in the corner of the box. Always check to make sure that the rug does not have leg straps or that there is an under-rug which needs unbuckling. The rug and blanket can then be grasped either side of the withers and folded back to the tail. The fold is then held and both rug and blanket are drawn off over the tail. Pulling the rugs off sideways is uncomfortable for the horse and pulls against the coat. The rug and blanket can then be folded and put with the roller.

It is appreciated if the rugs are put ready for the horse's return in such a way that the blanket is folded on top and can be picked up and put straight onto the horse without juggling it and dropping it in the bedding.

In cold weather if there is to be any delay before riding, the rug may be folded back enough to put the saddle on and then folded back over the saddle. If left unattended the horse must be tied up.

Storing rugs

In the spring winter rugs must be mended, cleaned and put away in store; dirty rugs rot and break. Major repairs will require that the rug is sent away to the local saddler to be stitched by machine, but simple repairs such as mending fillet strings or small rips can be repaired by hand at home using a needle and thread. Prompt attention to minor tears will prevent them getting worse and possibly ruining the rug.

Depending on the material, rugs and blankets can either be washed at home or sent away for specialist cleaning. Before washing rugs all leather fittings should be oiled for protection. Some synthetic materials can go into a large domestic washing machine while jute rugs should be soaked in cold water in a trough or dustbin. After soaking, the rug should be scrubbed and thoroughly rinsed before being hung up to dry. Finally, all fittings must be re-oiled. Webbing rollers can be washed providing that the leather is not soaked; it is better to just soak the dirty part of the roller. Leather rollers and leather fittings should be washed clean and treated with a suitable leather dressing. Clothing can be stored in trunks or on shelves in a dry room protected by moth balls. They should be regularly checked for mice which may nest in the rugs or chew them.

Bandages

Bandages are placed around the horse's lower leg to give protection, warmth and support during exercise, travelling or after injury. They must be properly applied as they can cause serious damage if incorrectly put on.

Putting bandages on

Regardless of the type of bandage to be applied there are a few golden rules which will help make the job easier and more efficient:

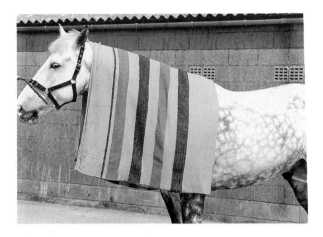

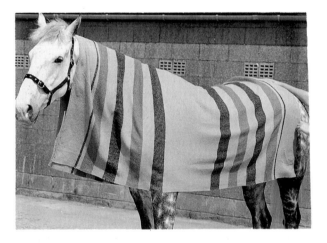

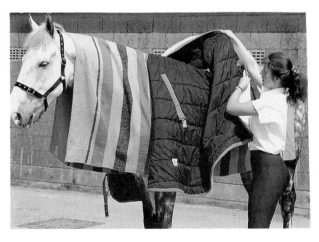

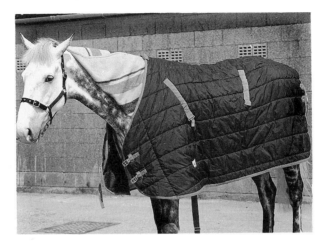

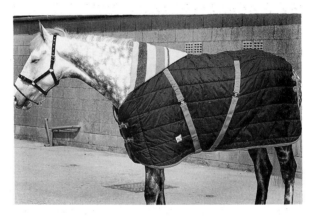

Figs 15.8–15.12 (*this page and opposite*) Putting on a rug and under-blanket.

- The bandage must have been correctly and firmly rolled up. The tapes must be flat and the bandage rolled towards where the tapes or Velcro are fastened.
- The bandage must not be too tight; there should be room to insert a finger in the top and bottom of a support or exercise bandage.
- The tension throughout the bandage should be even with no wrinkles and the tapes tied no tighter than the bandage itself.
- The bandage is ideally applied from front to back to avoid pulling too much on the tendons at the back of the leg.
- The padding underneath the bandage must always run in the same direction as the bandage and the edge of the padding must not lie

on the tendons or this will cause a pressure point and possible
damage.

- The tapes must be tied on the outside of the leg, not on the bone at
the front or on the tendons at the back.
- The tapes should be tied neatly in a knot or bow and the ends
tucked in to the tape and secured by sewing, insulating tape or
pulling one of the folds of the bandage over the tape. It is very
important that if insulating tape is used it is not pulled tighter than
the rest of the bandage.

Taking bandages off

Untie the tapes and unwind the bandage, moving quickly, passing the
unwound bandage from one hand to the other. Once the bandage is
off, feel the leg carefully to check all is well. The bandage should then
be shaken out, brushed or washed as necessary. Reroll the bandage
and store them in twos or fours.

Padding under bandages

Nearly all bandages are applied with some form of padding underneath. The exceptions are Sandown and some thermal bandages which
will be discussed later.

- *Gamgee* is cotton wool in gauze cover. Fresh from the packet it is
clean and gives good protection, especially wrapped round twice.
However, it is easily soiled and expensive. Its life can be prolonged
by blanket stitching the edges so that it can be washed and reused.
Gamgee is very popular for use over the top of wounds which
require bandaging and is frequently an important item of the first-
aid kit.
- *Fibagee* is felt-covered foam. It is easy to wash and durable,
making it popular for use under exercise and travelling bandages.
- *Leg wraps* are commonly used in the United States. They are thick
padded squares which are durable and give good protection, but
they are not suitable for use under exercise bandages.
- *Hay or straw* can be used for thatching legs to dry horses and keep
them warm.
- *Shaped tendon-protector shells* in a firm synthetic material may be
used under exercise bandages.

Fastening bandages

Bandages can be fastened by tapes sewn to the bandage. The tapes should be wide and flat; smoothing them while they are wet will save having to iron them later. A more modern alternative commonly found on stable bandages is Velcro. This must be kept clear of hay and straw or it will not fasten effectively. The two pieces of Velcro must also be long enough to allow sufficient overlap to fasten securely.

Types of bandages

Stable bandages

Stable bandages have several uses and it is important to be able to put them on quickly and correctly. They are used for:

- warmth
- drying off wet legs
- protection, for example, travelling bandages
- support for a sound leg
- keeping a dressing in place

They may be made of wool or synthetic material and are 10–12 cm (4–5 in) wide and 2–2.5 m (7–8 ft) long. Except for special thermal or Sandown bandages they are always fitted with padding underneath.

If the bandage is being used for keeping a poultice in place or for supporting an injured leg elastic bandages may be used with double gamgee. If the bandage is being used to protect the legs during travelling ensure that the gamgee extends well over the knee and coronet.

The procedure for fitting a stable bandage (Figs 15.13–15.17) is as follows:

- Place the padding round the leg. It should extend about 2 cm ($^3/_4$ in) over the knee and below the coronet.
- If the bandage is long enough start just below the knee or hock.
- If the bandage is short start just above the fetlock so that you are bandaging upwards towards the heart.
- Initially leave a vertical flap of bandage 10 cm (4 in) long. Then the first few horizontal turns secure the bandage.
- Each turn of the bandage should overlap half the width of the bandage.
- Complete the bandage.
- Tie the tapes in a neat bow and tuck the ends in.

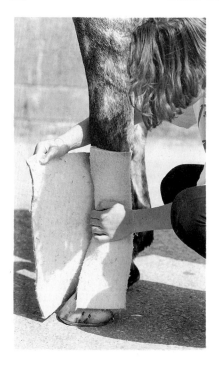

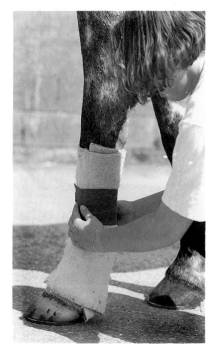

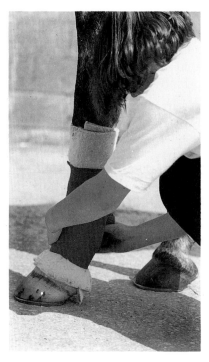

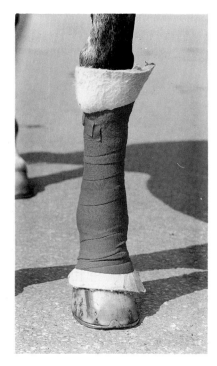

Figs 15.13–15.17 (this page and opposite) Putting on a stable bandage. This bandage is wrinkled and the turns are uneven; it should be reapplied.

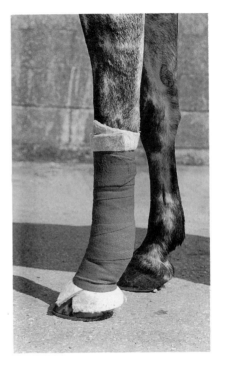

- If the bandage is for support, for example, for a tendon injury, use stretch bandage.

Exercise bandages

Exercise bandages may be fitted on the horse that is working to protect the leg in much the same way as a boot and to support the tendon. It is debatable how much help bandages are in actually preventing tendon strain, but they may help the leg cope with twists and turns.

Exercise bandages have considerable stretch and can be made of elastic, crepe or self-adhesive material. They should be 8–10 cm (3–4 in) wide and about 2 m (6–7 ft) long. It is essential that adequate padding is used under the bandage, for example, gamgee or a tendon-protector shell.

The principles of fitting an exercise bandage (Fig. 15.18) are the same as for fitting any other bandage except:

- They are applied more firmly.
- A longer flap is left initially, for security.

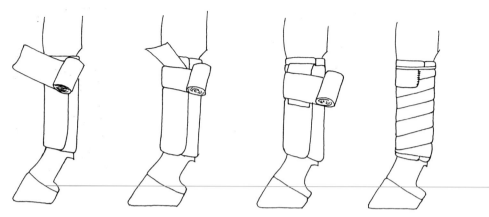

Fig. 15.18 Putting on an exercise bandage.

- They extend from below the knee to the fetlock joint (ergot).
- For competition purposes they are sewn or taped.
- They should not be left on for long periods.
- Overlap two-thirds of the bandage.
- Do not remove from a tired horse until he has stopped blowing.

Tail bandages

Tail bandages are made of stretch elastic or crepe material and are a little narrower and shorter than exercise bandages. They can be used on a pulled tail to improve the horse's appearance in which case the tail hairs are damped with a water brush before the bandage is put on. The bandage should not be left on any longer than four hours; otherwise the pressure may cause the tail hairs to turn white or fall out. The bandage should be applied firmly but not too tightly.

Tail bandages can also be used to protect the tail during short journeys. However, if the horse is travelling for more than four hours a tail guard should be used instead. Bandages can also be used to keep the tail hairs safely tucked away during clipping or when mares are being covered.

To put on a tail bandage (Fig. 15.19):

- If the tail is not plaited, damp it at the top.
- Stand behind the horse and hold up the tail or put the dock over your shoulder.
- Put the bandage under the tail leaving a 10 cm (4 in) flap.
- Secure the end of the bandage and then make one or two turns as high as possible.

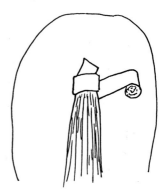
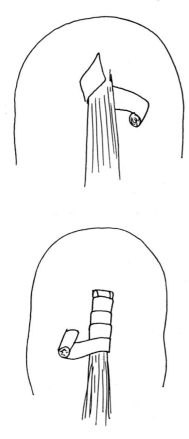
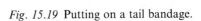

Fig. 15.19 Putting on a tail bandage.

- Bandage down the tail, overlapping about half the bandage at each turn.
- The bandage should reach the end of the dock.
- Wrap the tapes around the tail and tie to the side so that the horse cannot lean on the knot during travelling.

To remove a tail bandage undo the tapes and pull the bandage off with both hands. However, if the tail is plaited the bandage must be carefully unwound.

Boots

Boots are used to protect the horse's lower limbs from injury. Usually the injury is self-inflicted; the horse knocks or treads on himself with another foot. This knock may be due to the horse's conformation, action or shoeing, but could also be caused by fatigue, weakness, immaturity, thoughtless riding, stumbling on landing after a fence ('pecking'), deep going or a change in the ground under foot.

Types of boot

Brushing boots

Brushing boots are designed to protect the inside of the leg below the knee or hock, primarily the fetlock region which can be hit by the other foot at slower paces. The boots should be fitted slightly high to allow for them slipping while the horse is working and should be fastened from the top to the bottom, easing them gently into position. Synthetic boots with Velcro fastenings are very popular as inexpensive exercise boots (Fig. 15.20), while leather boots with buckle fastenings are more suitable for fast work (Fig. 15.21). The boot may be shaped to protect the underside of the fetlock.

Speedicut boots

Speedicut boots protect against high brushing wounds, just below the knee or hock, which can be sustained when the horse is galloping or being driven.

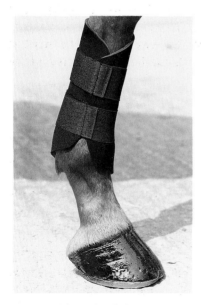

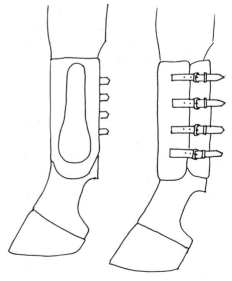

Fig. 15.20 Exercise boot with Velcro fastenings.

Fig. 15.21 Exercise boots with leather straps.

Over-reach boots

Horses are said to over-reach when a front foot stays on the ground too long and is struck by the inside edge of the hind shoe. This can occur when the horse is jumping and there is an extra effort on take-off or the horse lands in deep going and cannot get its front feet out of the way in time. A low over-reach results in a cut or bruise on the heel while a high over-reach or 'strike' may damage the tendons at the back of the leg.

Low over-reaches may be avoided by using over-reach boots; bell boots are synthetic boots which pull over the hoof or fasten round the pastern to protect the heel and coronet (Fig. 15.22). The boot must not be too long or the horse may tread on it and this type easily turns up in heavy going. A similar boot consisting of petals does not turn up and individual petals can be replaced if they get torn. A tough leather or fabric coronet boot is often used in polo to give added protection to the coronet. Over-reach boots can also be used to protect the horse from tread wounds caused by other horses during travelling or hunting. High over-reaches may be avoided by using brushing boots.

Yorkshire boots

Yorkshire boots are usually used to protect the hind fetlock from low brushing wounds, but their use has been largely replaced by the use of synthetic fetlock boots. They consist of a rectangle of thick material with a tape or Velcro two-thirds of the way down. The boot is wrapped round the leg, tied, eased over the fetlock and the top of the boot turned down (Fig. 15.23).

Rubber rings

A rubber ring with leather or a chain running through it can be fitted either above or below the fetlock (Fig. 15.24). Round the pastern it acts to stop the horse knocking the coronet while above the pastern it prevents brushing wounds. The ring is fastened by a buckle on the strap or chain running through the ring.

Sausage boots

A sausage boot is a large leather-covered padded ring which is fitted round the horse's front pastern to stop the horse bruising or capping his elbow while lying down with his feet tucked under his elbow (Fig. 15.25).

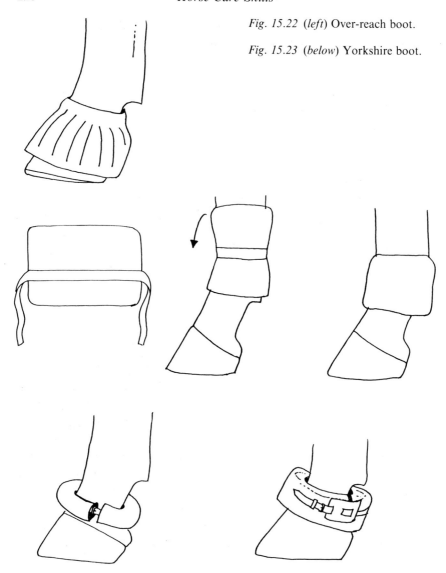

Fig. 15.22 (left) Over-reach boot.

Fig. 15.23 (below) Yorkshire boot.

Fig. 15.24 Rubber ring. *Fig. 15.25* Sausage boot.

Tendon boots

Tendon boots are similar in design to brushing boots, but they have added padding down the back of the leg to protect the tendons from injury should the horse strike into himself; they are used for fast work or jumping. Open-fronted tendon boots are often used for show jumping; the boot is left open at the front so that the horse is not encouraged to hit fences (Fig. 15.26).

Polo boots

Polo boots are similar to brushing boots, but they are made of heavy felt and extend down over the fetlock and may strap around the pastern (Fig. 15.27). They are designed to protect the fetlock and pastern from bruising by stick or ball.

Travelling boots

Travelling boots are an alternative to travelling bandages and are long padded boots designed to protect the horse from knee/hock to coronet. They are frequently shaped to fit over the joints of the leg (Fig. 15.28). They usually have Velcro fastening and care should be taken when they are first fitted to a horse as the restricted feeling may alarm the horse as he is asked to walk.

Knee boots

Knee boots are designed to protect the horse's knees when exercising on the roads or during travelling when they are used in conjunction with travelling bandages. They may be made of leather, heavy cloth or synthetic material and fasten well above the knee with the buckle on the outside. The top strap usually has a strong elastic insert to allow the boot to be fastened tightly enough to prevent it slipping without damaging the leg (Fig. 15.29). Once the top strap is done up the boot should be eased down to the top of the knee to check that it will not slip over the joint and then the lower strap should be fastened very loosely to allow the knee to flex without interference. This buckle fastens from back to front, which goes against the normal 'rules'.

Skeleton kneecaps or pads are sometimes used for road work and a horse may jump in kneepads which do not have a bottom strap.

Hock boots

Hock boots protect the point of the hock during travelling. There is a top strap with an elastic insert which holds the boot in place and a bottom strap which is fastened more loosely (Fig. 15.30).

Overboots

The overboot is a plastic galosh-type boot designed to fit over the horse's hoof (Fig. 15.31). It can be used on the unshod horse to protect the foot from wear or it can be used as an alternative to a poultice boot

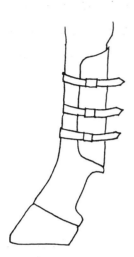

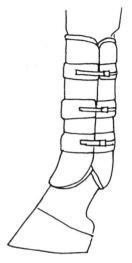

Fig. 15.26 Open-fronted tendon boot.   *Fig. 15.27* Polo boot.

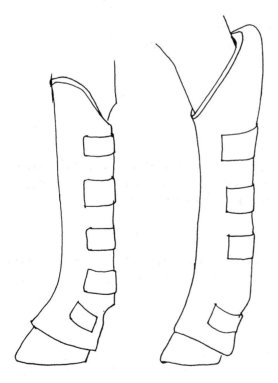

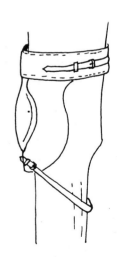

Fig. 15.28 Travelling boots.   *Fig. 15.29* Knee boot.

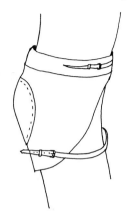

Fig. 15.30 (left) Hock boot.

Fig. 15.31 (bottom left) Overboot.

Fig. 15.32 (bottom right) Poultice boot.

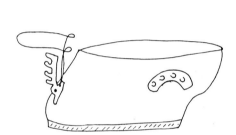

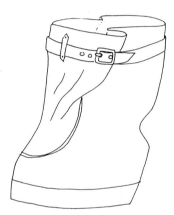

to keep a foot dressing in place. It is also useful for exercising horses during recovery from pus in the foot where the horse may have a tender place on the sole which the boot protects.

Poultice boots
A poultice boot is designed and shaped to accommodate the horse's hoof and lower leg and it is used for keeping foot poultices in place (Fig. 15.32).

Fetlock boots
This boot protects the inside of the fetlock and is sometimes used on the hind legs when show jumping to protect the horse from injury while discouraging him from hitting the fence (Figs 15.33 and 15.34).

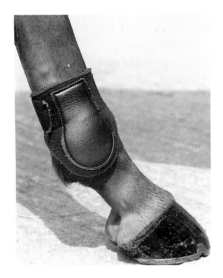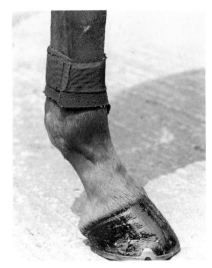

Figs 15.33 and 15.34 Fetlock boot.

Jacuzzi boots

This big rubber boot resembles an equine Wellington boot. When on, it has a hose attached and water circulates inside the boot to cool the horse's lower leg. It is used after strenuous exercise.

16 Preparing Horses for Use

Grooming

Another 'housework ' aspect of horse care is daily attention to the horse's feet and coat. There are several factors that make grooming so important:

- It promotes health by stimulating the blood supply to the horse's skin.
- It improves the horse's appearance, keeping him clean and tidy.
- It helps prevent disease by ensuring thorough daily inspection of the horse's whole body.
- It allows the handler to become familiar with the horse. It is often subtle changes in behaviour that indicate the early signs of illness; the groom should notice these changes first.
- It is a strong contact part of the horse/human relationship.

The grooming kit
The grooming kit consists of several items each of which have a specific use (Fig. 16.1).

The grooming kit must be kept clean and if it is being used on several horses it is likely that the brushes will need a weekly wash in warm soapy water. They should be thoroughly rinsed and left to dry before being returned to the grooming box.

Dandy brush
This brush has coarse, stiff bristles and is used for removing mud and dried sweat from the body and limbs. It should not be used on any horse's head and only with discretion on the body of a thin-skinned horse or clipped horse. The hairs of the tail should not be brushed out with a dandy brush or the tail will become thin. It is very useful for grass-kept horses and is the brush used for the first stage of grooming.

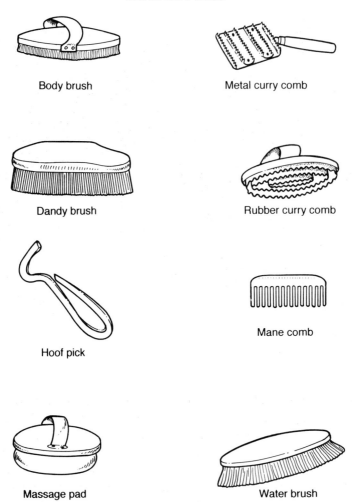

Body brush

Metal curry comb

Dandy brush

Rubber curry comb

Hoof pick

Mane comb

Massage pad

Water brush

Fig. 16.1 Items of the grooming kit.

Body brush

The bristles of the body brush are shorter and softer than the dandy brush. It is used to remove grease and dirt from the coat (Fig. 16.2). The brush is held in the left hand when grooming the near side of the horse and changed into the right hand for the off side. It is used with a circular action to get deep into the coat and loosen the grease, followed by a long stroke to remove the dirt. The body brush is used to clean the horse's head.

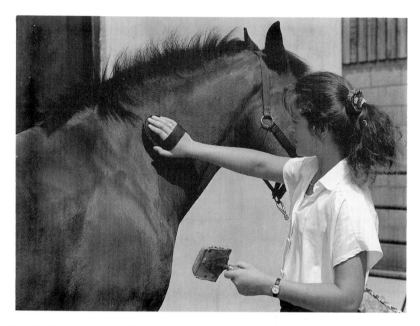

Fig. 16.2 Using the body brush.

Curry comb

The curry comb is held in the other hand and used to clean the body brush; the body brush is swept over the curry comb every four or five strokes. The accumulated dirt is tapped out of the curry comb at regular intervals. The metal curry comb with rows of teeth is only ever used to clean the body brush; using it on the horse's body would cause considerable discomfort. However, the rubber or plastic curry comb can be very useful for removing dirt and hair when the horse is shedding his coat.

Water brush

The water brush has fairly long soft bristles and is used to dampen or 'lay' the mane and tail before plaiting or to encourage the mane to lie flat or before applying a tail bandage. It can also be used to scrub the legs or feet clean.

Sponge

Several sponges will be needed: one for the eyes, nose and lips, one for the dock and sheath (these should be marked so that they are not mixed up), and a large sponge for washing the horse down or removing stable stains. These sponges should be kept for use on the horse and not find their way into the tack cleaning kit!

Wisp

A thorough grooming may include the horse being strapped or wisped. This consists of stimulating the blood flow to the muscles and thus increasing muscle tone, by gently banging the muscles of the neck, shoulders and quarters (Fig. 16.3). It is similar to patting the horse, but a steady rhythm is established using more weight behind the 'bang', and as the horse anticipates the next blow he tenses his muscles. The wisp may be a stuffed leather pad or a traditional wisp made from a length of twisted hay or straw. If the horse is not accustomed to the process, it should be introduced very gently.

Mane comb

A metal or plastic comb is used to comb out the mane, for pulling the mane and tail and for preparing the mane and tail for plaiting.

Stable rubber

This is a linen cloth similar to the type of tea-towel used for drying glasses. It is used slightly damp to wipe over the horse at the end of

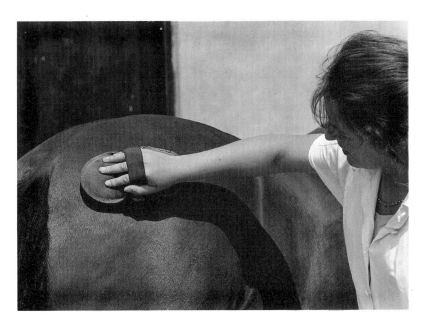

Fig. 16.3 'Strapping' or 'wisping' a horse.

grooming to remove any dust. It can also be used when strapping the horse to wipe the coat flat in between 'bangs' or used instead of the wisp as a folded pad.

Hoof pick

The hoof pick is perhaps the most important item of the grooming kit and yet the one most likely to disappear! It is used to remove mud and stones from the foot and may have a brush on one end to thoroughly clean the underside of the hoof. It should be used from heel to toe, following the contours of the frog (Fig. 16.4).

Sweat scraper

The sweat scraper is used to remove excess sweat or water from the horse's coat after exercise or washing the horse (Fig. 16.5).

The grooming routine

Horses are usually groomed twice a day: a quick brush over in the morning to make them respectable enough to go out on exercise and then a thorough groom in the afternoon or after exercise.

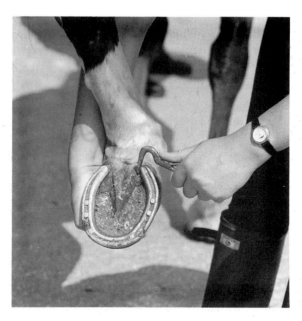

Fig. 16.4 Picking out the foot.

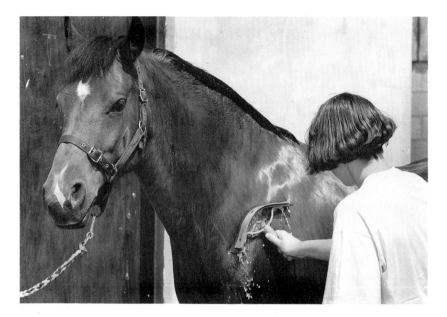

Fig. 16.5 Using a sweat scraper.

Quartering

Quartering is the grooming given first thing in the morning as part of the early morning routine. After the horse has finished his feed and has been given a haynet the horse is tied up and the feet are picked out. The rugs are turned back and any stable stains brushed or sponged off and dried, paying particular attention to the knees, hocks, under the stomach and other areas that may have got dirty when the horse lay down. The rugs are replaced so that the horse does not get cold and the eyes, nose and dock are sponged. Finally the horse's mane is brushed and any bedding removed from the tail. This quick groom makes the horse comfortable and tidy enough to go out on exercise.

Full grooming of the stabled horse

The thorough grooming of a horse is best done after exercise when the horse is warm and the pores of the skin are open. In some competition and hunting yards it is done as part of the afternoon yard routine if all the horses have been exercised in the morning. However, on competition or hunting days it may take the place of quartering in the morning. An efficient groom should be able to complete the task in about 30 minutes, allowing an extra 20 minutes if the horse also needs to be strapped. Obviously grooming will take longer if the horse is very dirty or if the worker is inexperienced.

The horse should first be tied up either in the stable or outside if the weather is suitable, making sure that the yard gate is closed and that the tying up place is safe. In warm weather the horse's rugs can be removed, but in winter a blanket should always be thrown over the part of the horse that is not being groomed.

The horse's feet should be picked out from heel to toe removing all debris and checking for thrush (a fungal infection of the frog) and that the shoes are not loose or worn. The feet can all be picked out from the near side if the horse is accustomed to this practice and the debris may be caught in a skip. If the feet are dirty they should be scrubbed clean over a bucket of water, using a water brush or old dandy brush. Once they are dry, a hoof dressing may be applied.

The next step is to remove any dried mud or sweat from the horse using a rubber curry comb or a cactus cloth for sensitive horses. If the mud or sweat is still damp or if the horse is very sensitive it may be better to sponge the areas clean with warm water and then towel dry the horse.

A thorough grooming includes using the body brush to remove dirt and grease from the horse's skin and coat. Starting on the near side behind the ears, the body brush should be held in the left hand and the curry comb in the right hand. The full strength of the arm should be used to penetrate the coat, working in the direction of hair growth with straight and circular movements. Periodically the body brush should be cleaned on the curry comb and when necessary the curry comb tapped on the floor near the door to get rid of the accumulated dirt. This dirt must be swept up later. When moving round to the off side the brushes should be changed to the other hand and the procedure repeated.

It is a good idea to put the curry comb sharp side down in a safe place when brushing the legs. This allows you to crouch (never kneel or sit) beside the horse's leg and hold the leg steady with the free hand. Holding the tail when brushing a hind leg will help deter the horse from lifting a leg. Remember to stand close to the horse and be firm and positive in your movements.

Once the body and legs have been brushed, the body brush should be used to brush the mane, firmly brushing a few hairs at a time to get right down to the crest. If the mane is tangled a mane comb or plastic curry comb can be used, taking care not to pull out or break the hairs. The mane can be 'laid' by brushing the hairs into place with a damp water brush.

The horse should be untied to brush the head in case he tries to pull back. First brush the front of the face and then undo the headcollar and replace it round the neck and gently brush the rest of the head while steadying the horse with the other hand. Take care to be thorough and not to knock any bony parts. Once completed, replace the headcollar and tie the horse up again.

If the horse needs to be strapped, wisp or bang him for about 20 minutes at this stage in the grooming routine as previously described.

If the weather is cold, once brushing or strapping has been completed the horse can be wiped over with a damp stable rubber and rugged up. The horse should then be untied and a clean sponge used to wipe the eyes, muzzle, mouth and nostrils. The horse can be tied up again and a second sponge used to clean under the dock. Many horses do not like this much so stand to one side, firmly raise the tail and gently but firmly clean the area, rinsing the sponge as necessary.

The tail can now be brushed or fingered through, depending on personal preference and the thickness of the horse's tail. A dandy brush, especially used on a dirty tail, will pull and break the hairs, rapidly thinning the tail. One hand should hold the end of the dock and a few hairs should be separated out at a time removing tangles and bedding. If the horse has a pulled tail the top of the tail can be damped and a tail bandage put on. If not already done the horse's feet should be oiled, the mane laid and the horse finally rugged up, untied and the headcollar removed. Remember to shake out the blankets and rugs before replacing them.

Safety is a prime consideration at all times when grooming. Take care that you do not put yourself in potentially hazardous positions and that jewellery and perfume are not worn; some perfumes make stallions lustful! If you are susceptible to dust a face mask may be worn when grooming to help prevent allergic reactions such as asthma.

Grooming the grass-kept horse

The horse kept at grass needs the grease in the skin and coat to waterproof and protect him from wet weather. This means that he should be cleaned of mud and sweat, but not thoroughly brushed in the same way as a stabled horse.

When brought in from the field the horse should be tied up and the feet picked out and washed, checking the state of the shoes and feet and looking for conditions such as cracked heels. If necessary the feet can be oiled when dry. The mud should be removed from the coat using a dandy brush or plastic curry comb on the body and paying particular attention to the saddle and girth areas which may rub if mud is left behind. The head should be carefully brushed with a body brush, first untying the horse. Sticky sweat marks should be sponged off as should wet muddy legs. The eyes, nose and dock should be sponged and the mane cleaned with a dandy brush or plastic curry comb. The tail can be brushed out with the body brush or fingered through if it is clean. If the tail is dirty it should be washed first.

Cleaning the sheath

Greasy dirt naturally accumulates inside the horse's sheath and some geldings need this area washed regularly to prevent a build up which results in a strong smell and possible risk of infection. The sheath can be washed using warm water and a mild soap with the hands protected by rubber gloves. An assistant may be needed to restrain the horse, either just holding him or picking up a front leg, as some horses may kick out until accustomed to the procedure.

Preparing a horse for competition

Washing the mane (Fig. 16.6)

As always it is important to be organised and the first thing is to gather all the equipment needed: warm water, horse shampoo, a large sponge, towel and sweat scraper. The horse should wear a headcollar, but should not be tied up in case he pulls back. The mane should be wetted with the sponge and a small amount of shampoo worked into the forelock. To prevent the shampoo going in the horse's eyes it may be useful to pull the forelock back between the ears. Gradually work down the mane using the fingers to thoroughly clean the crest. The mane should then be rinsed using the sponge until all the shampoo has been removed. Sweat scrape both sides of the neck and towel dry the ears before brushing out the mane and leaving to dry.

Washing the tail

Collect the washing equipment as before, put on a headcollar and tie the horse up. You may need an assistant for a young or nervous horse. The top of the tail should be soaked using the sponge and the end of the tail immersed in the bucket of water; if the end of the dock goes into the water the horse may drop his hindquarters suddenly. Shampoo should be worked into the tail and rinsed out as before. Excess water can be removed by gently swinging the end of the tail in a circle; stand to one side of the horse when doing this. The tail can then be

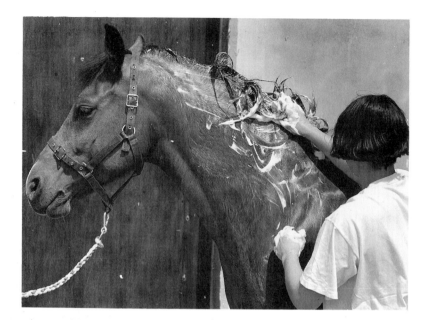

Fig. 16.6 Washing the mane.

brushed or fingered through. Spray preparations to prevent tangling can be applied at this stage.

Bathing the horse
Light-coloured or muddy horses may have to be bathed prior to a competition. To prevent the horse becoming chilled choose a fine day, work quickly and dry the horse off rapidly. If the weather is chilly use warm water; a hose can be used on warm days. Hosing should be introduced carefully as the horse may be alarmed; trickle a gentle stream of water on the horse's front foot, gradually working up the leg until the horse accepts the feel of the water. Wash and dry the head first with the horse untied. Then tie him up to be washed, shampooed and rinsed. Then scrape dry and towel off, paying particular attention to the lower legs and heels. The legs may be bandaged to help them dry and, depending on the weather, the horse lunged or walked, with or without rugs, to dry off and keep warm.

Washing the legs
Many people wash their horses legs on return from exercise or if they are muddy after being turned out in the field. Care must be taken as

constant washing removes protective grease from the skin resulting in cracked heels and mud fever. If the legs are to be washed use plenty of water and either let the legs 'drip-dry' in a deep clean bed or towel dry and apply stable bandages. The motto is – do it properly or not at all! Barrier cream on the heels and underside of the pastern can help keep the skin soft.

Care of the horse after fast exercise

The hot and sweaty horse needs prompt efficient attention to help his body systems recover effectively. Once the horse has pulled up and the rider has dismounted, the stirrups should be run up and the girths and noseband loosened. If the weather is cold a rug should be thrown over the horse. The horse should be walked until calm and he has stopped blowing. The tack, including boots and bandages, can then be removed and a headcollar put on to restrain the horse while sponging down. In cold weather stand the horse in a sheltered place and use warm water on only the sweaty and muddy areas. In warm weather stand the horse in the shade and use cold water or hose the horse down. Pay particular attention to the bridle and saddle areas.

Surplus water should be removed with a sweat scraper and in cold weather the horse can be towelled dry and an appropriate number of rugs and type of rug put on before the horse is walked dry. For example, the horse may wear a sweat sheet covered by a stable rug with the front folded back and secured by a roller. Alternatively, the horse can be 'thatched' – an inside-out stable rug is placed over straw and held with a roller. If the weather is hot the horse may only need a sweat sheet with a cotton sheet over the top.

Pick out the feet, wash them and remove studs if necessary before putting the horse in the stable. Check the horse after 30 minutes by feeling the ears to see if he is warm. If he is cold and the rugs are damp change them for dry ones to help him dry off and keep warm. If the horse is dry, brush him off and put on his normal rugs.

Improving the appearance of a horse

Not content with rearranging the horse's way of life, we also alter the way the horse looks, tidying the mane, tail, feathers and coat to suit

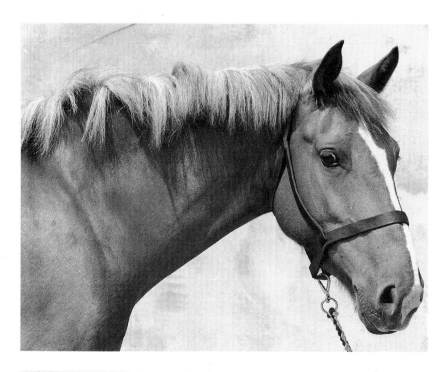

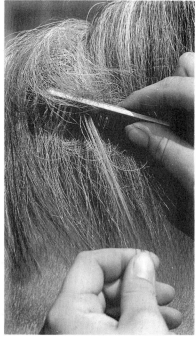
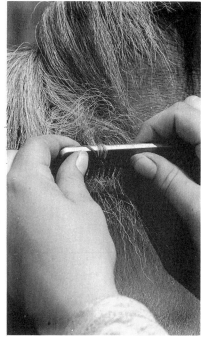

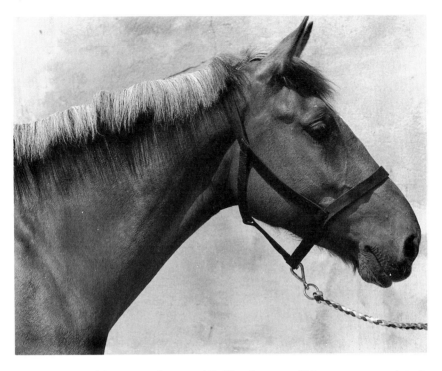

Figs 16.7–16.10 (*this page and opposite*) Pulling the mane. This mane now needs to be put into stable plaits to make it lie evenly.

fashion and the job the horse has to do. Thus, the competition horse and hunter has his mane and tail pulled, feathers and whiskers trimmed and his coat clipped.

Pulling the mane (Figs 16.7–16.10)
The horse's mane is pulled for several reasons:

- to improve appearance
- to thin and shorten the mane
- to make the mane easier to plait
- to encourage the mane to lie flat

However, Arabs and Mountain and Moorland ponies do not have their manes or tails pulled.

If possible pull the mane after exercise or on a warm day; the pores of the skin will be open making it less painful for the horse when the hairs are pulled out. Some horses object quite strongly to the process and a handler may be necessary to restrain them. Thoroughbred-type horses tend to have fine manes which are easy to pull while part-bred horses can have very thick manes which are tough to pull. Do not wash the mane first as the hairs become too slippery to hold onto and pull effectively. The mane should be pulled so that it lies on the right (off) side of the neck. If it is reluctant to do so, loose stable plaits left in for a day or two followed by regular brushing and damping down will help train the mane.

Method

(1) Comb the mane thoroughly to remove all tangles.
(2) Separate out a few hairs from the underneath of the mane and run the comb up to the roots and remove them with a sharp pull.
(3) Repeat this process until the mane is of the desired thickness and length. Any remaining long hairs from the top of the mane can be shortened by breaking off the ends with the fingers. The forelock is pulled last.
(4) Remove the underneath hairs to ensure that the mane lies flat and grows evenly.

Plaiting the mane (Figs 16.11–16.15)

The horse's mane is plaited to make the horse look smart for competitions, to show the horse off in the show ring or to prospective buyers or to make the mane lie tidily on the correct side.

Equipment

Before starting to plait, the necessary equipment should be collected together. This includes a mane comb, water brush, water and something to stand on. The mane can be secured with thread of a suitable colour, traditionally the preferred method, or with rubber bands. If using thread, a pair of scissors and several needles will also be required. The needle should be of the thick, blunt-ended type used for sewing with wool.

Before starting

It is advisable not to plait the horse in a bedded stable in case a needle is dropped and lost. If this happens, the bedding in the area should be removed, the floor swept and fresh bedding put down. Before starting, it is a good idea to thread several needles with enough thread to do two plaits to save having to rethread the same needle and to place them securely in a piece of thick fabric within easy reach. Plaiting aprons with large front pockets are useful.

Method

(1) Comb out the whole mane and dampen it down using the water brush.

(2) Starting at the poll, divide the mane into as many plaits as required. Tradition used to demand seven or nine plaits, but the modern trend is for many small plaits. A thin neck benefits from larger plaits placed high on the crest while a fat neck can be disguised by smaller tight plaits.

(3) Using the mane comb to keep the remaining mane out of the way, divide the section nearest the poll into three equal bunches and plait down to the end. Pull the hair tightly at the beginning of the plait or the finished plait will look loose and fluffy.

(4) Once the end of the mane is reached, secure by wrapping the thread around it. There are various ways of making the actual plait. One way is to turn the end of the plait under, rolling the plait up towards the neck. Each turn may have to be stitched to keep the plait tight and secure. The plait can then be finished by pushing the needle through the whole plait from underneath and snipping off the thread. This way no thread will be seen. Alternatively, once the ends of the mane are secured the plait can be folded under to bring the end up to the roots of the mane, sewn and then folded again. If the mane is the correct length this will result in a tight ball at the top of the neck. If extra security is needed the needle can be pushed up through the middle of the plait and the thread taken around the plait alternately to the left and right before cutting the thread as close to the plait as possible.

(5) Work down the mane until it is all plaited.

(6) The forelock is done last and can be plaited as the mane or in a similar way to a tail plait (see overleaf). If the horse is restless or head-shy, untie him and get a helper to keep him still.

Removing plaits

Take care when removing plaits; it is all too easy to cut the mane. Use small scissors or an unpicking tool working in the direction of the hair. In time you will be able to use very little thread and remove the plaits

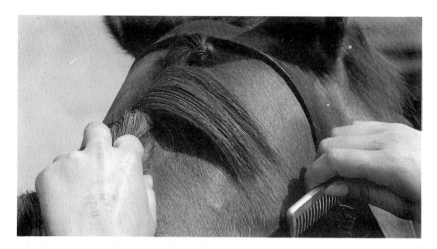

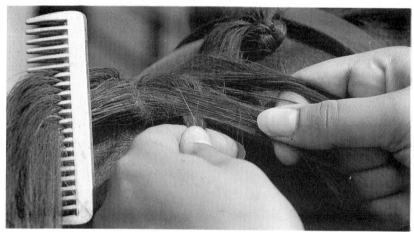

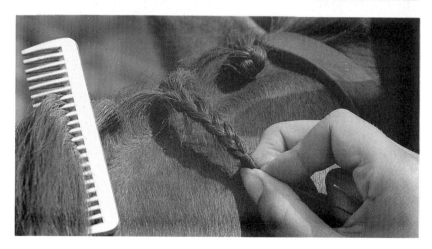

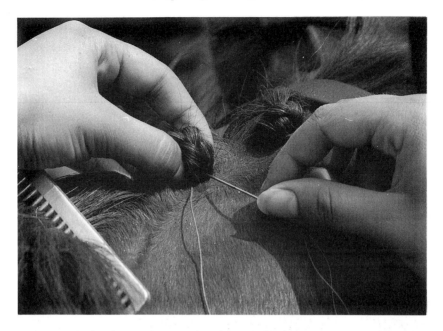

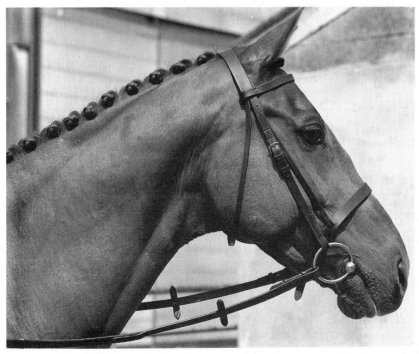

Figs 16.11–16.15 (*this page and opposite*) Plaiting the mane.

with two or three snips. Undo the plait with your fingers and damp down the mane to remove the curl.

Pulling the tail (Figs 16.16 and 16.17)
The horse's tail is pulled for several reasons:

- to improve appearance
- to show off the quarters
- to avoid having to plait the tail

If possible, pull the tail after exercise or on a warm day; the pores of the skin are then open making it less painful for the horse when the hairs are pulled out. Some horses object violently to the process and a handler may be necessary to restrain them. It is likely that the horse will bleed where each hair is pulled out and it may be better to spread the process out over several days.

Method

(1) Brush the tail thoroughly to remove all tangles and comb out the top.
(2) Separate out a few hairs from the side of the dock, run the comb up to the roots and remove them with a sharp pull.
(3) Repeat this process down each side of the dock until the tail is neat and tidy. Any long hair in the middle of the dock can be shortened or pulled to match the sides.
(4) Side hairs should lie flat and neatly against the dock.

Once the tail has been pulled it can be kept tidy by regular damping and bandaging. As the hairs grow they can be removed on a regular basis – tweaking out a few every day keeps the tail smart without making the horse resentful.

Plaiting the tail (Figs 16.18–16.22)
A full tail may be plaited for competition or hunting. The equipment needed is the same as for mane plaiting.

Method

(1) Wash and brush out the tail.
(2) Separate out a few hairs from either side of the dock and some from the middle of the dock to make the third strand of the plait.

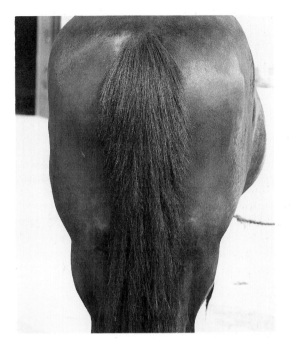

Fig. 16.16 Unpulled tail.

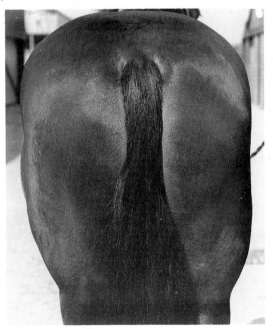

Fig. 16.17 The same tail pulled.

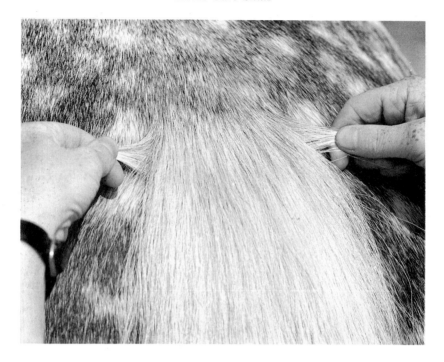

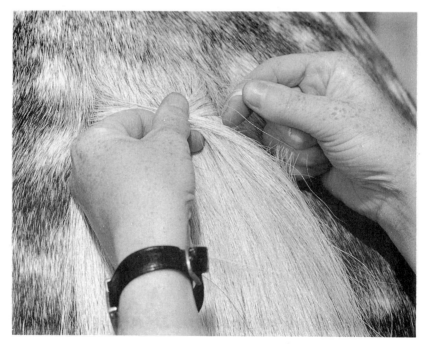

Figs 16.18–16.22 (*this page and opposite*) Plaiting the tail.

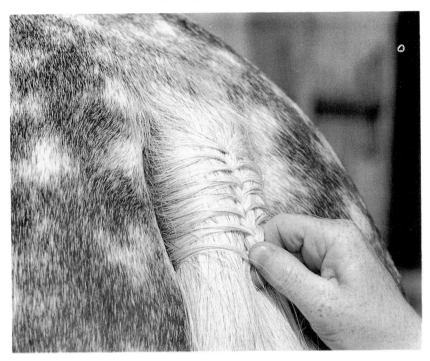

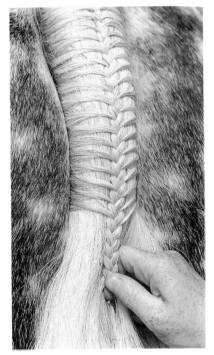

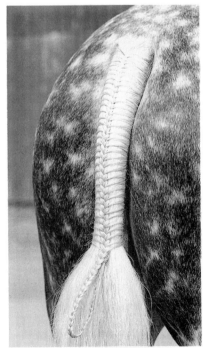

(3) Plait down the tail incorporating a few hairs from the side of the tail each time. Make sure that the hairs are pulled as tight as possible.

(4) Continue the plait two-thirds of the way down the dock and then continue plaiting without taking any more hair.

(5) When the end of the hair is reached, sew it, loop it up underneath and stitch it firmly into place.

A bandage can be put on top of the plait to keep it tidy or for travelling. However, the bandage must not be pulled off but carefully unrolled.

Putting up a tail

Tails may be put up for cross-country, hunting and polo to keep them out of the way. Plait the tail all the way down to the end and secure with a band or thread. Then turn up the plait to just below the dock, double it over and tape or stitch it into place.

Quarter marks

These are patterns of hair, set at angles to the normal lie of the coat. For example, the hair on the quarters can be brushed horizontally towards the tail to make the quarters look longer, while the hair on the barrel can be brushed vertically downwards to make the back look shorter and the girth deeper.A short comb, a pattern sheet or a brush can be used to create the patterns.

Clipping

Horses are clipped to remove excess coat; this usually means the thick winter coat that grows in October and lasts until about March.

Reasons for clipping

- To avoid heavy sweating and loss of condition.
- So that the horse can work longer and faster without distress.
- To make the horse easier to clean.
- To dry the horse off quicker thus avoiding chills.
- To improve appearance.

When to clip

The first clip is usually after the horse's winter coat has established in early October. After this the horse may need reclipping as often as every three weeks until Christmas. Horses are not usually clipped after the end of January, once the summer coat has started to grow, as this may spoil the growth of the summer coat. However, performance horses may be clipped in summer to prevent overheating.

Types of clip

Full clip

With a full clip the whole coat is removed. A full clip is used for horses that grow a thick coat or for performance horses, for example show jumpers, in the summer. A triangle is left at the top of the tail to avoid clipping the tail hairs.

Hunter clip (Fig. 16.23)

With a hunter clip all the hair except that on the legs and saddle patch is removed; the hair on the legs gives protection from thorns, mud fever and cracked heels, while the saddle patch is left on to avoid saddle pressure. A hunter clip is used for horses in hard work that are going to sweat heavily.

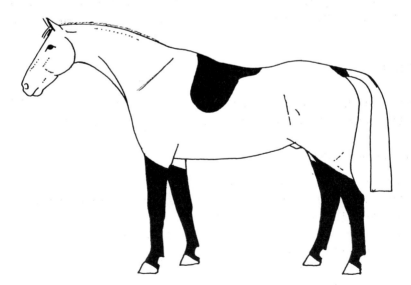

Fig. 16.23 Hunter clip.

Blanket clip (Fig. 16.24)

With a blanket clip hair is removed from the neck and belly leaving a 'blanket' over the back and quarters. A blanket clip is used for horses that feel the cold or are likely to be standing about, for example riding-school horses. It is also used as a first clip for eventers being got fit during the winter months and is useful for young horses that are unlikely to be working too hard.

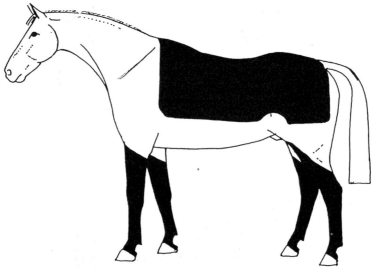

Fig. 16.24 Blanket clip.

Trace clip (Fig. 16.25)

With the trace clip hair is removed from the bottom of the neck, top of the legs and the belly. The head is often left unclipped. A trace clip is useful for horses that are turned out during the day in New Zealand rugs and need some protection from the cold.

Chaser clip (Fig. 16.26)

A chaser clip is a very high trace clip including the head, so called as it is sometimes used for National Hunt horses as it looks smart but still keeps the back warm.

Dealer clip (Fig. 16.27)

With a dealer clip the hair is removed below a line from the stifle, along the bottom of the saddle flap, up the neck and down the side of the face. A dealer clip is a quick clip which makes a horse look

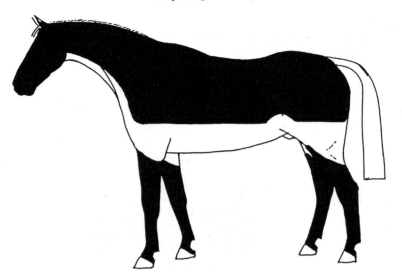

Fig. 16.25 Trace clip.

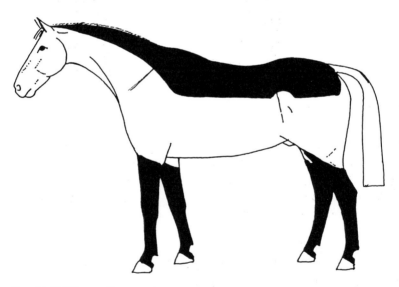

Fig. 16.26 Chaser clip.

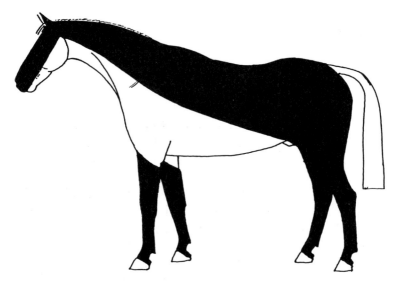

Fig. 16.27 Dealer clip.

presentable, allows it to work and yet still leaves plenty of coat for
protection.

Before clipping

Make sure that the clippers have been serviced, are in good working
order and have sharp blades. Resharpen blades as soon as they
become blunt and keep them in pairs in oiled cloth to prevent rusting.
Start with a clean horse – a muddy or greasy coat will soon blunt the
blades. Having decided which clip to give the horse, it is a good idea to
measure lines with string and mark them with chalk. This will ensure
that the lines of the blanket and trace clip are even on both sides of the
horse. Finally, bandage the tail and put stable plaits in the mane to
keep them out of the way.

Clipping equipment

- Clippers and spare blades
- Oil
- Soft brush
- Paraffin
- Extension lead
- Circuit breaker
- Soft rag

- Rugs and grooming kit
- Assistant
- Twitch
- Dog clippers for head

The clipping procedure

(1) The handler should wear suitable clothing and the horse should be clipped in a well-lit box. A box with a non-slip rubber floor is ideal although some horses are less frightened if clipped in their own stable.

(2) Assemble the clippers with correct blade tension, oil the clippers and blades and wipe off excess oil. If the horse has not been clipped before allow him to become accustomed to the smell and sound of the clippers before starting to clip.

(3) Start clipping in a safe place on the horse, for example the shoulder. This area is flat and not too sensitive. Move the clippers against the direction of hair growth.

(4) Use long sweeps with firm pressure, moving the skin as necessary in awkward places such as the elbows. An assistant is useful to hold up a front foot so that the skin around the elbow and chest is stretched – this will help avoid nicking the horse.

(5) During clipping keep the air filters clean and oil the blades regularly, checking that they are not hot.

(6) As you remove the hair, keep the horse warm by throwing a rug or blanket over him.

After clipping

Once the clip is completed brush the horse off and wipe over with a damp stable rubber to remove any short hairs left behind. Then rug the horse appropriately. Dismantle, clean and oil the blades and clippers and store them safely. Wipe clean the cables and leads before putting them away. Collect up the clipped hair in a skip and dispose of it.

17 Saddlery

Horses are fitted with saddles, bridles and martingales to enable the rider to sit on the horse securely and to have control. It is important to know about fitting a saddle and bridle and to be able to put them on the horse safely, quickly and efficiently.

Bridles and bits

Bridles can be classified into five families:

- the snaffle
- the double bridle
- the pelham
- the gag
- the bitless bridle

Under different competition rules, some bits or bridling arrangements may not be allowed, particularly in dressage and Pony Club show jumping.

The leather of the bridle should be of a suitable size and weight for the horse; for example, for showing and dressage light-weight leather may be used while for hunting and eventing heavier leather would be advisable.

Parts of the bridle
The parts of the bridle are basically the same for all types of bridle (Fig. 17.1) and consist of:

- *Headpiece and throatlash.* The throatlash should be fitted to allow a hand's-width between it and the horse's jaw; if too tight it will be uncomfortable when the horse flexes at the poll.

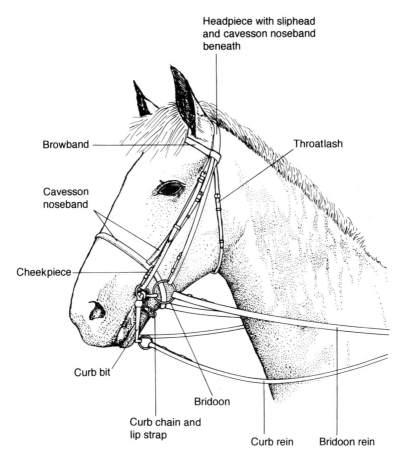

Headpiece with sliphead
and cavesson noseband
beneath

Browband

Throatlash

Cavesson
noseband

Cheekpiece

Curb bit

Bridoon

Curb chain and
lip strap

Curb rein   Bridoon rein

Fig. 17.1 Parts of the bridle.

- *Browband.* This prevents the headpiece slipping back.
- *Cheekpieces.* These attach to the headpiece and hold the bit in place.
- *Noseband.* A simple snaffle bridle has a cavesson noseband which is fitted so that it lies about 2.5 cm (1 in) below the projecting facial crest running down the side of the horse's head. It may be fastened so that two fingers can be inserted between the noseband and the horse's nose or it may be tightened to prevent the horse opening the mouth.
- *Reins.* These attach to the bit and allow the rider to control the horse. Reins may be plain leather, rubber-covered, laced, plaited or made of web with finger slots of leather placed at intervals

(Continental reins). Reins measure from 1.3 m (4 ft 3 in) long for
ponies to 1.5 m (5 ft) long for horses and the width varies
according to use.
- *Bit*. (This is discussed in more detail below.)
- *Bridoon sliphead*. In the case of a double bridle the bridoon bit has
  its own support; its off-side cheekpiece attaches to a strap which
  passes through the browband and becomes the cheekpiece on the
  near side.
- *Bridoon rein*. This rein attaches to the bridoon bit and is thicker
  and sometimes slightly shorter than the curb rein.
- *Curb rein*.
- *Curb chain*. The curb chain attaches to the curb bit and may be
  made of metal, leather or elastic.
- *Lip strap*. The lip strap is a narrow leather strap used to keep the
  curb chain in place. It prevents the curb chain from being lost.

The action of bits
Bits act on one or more of seven parts of the horse's head (Fig. 17.2):

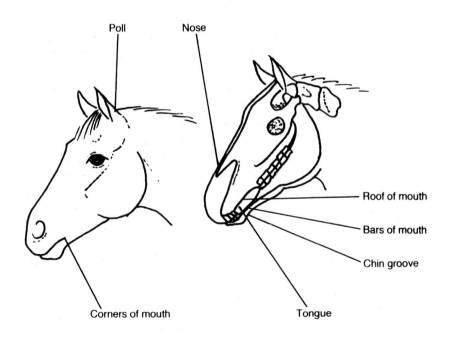

Fig. 17.2 Points of action of a bridle.

- corners of the mouth
- bars of the mouth
- tongue
- poll
- chin groove
- nose
- roof of the mouth

The action of the bit is affected by:

- the shape of the bit
- the shape of the horse's mouth
- how the horse carries his head and how the rider carries their hands
- martingales, nosebands and other devices

The snaffle

The snaffle is the most straightforward bit with either a jointed or straight mouthpiece. It acts on the corners of the mouth with an upwards action thus raising the horse's head. The jointed mouthpiece has a more direct squeezing action while the mullen or half-moon mouthpiece has more action on the tongue. However, as the horse learns to accept the bit and flexes at the poll the snaffle acts increasingly on the lower jaw; a drop noseband can accentuate this action.

There are many types of snaffle varying in action and severity (Figs 17.3–17.5). A loose-ring snaffle encourages the horse to mouth the bit and salivate, resulting in a softer contact. A fixed-ring or eggbutt snaffle has a more direct action, but may encourage the horse to lean on the bit and constant pressure will reduce the blood supply to the horse's mouth resulting in poor contact. A horse that is reluctant to take the bit or one that moves the bit too much may go well in a Fulmer snaffle which has cheeks secured to the cheekpieces by short straps called cheek retainers. The French link has a curved spatula in the centre which allows more room for the tongue. Jointed rubber and nylon bits (Fig. 17.4) are useful for young horses which may resent a metal mouthpiece, while mullen mouth snaffles are mild, allowing room for the tongue for horses that cannot cope with a jointed bit.

Generally speaking, a bit with a thick mouthpiece, such as the German snaffle, is mild as it spreads the pressure over a larger area while thin mouthpieces are more severe. Snaffles can also be made more severe by twisting the mouthpiece, as in a twisted snaffle, by

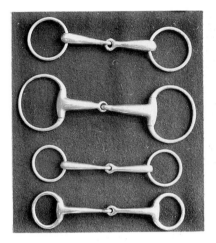

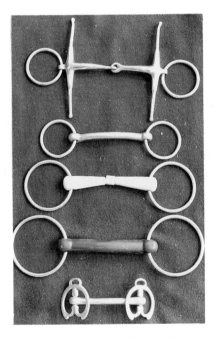

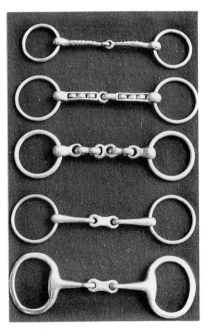

Fig. 17.3 A selection of snaffle bits. From top: jointed German loose ring; jointed German eggbutt; loose ring bridoon; eggbutt bridoon.

Fig. 17.4 A selection of snaffle bits. From top: Fulmer (or Australian) loose ring; mullen mouth (metal): jointed nathe; rubber mullen mouth; horseshoe cheek mullen mouth stallion show bit.

Fig. 17.5 A selection of snaffle bits. From top: wire ring twisted bridoon; Magenis; Waterford; loose ring French link; eggbutt French link.

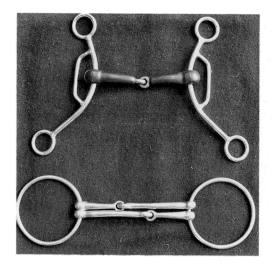

Fig. 17.6 (top): American gag; *(bottom)*: W-mouth snaffle.

having rollers on the mouthpiece, as in the Cherry roller or the Magenis, or by having extra joints, as in the Waterford or the W-mouth (Fig. 17.6).

Snaffle bits are measured between the rings when laid flat. In the horse's mouth they should fit snugly with about 0.5 cm ($^1/_4$ in) projecting either side of the mouth. If the bit is too narrow it will pinch the horse's lips; if too wide it will slide across the horse's mouth and the joint lying low on the tongue will encourage the horse to try and put his tongue over the bit. An approximate guide to the size of jointed snaffle needed for different horses is:

14.4–15 cm (5$^3/_4$–6 in)   hunter
13.1–13.75 cm (5$^1/_4$–5$^1/_2$ in)   14.2–15 hh and thoroughbreds
11.9–12.5 cm (4$^3/_4$–5 in)   less than 14.2 hh (ponies)

Mullen mouthpieces need to be about 0.75–1.25 cm ($^1/_4$–$^1/_2$ in) narrower to fit correctly.

The double bridle

The double bridle consists of a curb bit used in conjunction with a snaffle or bridoon (Fig. 17.7). This sophisticated arrangement works on many areas of the horse's head giving a fine degree of control. This means that a double bridle should only be used by trained riders on horses that work correctly in a snaffle bridle.

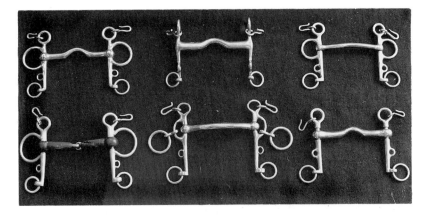

Fig. 17.7 A selection of curb bits (*from top, left to right*): Hartwell pelham (with port); fixed cheek Weymouth; mullen mouth pelham: jointed rubber pelham; Rugby pelham; slide cheek Weymouth.

The bridoon is normally jointed and is thinner and lighter than a snaffle (Fig. 17.3). The curb bit is unjointed with an upward curve called a port which accommodates the tongue so that the bit can work directly on the bars of the mouth. A long-cheeked curb bit is more severe than one with short cheeks as the amount of leverage is much increased. The bridoon acts on the lips and corners of the mouth to raise the horse's head while the curb acts on the bars of the mouth, the poll and the chin groove to flex the poll.

The Weymouth may have fixed cheeks, used in conjunction with an eggbutt bridoon, or a slide mouth, used with a loose-ring bridoon. The curb chain should be adjusted so that it comes into play when the bit is at a 45-degree angle to the mouth.

The pelham

The pelham (Fig. 17.7) is a compromise between the snaffle and the double bridle being a curb bit with one mouthpiece and a top snaffle rein and a bottom curb rein. The action is on the corners of the mouth (snaffle rein), poll and chin groove (curb rein), but the action tends to be indistinct, particularly when roundings are used to allow the use of one rein. (A rounding is a loop of leather running between the two rings of the bit.) The mouthpiece may be straight or jointed, and a vulcanite pelham with its mild mouthpiece and curb action is often useful for horses with good mouths that are strong, for example, over cross-country.

The curb chain should be adjusted so that it lies comfortably in the chin groove and comes into play when the tension on the curb rein increases and pulls the cheeks of the curb bit to an angle of 45 degrees. The curb chain then tightens and has a downward and backward pressure on the lower jaw. Attaching the curb chain through the top rings of the bit allows the curb to have a more direct action and helps stop the curb chain rising up out of the chin groove.

Curb chains are made of a series of linked metal rings which may be single or double (Fig. 17.8). Double linked chains spread the pressure over a larger area and are probably preferable to the more severe single link chains. Curb chains may also be made of elastic or leather. Provided that the leather is kept soft and supple they are less likely to cause rubbing than metal curb chains.

An important member of the pelham group is the Kimblewick (Fig. 17.9) which uses a single rein and is frequently seen on strong ponies. However, horses can learn to lean on this bit and it should not be over-used.

The gag

The gag is a type of snaffle but the rings of the bit have holes in them allowing an extended cheekpiece to pass through and attach to the rein (Fig. 17.10). This means that when the reins are pulled the bit is pulled up in the horse's mouth encouraging the head to be raised. The gag usually has a second rein attached to the bit ring in normal fashion so that the gag rein need only be used when necessary. The gag can be severe and is best used by those who are skilled.

The American gag is useful for strong horses (Fig. 17.6). The rein is attached to the bottom ring and when tightened can exert a very powerful pressure on the poll which acts to lower the head. The leverage is increased by the length of the cheekpiece above the mouthpiece.

The bitless bridle

A bitless bridle acts on the horse's nose and chin groove and is useful for horses with mouth problems (Fig. 17.11). However, it can be severe and should be used with care. The nose and curb pieces must be well padded to avoid rubbing.

Fitting a snaffle bridle

- The browband should fit snugly round the horse's forehead without pinching the base of the ears.

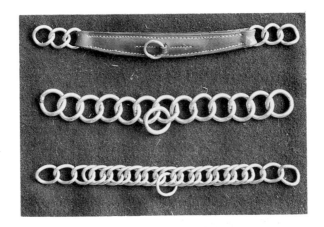

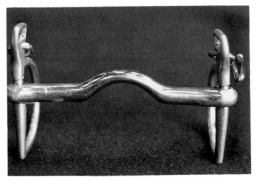

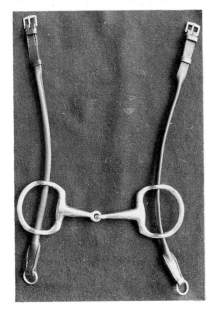

Fig. 17.8 (*top*) A selection of curb chains. From top: leather; single link; double link.

Fig. 17.9 (*middle*) Kimblewick.

Fig. 17.10 (*bottom*) Gag.

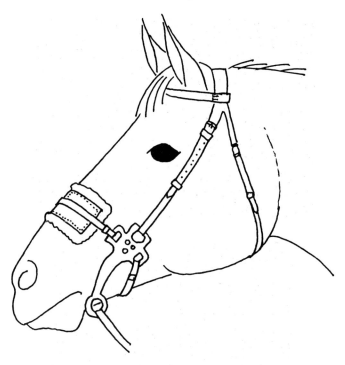

Fig. 17.11 A simple type of bitless bridle.

- The buckles of the cheekpieces onto the headpiece should be an even height on both sides and preferably just above eye level.
- The bit should just wrinkle the corners of the mouth with 0.5 cm ($\frac{1}{4}$ in) showing either side – the bit should be pulled straight in the horse's mouth to check its width. The mouth should be opened to check that the bit clears the tushes (the canine teeth found in geldings and stallions lying between the incisors and molars).
- It should be possible to fit a hand between the throatlash and the jaw (Fig. 17.12).
- A cavesson noseband should lie two fingers (2.5 cm (1 in)) below the cheekbone (Fig. 17.13) and allow two fingers between it and the jaw when tightened.

Fitting a double bridle (Fig. 17.14)
A double bridle is fitted as a snaffle bridle except:

- The bridoon has a separate headpiece which buckles on the off side

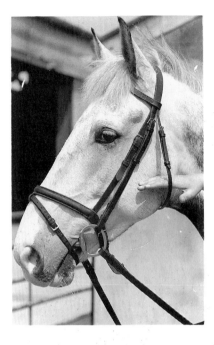

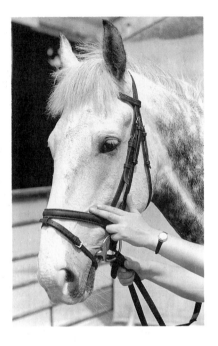

Fig. 17.12 Fitting a snaffle bridle: throatlash.

Fig. 17.13 Fitting a snaffle bridle: noseband.

a little below the buckle of the main headpiece. The bridoon should slightly wrinkle the lips.

- The curb bit is fitted to lie below the bridoon so that it can work separately, but it must not be so low as to interfere with the tushes.
- The curb chain is hooked on to the off side and twisted clockwise so that the lip strap ring hangs down. The flat ring of the curb chain is put on the near-side hook and the selected link is picked up, maintaining the twist to the right and placing it on the hook. If the curb chain is shortened more than three links, equal numbers of links should be taken on each side. The chain must lie flat in the chin groove and remain flat when the curb is used. Double link chains or ones made of leather are most satisfactory.
- The lip strap is buckled on the near side having been passed through the loose ring on the curb chain.

Fitting a pelham

The bit should lie close to the lips without causing them to wrinkle (Fig. 17.15). The curb chain should lie in the chin groove and can be

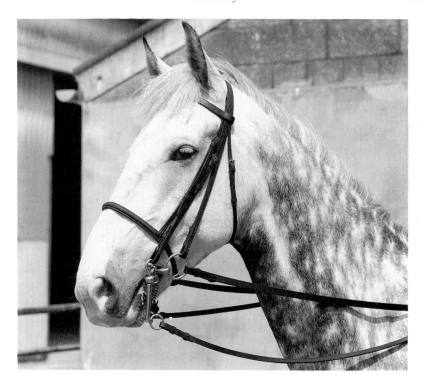

Fig. 17.14 A double bridle correctly fitted.

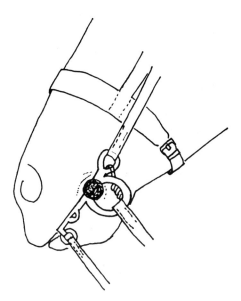

Fig. 17.15 A vulcanite pelham correctly fitted.

placed through the top rings of the bit to prevent chafing. Note that the curb chain hooks should open outwards away from the horse's face to avoid injury.

Nosebands

Drop noseband (Fig. 17.16)
This noseband fits around the nose below the bit and is designed to prevent the horse opening the mouth and thus evading the bit. It should be fitted so that the front lies on the bony part of the nose; if too low it will interfere with breathing. The noseband should be attached to the cheeks to prevent it flopping downwards onto the horse's nostrils. It must not be fitted too tightly and must allow flexion and movement of the jaw.

Grakle noseband (Fig. 17.17)
This has two straps which cross over the nose and below the bit in a figure of eight. It is designed to prevent the horse crossing the jaw and it is less likely to affect breathing than the drop noseband. It is fitted so that the headpiece ends just above the facial crest running down the side of the horse's head. The two straps are stitched together or pass through a leather pad.

Flash noseband (Fig. 17.18)
This consists of a cavesson plus a strap which passes through a loop on the front of the noseband and does up under the bit. Again it is less likely to affect breathing than a drop noseband and it also allows the use of a standing martingale.

Kineton noseband (Fig. 17.19)
This noseband transfers the bit pressure to the nose and is used on strong horses. It consists of two metal loops attached to each other by an adjustable strap. Each loop fits around the bit ring next to the horse's face so that the centre strap rests on the bony part of the nose. When the reins are pulled the pull is transferred via the bit to the nose.

Martingales

Competition rules frequently limit the use of martingales and schooling aids. These rules often apply at the venue as well as during the competition.

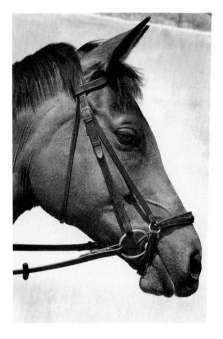

Fig. 17.16 Drop noseband.

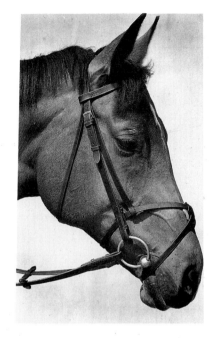

Fig. 17.17 Grakle noseband.

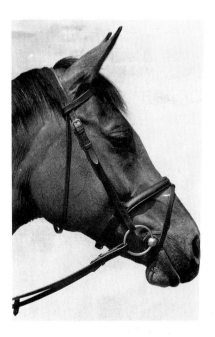

Fig. 17.18 Flash noseband.

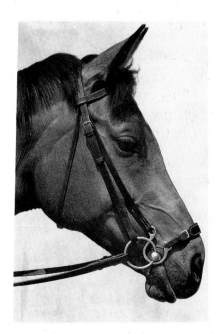

Fig. 17.19 Kineton noseband.

Standing martingale (Fig. 17.20)
A standing martingale has a neck strap through which passes a leather strap with a loop at either end; one end attaches to the girth, the other to a cavesson noseband. The martingale holds downwards on the horse's nose so that the horse does not lift his head beyond the point of control. The martingale should be adjusted so that it does not interfere with the horse when he is carrying his head in an acceptable fashion, nor should it tie him down and prevent him jumping spread fences effectively. When standing in a relaxed position it should be possible to push the martingale up into the horse's gullet.

Running martingale (Fig. 17.21)
A running martingale has the reins passing through the rings of the martingale thus helping to keep the pressure on the bars of the horse's mouth when the head is raised. Correctly fitted the martingale should only come into play when the horse raises his head above a permitted level. The rings of the martingale should nearly be able to reach the withers. A bib martingale has a centre-piece of leather to prevent the horse getting caught up in the branches of the martingale. Rein stops must be fitted on the reins to prevent the martingale rings getting caught on the rein fastening to the bit.

Irish martingale (Fig. 17.22)
An Irish martingale or rings is a short strap with rings like a pair of spectacles, designed to prevent the reins coming over the head in the event of a fall.

Market Harborough martingale (Fig. 17.23)
This has a normal martingale body which splits in two, passes through the bit rings and fastens onto the rein. Its action exerts a strong downward pull on the bit when the horse throws his head up.

Breastplate (Fig. 17.24)

Breastplates are used to stop the saddle slipping back. A hunting breastplate is similar to a martingale with straps running back to fasten to the saddle 'D's'. Care must be taken not to fit them too tightly as they can cut into the horse's chest when jumping. Standing and running martingale attachments can be fitted to the breastplate. An Aintree breastplate is used for racing; this fastens around the chest and is kept in place by a strap over the withers.

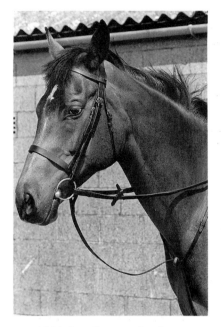

Fig. 17.20 Standing martingale.

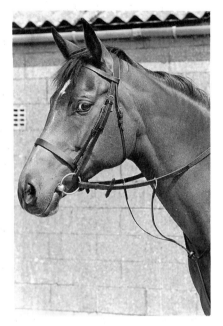

Fig. 17.21 Running martingale.

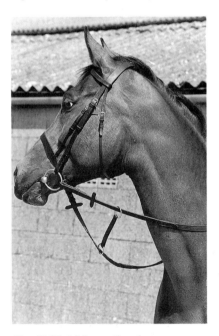

Fig. 17.22 Irish martingale.

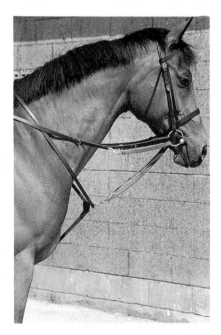

Fig. 17.23 Market Harborough martingale.

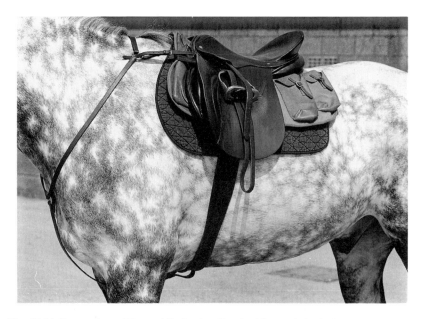

Fig. 17.24 Breastplate. (The saddle is also fitted with a weightcloth.)

Schooling aids

Most schooling aids are designed to teach the horse to lower and stretch the head and neck, thus stretching the muscles of the back and allowing the horse to engage the hindquarters. Schooling aids are common throughout much of Europe and elsewhere in the world. However, if misused they can cause accidents and so must only be employed properly by those trained and skilled in their use.

Draw reins (Fig. 17.25)
Draw reins start at the girth, pass between the front legs, through the bit rings and back to the rider's hands. Each rein passes from the inside to the outside of the bit ring. Draw reins should be used with a normal rein placed above the draw rein. The draw rein may also be fitted so that it runs from the girth straps of the saddle, through the bit rings and back to the rider's hands.

Chambon (Fig. 17.26)
The Chambon runs from the girth, between the horse's front legs to the poll and then down to the bit to put pressure on the poll and induce a lowered head carriage. It is used on the lunge with a mild snaffle bit.

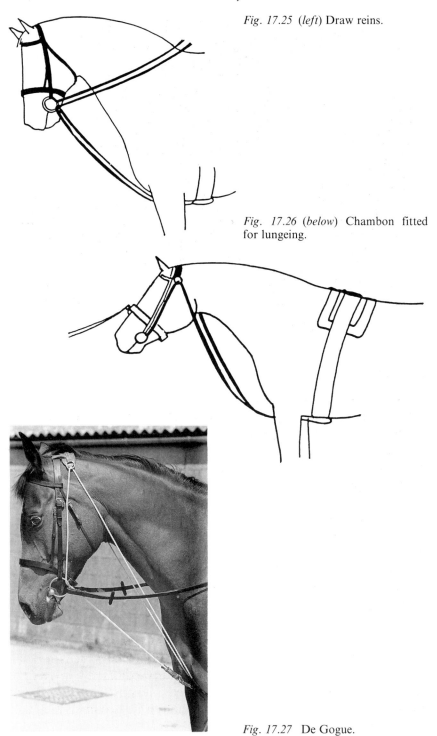

Fig. 17.25 (*left*) Draw reins.

Fig. 17.26 (*below*) Chambon fitted for lungeing.

Fig. 17.27 De Gogue.

De Gogue (Fig. 17.27)

The De Gogue is more advanced than the Chambon and can be used for ridden work as well as on the lunge. On the lunge the De Gogue has a strap running from the martingale body to the poll, to the bit and back to the martingale or saddle 'D', forming a triangle. For riding, instead of passing from the bit back to a fixed position, a rein is attached.

Saddles

Parts of the saddle (Fig. 17.28)

Saddle tree

This is the framework of the saddle and its size and shape depends on what the saddle is to be used for. Traditionally it is made of beechwood but now tends to be made of laminated wood, bonded and moulded, giving a lighter and stronger tree. Racing saddles may have light, fibreglass trees.

The tree may be either rigid or spring: a rigid tree gives strength and solidity; a spring tree (Fig. 17.29) has two flat panels of steel from pommel to cantle and allows the rider more direct communication with the horse underneath them. However, it may tend to concentrate the rider's weight onto a small area and is generally used with a numnah.

Stirrup bars

These are made of forged steel which is riveted to the points of the tree. A hinged safety catch is usually fitted and must never be used in the up position. The bars are placed forward in jumping saddles and further back in dressage saddles.

Seat

Initially webbing is fixed from pommel to cantle and then covered in stretched canvas or linen to form the seat shape. Wool or foam is placed on top as a padding and finally the whole is covered in leather with skirts to cover the stirrup bars.

Saddle flaps

Saddle flaps and girth straps are then added. If the first two straps are fitted to the same webbing piece and the third is independent then the

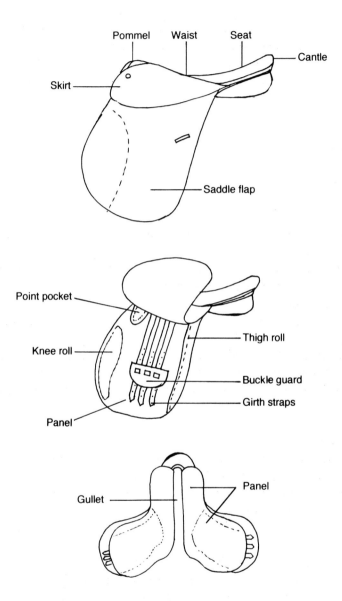

Fig. 17.28 Parts of the saddle.

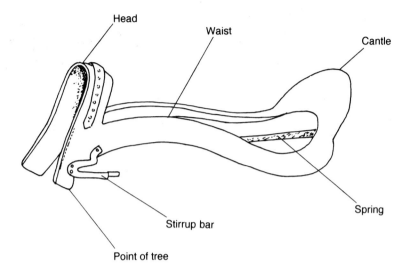

Fig. 17.29 Parts of the spring tree.

girth should be attached to the first and third straps. Dressage saddles may have long girth straps.

Panels
A full panel gives a greater weight-bearing surface and, combined with a wider-waisted saddle, is better for the horse. Thigh and knee rolls are also added to some saddles to help the rider's position. Short or half panels tend to be used on some pony saddles or on show or polo saddles.

Lining
Old saddles may have serge or linen lining, but more commonly saddles are now leather-lined.

Types of saddle

Jumping (Fig. 17.30)
The jumping saddle has forward-cut flaps and knee and thigh rolls to help the rider stay in balance in a forward position. A show-jumping saddle may have a deep seat while a cross-country saddle may have a flatter seat to allow a greater range of movement by the rider.

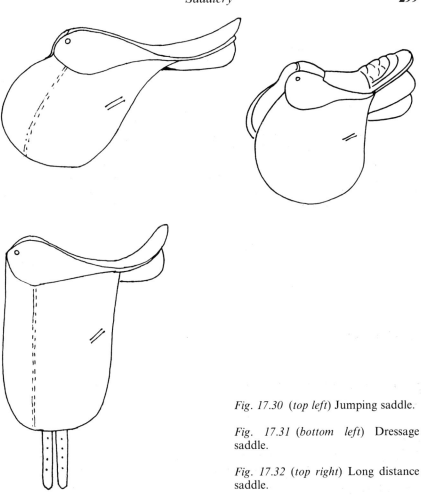

Fig. 17.30 (top left) Jumping saddle.

Fig. 17.31 (bottom left) Dressage saddle.

Fig. 17.32 (top right) Long distance saddle.

Dressage (Fig. 17.31)
This saddle helps the rider to achieve a deep seat and a long leg and is straighter cut with a long saddle flap. It may have large thigh rolls.

Working hunter
The working hunter saddle is a straight cut show saddle but with knee rolls for showing in working hunter classes.

General purpose
This is more forward cut than a dressage saddle, but still allows the rider to ride with a longer stirrup. It is designed to suit all disciplines, and is also called an event saddle.

Showing

This saddle is designed to show off a horse's shoulder and is only slightly forward cut with a half panel and a relatively flat seat. It is worn without a numnah. Some showing saddles also have a plain flap, no knee roll and a full panel.

Long distance (Fig. 17.32)

This saddle is designed like cavalry and Western saddles to spread the rider's weight over a greater area.

Racing

This is a light-weight saddle with a sloping head and very forward-cut tree. The design varies from the flat race saddle weighing a couple of kilos, or even less, to the more substantial National Hunt saddle.

Polo

This has a reinforced pommel with short panels and long sweat flaps. There are no knee or thigh rolls so that the player can move freely in the saddle.

Accessories

Girths

Leather girths come in three main designs: three-fold, Balding and Atherstone (Fig. 17.33). The shape of the latter two allows the horse's elbow to move while minimising the risk of rubbing. The three-fold girth has a material insert between the folds which should be kept well oiled. It is fitted so that the fold faces the rear. All three girths may have elastic inserts at the ends of the girth before the buckles to allow the horse's chest to expand while galloping.

The Lonsdale girth is a short girth to fit on dressage saddles with long straps. Care must be taken that the buckles are not fitted where they may chafe the horse.

Synthetic girths are popular, being much cheaper than leather ones. Other girths include string, lampwick and webbing.

All girths must be kept scrupulously clean and regularly checked for wear, particularly where the buckles attach.

Stirrup leathers

These must be of the best quality and regularly checked for safety. The

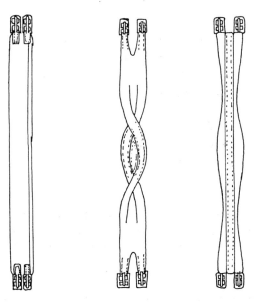

Fig. 17.33 Girths *(from left)*: three-fold; Balding; Atherstone.

length and weight of leather will depend on the rider with buffalo or rawhide being the strongest but also the most prone to stretching.

Stirrup irons (Fig. 17.34)
These should be made of stainless steel; nickel is soft and potentially dangerous. The size and weight of the iron must be suitable for the weight of the rider and the discipline, with clearance either side of the foot. Too big an iron is as dangerous as one that is too small. The bent leg (Simplex) safety stirrup is designed for riders who like to have their foot well forward in the iron. Children often use a safety iron which has a thick rubber band replacing the outside of the iron. If the child falls off the rubber band pops off so there is no risk of being dragged. This stirrup is essential with the child's felt pad saddle with 'D's instead of bars. Racing irons are made of light-weight stainless steel or aluminium. Rubber treads are often fitted to the stirrup iron to help the rider keep their foot in the stirrup.

Buying and fitting saddles
The importance of a good fitting saddle for the comfort, well-being and performance of both horse and rider is now recognised, and as a general rule it is wise to buy the best you can afford. For the large

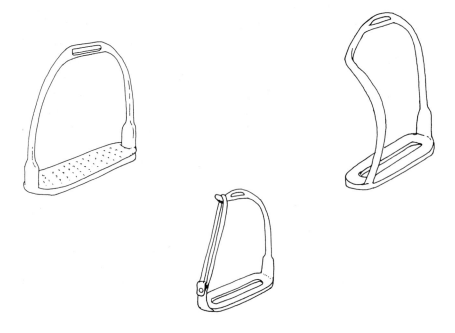

Fig. 17.34 Stirrup irons: *(left)* stirrup with stirrup tread; *(bottom)*Peacock safety stirrup; *(right)* bent leg (Simplex) safety stirrup.

majority of saddle purchasers the services of a competent and experienced saddle fitter should be sought to ensure that a really good fit is obtained.

Saddle fit very much depends on the horse's breeding. For example, a thoroughbred nearly always has a high narrow wither thus requiring a narrow fitting saddle to avoid the saddle resting on the withers. Cobs and hunters generally require a fairly straightforward wide fit, but breeds such as Arabs and the New Forest ponies have problems all of their own, to the extent that 'Arab' and 'Forester' saddles have now been developed to cope with their shape.

Remember that the horse's shape changes as it matures and becomes fitter. The shape of the saddle also changes as the padding flattens.

Examining a saddle
The tree should be tested for breakage and damage which may be on one or both sides of the tree. If the front arch is damaged it may widen

and come down on the withers. To test the tree place the hands either side of the pommel and try to widen and move the arch or hold the cantle and grip the pommel between the knees. Any movement or cracking sound indicates damage. If the waist is damaged there will be movement when the pommel is placed against the stomach and the cantle pressed up towards the pommel. There is always some give in the seat of a spring tree saddle, but it should spring back into place when released. The cantle should be rigid and any movement would indicate damage. The saddle should be examined for any uneven padding or outline and then placed on a saddle horse to check that it sits evenly.

Once on the horse the width of the gullet should be checked; there must not be any pressure close to the vertebrae. The saddle should sit evenly and level with no tilt towards the cantle or pommel which would unbalance the rider. The panels underneath should be in close contact with the horse's back for the whole length of the saddle. The riders weight should be evenly distributed over the lumbar muscles but not the loins and the saddle must not interfere with movement of the horse's shoulder.

When the rider is on, it should be possible to place three fingers under the pommel, and the horse should be ridden for a few mintues to check that the saddle has not dropped any further. This often happens, especially with a narrow horse. With a new saddle it should be possible to place four fingers under the pommel to allow for the saddle to drop as it is worn in. There must be ample clearance under the cantle and along the gullet and daylight along the gullet when viewed from behind (Fig. 17.35). The saddle must not rock from front to back as this indicates that pressure is not being evenly spread along the length of the saddle. Additionally, the horse should be checked ridden; any undue movement in the saddle will show up then, particularly during rising trot.

Tacking up

(1)   Collect the saddle, bridle, martingale and boots (if worn). Check that the throatlash and noseband of the bridle are undone and carry the bridle so that the reins are clear of the ground. Check that the saddle has a girth and numnah attached and carry it over your lower arm with the pommel towards the elbow.

(2)   Put the equipment in a safe place outside the stable and catch and

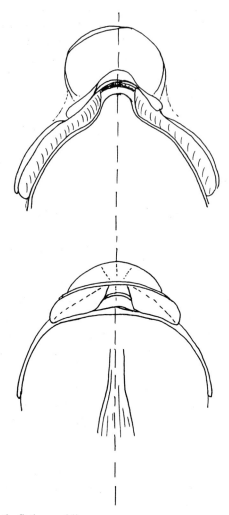

Fig. 17.35 A correctly fitting saddle.

    tie up the horse. Remove any rugs, clean the horse as necessary and pick the feet out.

(3)   Put on the boots if appropriate.

(4)   If a martingale is used fit it before the saddle; untie the horse and pass the neckstrap over his head from the near side. Then tie the horse up again and put on the saddle remembering to put the girth through the loop of the martingale.

(5)   Put on the saddle before the bridle in order to allow the horse's back to warm up. With the saddle usually on the left arm,

approach the horse from the near side and pat his back. Then using both hands place the saddle on the withers and slide it back into position. Straighten the numnah, pull it up into the arch of the saddle and attach the girth to the same two straps on both sides, before moving to the off side and fastening the girth, checking that the skin is not wrinkled. Ensure that the stirrup bars are down for safety's sake.

(6) If the weather is cold replace the rug. If the horse is restless fasten the buckles and roller.

(7) Put on the bridle (Figs 17.36–17.38). Carry the bridle and reins over the left arm with the browband nearest the elbow. Hold the bridle up against the horse's head to ensure that the fit is approximately correct. Then standing on the near side behind the horse's eye, reassure the horse, untie him and unfasten the headcollar, maybe placing it round the horse's neck. Pass the reins over the head and, holding the headpiece with the right hand, place the left hand under the bit, guiding it to the horse's mouth. Gently open the mouth by placing the first finger in the gap between the horse's incisors and molars. As the horse opens his mouth, slip the bit in and simultaneously lift the bridle with the right hand. Use both hands to put the bridle over the ears and to tidy the mane and forelock. Adjust the fit as necessary and then fasten the throatlash and noseband and replace the keepers. Put the headcollar back on over the bridle. If it is a double bridle ensure that the bridoon is on top and in front of the Weymouth.

Leaving a saddled horse

The horse should be tied up with the reins made safe; they may be doubled round the horse's neck, twisted and looped through the throatlash or slipped under a stirrup leather.

Untacking

On dismounting, run up the stirrup irons and loosen the girth. Take the reins over the horse's head and lead him into the stable, making sure to turn the horse round and close the stable door. Some stable yards insist that a headcollar is then placed round the horse's neck leaving the rope untied. Then unfasten the noseband and throatlash and release the martingale from the girth. Ease the bridle over the horse's head, steadying his nose and allowing him to drop the bit in his

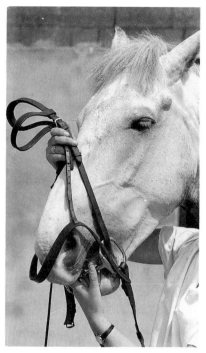

Figs 17.36–17.38
Putting on a bridle.

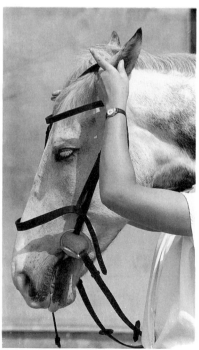

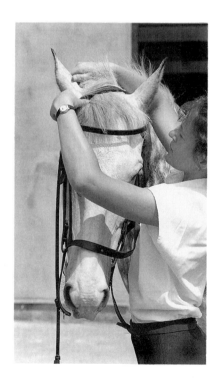

own time. Put the bridle over your left arm, put on the headcollar and tie the horse up. Unfasten the girths and lift the saddle over the horse's shoulder, putting it on your left arm. Turn muddy girths before placing them over the saddle. Then place the saddle on the stable door or on the ground with the pommel towards the ground and the cantle, protected by the girth, against the wall. Lastly remove the boots.

Care of the horse after untacking

After the horse has been untacked pick out the feet and, if necessary, wash off the hooves and heels. Check the legs for heat and swelling. Sponge the saddle and bridle areas to remove sweat marks, at the same time checking for rubs. Then brush the horse and replace the rugs.

18   The Theory of Feeding

We have taken horses from the wild and completely changed their lifestyle; instead of roaming freely, eating and browsing plants, herbs and leaves of their choice we have enclosed them in fields and stables. They are dependent on us for all their food and water requirements and it is important to supply these requirements properly if the horse is to remain healthy and do the work we demand.

Feeding practice

The horse prefers a diet based on roughage and one that is free from moulds or taint. Its digestive system is designed for a small intake at frequent intervals. If the horse is fed two large feeds a day, the food will be less well utilised and therefore money is wasted. Moreover, although the horse appreciates some variety, it does not like sudden change, particularly of the roughage part of its diet. This is because the roughage is broken down in the horse by bacteria which develop to meet a particular need. If there is a major change in diet, the bacterial population will change, but this takes time.

Within the gut, cereal-based foods tend to form a mass like bread dough, which the digestive juices have difficulty in penetrating. Digestion is more efficient if cereals are mixed with roughage. The inclusion of a little bran, dried grass, nuts or soaked sugar beet with the cereals can aid digestion. Chaff (chopped hay or straw) may also be included. It is a useful aid to digestion to offer the stabled horse a small amount of hay before the morning corn feed. The hay will go into the stomach ahead of the corn and help to break up the 'dough'.

Oat and barley straw are as nutritious as low-quality hay. Straw can therefore usefully supplement the diet of ponies wintering outside. However, neither hay nor straw supplies an adequate diet without supplement: feed blocks are useful in this respect.

Concentrate feeds based on corn are important highlights of the day for the stabled horse, and are best given at regular times. The horse is, of course, capable of being flexible in feeding arrangements when away from home. Because the horse has a keen sense of smell, all feed containers must be kept scrupulously clean and mangers must be checked before the next feed is put in.

The vital nutrients

In order to design a balanced ration it is necessary to understand what nutrients the horse requires. The six necessary ingredients of the horse's diet are water, carbohydrates, fats, proteins, minerals and vitamins.

Water

Water is essential in the horse's diet: foals contain 75–80% water and older horses contain about 70% water. It is obviously vital that the water level is maintained and horses will die relatively quickly if deprived of water. Water has a number of essential functions:

- Regulation of body temperature and sweating.
- It is the medium in which essential chemical reactions take place.
- As a transport medium within the body.
- To give shape to body cells.
- To excrete waste products as urine.
- As the basis of milk for lactating mares.

In the wild horses tend to drink at dawn and dusk but stabled horses need more water because they are eating dry feed. A stabled horse will normally drink 20–40 litres (5–10 gallons) depending on how much work he is doing, his feed and the climatic conditions.

Water should be free from taint, poison and disease. At competitions it is better to take your own water or use a tap rather than let the horse drink from a public trough where he may pick up infection. In the stable yard, if the buckets are filled from a trough use a dipper bucket to avoid the trough being contaminated by the dirty bottoms of buckets that have been in the stable. All troughs, drinkers and buckets must be kept clean and emptied and scrubbed out regularly. Horses will refuse soiled or stale water so it is better that buckets are emptied and refilled rather than topped up.

Except when he comes in hot and tired a horse should have free access to fresh water at all times. Buckets must be refilled before feeding a concentrate feed so that the horse has the opportunity to quench his thirst before eating; a deep drink after a meal could wash food through the stomach, although the shape of the stomach makes this unlikely.

The performance horse should not be deprived of water for more than 30 minutes before exercise. He is unlikely to gorge himself with water if he has free access to water. It is better not to allow the horse free access to water after heavy exercise, but to give little and often until respiratory rates are back to normal. When horses are dehydrated after heavy sweating during exercise or travelling, they should be offered electrolytes (body salts) dissolved in the water once they have started drinking. The tired horse, such as the hunter on his return to the stable, may be offered a little 'chilled water', which is water with the chill taken off it.

Carbohydrates

Nature's perfection is clearly seen in the relationship between animals and plants. Plants take up water from the ground together with carbon dioxide from the air, and, with the aid of energy from the sun, combine these two simple products into a more complex energy-storage product called carbohydrate. The animal eats the plant, utilises the carbohydrate within the muscle, and the energy is released in the form of body heat and activity. Carbohydrates can be divided into two groups:

- *Simple carbohydrates* – including starch, glycogen and sugars.
- *Complex carbohydrates* – including cellulose and lignin.

Simple carbohydrates

Starch and sugars are found in plants and grains; starch is the plant's form of stored carbohydrate. The simple carbohydrates are digested mostly in the small intestine of the horse; they are broken down and absorbed into the blood stream and transported to the liver, mainly in the form of sugars. Glucose, a simple sugar, is the ultimate source of energy for most cells in the horse's body. Glucose is stored as glycogen but the amount of glycogen that can be stored is limited, so excess glucose is converted to fat and stored in fat or adipose tissue.

Young plants, such as grasses, contain large amounts of sugars and simple carbohydrates, whereas grains such as oats, barley and maize, contain high levels of starch.

Complex carbohydrates
Cellulose is found in all plant cell walls; the horse does not have any digestive enzymes capable of breaking down these walls to release the valuable carbohydrate contained within them. However, the bacteria and micro-organisms living in the horse's caecum and large intestine can break down and digest cellulose. Cellulose is broken down by the bacteria, the breakdown products are absorbed into the horse's bloodstream, taken to the liver and converted to glucose. This is why a horse can survive on a diet of grass.

Cellulose is the fibrous part of the horse's diet, found in grass, hay, silage, etc. This fibre is vital for normal and healthy functioning of the horse's gut. Lignin is another complex carbohydrate found in stemmy materials; this cannot be broken down in the gut by the horse or its resident bacterial population, it is indigestible and is excreted in the faeces.

Carbohydrates, either as cereals or roughage, form the largest part of the horse's diet and provide the horse with energy.

Measuring the energy in food
Human food is often measured in calories; a calorie being a measure of the amount of energy in the food. However a calorie is a small unit and is often expressed in thousand calorie units called kilocalories. Read your yoghurt pot to discover the quantity of energy in the yoghurt and you will find that it is usually expressed in kilocalories. A joule is another common unit for measuring energy and is used in horse nutrition. There are 4.2 joules to a calorie. It is more convenient, however, to use a much larger unit, the megajoule (1 megajoule = 1 000 000 joules). Consequently we can express the energy value of horse feeds in megajoules (MJ) per kilogram of food. As a horse cannot extract absolutely all of the energy from its feeds, it is more useful to show only the amount of energy which it can digest: this is expressed as Digestible Energy (DE). Thus, typically, oats contain about 14 MJ of DE per kilogram, whereas horse and pony cubes may only contain 10 MJ of DE per kilogram. You would therefore have to feed 1.4 kg of cubes to supply your horse with the same energy as 1 kg of oats; conversely 0.7 kg of oats would replace 1 kg of cubes.

The energy requirement of your horse will depend on many factors but principally his size and the amount of work he is doing. Once these are known it is fairly simple to work out his energy requirements in terms of megajoules per day, and hence how much feed he must get.

Fats

Horse diets contain about 4% fat and it is a relatively minor source of energy compared to carbohydrate. Fat is, however, a useful fuel store. Fat also acts as a protective layer under the skin and around the internal organs and it is essential for good skin and coat condition. Typically the horse's body contains about 17% fat.

Fats contain over twice as much energy as carbohydrates, but there are limitations in its conversion to energy and horses have to be 'trained' to utilise more of it. Carbohydrates are still the main energy source for horses.

Protein

Protein makes up the majority of body tissues in forms as diverse as muscle, hair and hoof. Protein is needed in the diet for body building and tissue repair; thus the percentage of protein required in the diet of young, growing horses is highest, but this requirement declines gradually as the horse reaches maturity, when only enough protein to replace worn out body tissue is needed. Higher levels of protein are also needed by the pregnant and lactating brood mare.

Proteins are made up of simple building blocks called amino acids. More than 20 amino acids occur in the horse's diet and some amino acids are also produced in the horse's body to take the place of the amino acids that may be lacking in the diet. However, some of these amino acids are made at a rate that does not meet the demands of the horse's system. These are known as 'rate-limiting amino acids' and may have to be supplemented in the diet, the most important being: *lysine*, *methionine* and *tryptophan*. Some proteins will contain higher proportions of rate-limiting amino acids than others; these are high quality proteins and are important when feeding the growing horse. Feeds high in protein are peas and beans, soya bean meal, milk powder and high protein compound feeds.

The amino acid most likely to be deficient in the horse's diet is lysine, deficiency of which will severely affect protein synthesis in the horse's body and poor growth will result. *All cereals are low in lysine.*

Except during starvation, proteins are of little importance as an energy source; contrary to many a horse-owner's belief, working adult horses do not require a high protein ration. Look after the energy and the protein will look after itself.

Measuring the protein in food

Foods can be chemically analysed to give the percentage content of crude protein which is the value you see written on bags of compound feeds. This value is only a guideline as it gives you no idea how digestible that protein is, nor any guide to protein quality. Thus bran has a high crude protein value but low digestibility and a poor balance of amino acids.

Minerals

Earlier this century there was less intensive production from the land than is the case today. Fertilisers, weedkillers and highly productive varieties of plants were then in their infancy. Until quite recently, crops contained more weeds and herbs than modern crops. Weeds and herbs have a good mineral balance, whereas modern, fast-grown, clean crops require supplementing by minerals when fed in some circumstances, for example in the case of young stock.

In general, the stable-fed horse needs extra salt. It is also important that the balance of the minerals (notably calcium and phosphorus) is kept at a reasonable level or weak bones will result. For example, bran is very bad in this respect. It is too high in phosphorus and also contains a substance that inhibits calcium uptake. Bran needs balancing with ground-up limestone to provide extra calcium.

The modern horse is often stabled with limited access to grass and fed a variety of conserved, processed and heat-treated feeds. The vitamin levels of these feeds will have suffered by these treatments, consequently a mineral and vitamin supplement should be provided if the horse is being fed a traditional hay, oats and bran diet. If a good quality compound feedstuff is used, as specified by the manufacturer, a supplement may not be necessary.

The horse's diet usually contains sufficient magnesium, manganese, fluorine, iodine and cobalt but may be lacking in calcium (Ca), phosphorus (P), sodium (Na), chlorine (Cl) and in some circumstances, iron (Fe), zinc (Zn), sulphur (S), copper (Cu) and selenium (Se). Some geographical areas have deficiency problems and hay and cereals grown there may need supplementing. Other areas have problems of excess, whether in the soil itself or as a result of pollution.

Vitamins

Vitamins are a complex group of organic substances that are essential, in small quantities, for normal body function. The bacteria in the horse's hind gut can synthesise some B vitamins in adequate quantities but most vitamins need to be supplied in the diet.

Table 18.1 Minerals.

Name	Functions	Deficiency signs	Sources
Calcium (Ca)	(1) Bone growth, maintenance and development. (2) Blood coagulation. (3) Lactation. (4) Nerve and muscle function.	Bone disorders implicated in the onset of azoturia. Increased blood clotting time.	Green leafy food, especially legumes, e.g. alfalfa. Cereals and bran are poor sources; horses on high cereal diets need additional calcium, e.g. ground limestone or calcium gluconate.
Phosphorus (P)	(1) Closely related to calcium in bone. (2) Energy metabolism.	Bone abnormalities. Subnormal growth in young horses.	Cereal grains, e.g. oats, bran, barley.

It is vital that the ration fed to your horse has a calcium to phosphorus ratio of between 1.6:1 and 2:1 in terms of available minerals.

Name	Functions	Deficiency signs	Sources
Sodium (Na)	(1) Acid-base balance. (2) Body fluid regulation. (3) Transmission of nerve impulses. (4) Absorption of sugars and amino acids from the gut.	Body dehydration, poor growth, reduced utilisation of digested proteins and energy.	Most natural feedstuffs are low in sodium thus the diet should be supplemented with common salt (NaCl), e.g. a salt or mineral lick in the manger.
Chorine (Cl)	(1) Closely associated with sodium and potassium. (2) Body fluid regulation.	Where the requirements for sodium are met it is unlikely that chlorine will be deficient.	
Copper (Cu)	(1) Interacts with sulphur and molybdenum. (2) Formation of bone, cartilage, elastin and hair pigment. (3) Utilisation of iron during production of haemoglobin and red blood cells.	Anaemia, poor growth, hair depigmentation, weight loss. Implicated in some bone disorders.	Copper in feedstuffs is directly related to the copper in the soil on which the feed was grown as well as feed type. High levels in seeds and seed by-products.
Zinc (Zn)	(1) Normal cell metablism. (2) Enzyme activator and antagonist.	Rare but may reduce appetite and growth. High zinc levels interfere with copper utilisation, associated with lameness and bone abnormalities, especially epiphysitis.	Yeast, bran and cereal germ.
Iron (Fe)	(1) Normal haemoglobin and red blood cell production.	Anaemia.	Most natural feeds, except milk. Horses fed a normal diet are unlikely to be deficient, unless heavily parasitised.

Table 18.1 *contd*

Name	Functions	Deficiency signs	Sources
Selenium (Se)	(1) Maintenance of normal muscle. (2) Closely related to vitamin E as cell membrane stabiliser and protector.	Pale, weak muscle in foals and occasionally in adult horses – white muscle disease. Excess mane and tail hair loss, hoof deformities, joint stiffness, lethargy, anaemia and weight loss.	Linseed or commercial product.

What to feed

In order to make a decision about what to feed, the horse owner has to take many things into consideration, for example:

- cost
- availability
- the horse's nutrient requirements
- quality
- the nutrient content of the feed

Table 18.2 Vitamins

Name	Function	Deficiency signs	Sources
Vitamin B$_1$ (thiamin)	(1) Enzyme co-factor. (2) Synthesised in horse's gut.	Rare unless consistently fed poor quality hay or has eaten bracken (*Pteridium aquilana*) which contains a B$_1$ antagonist. *Symptoms:* poor growth, weight loss, incoordination, abnormal reflex activity.	Yeast, alfalfa, green leafy crops, peas, beans, cereal germ. Bracken poisoning can be remedied by removing bracken from diet and giving large doses of B$_1$.
Vitamin B$_2$ (riboflavin or lactoflavin)	(1) Cannot be synthesised by horse. (2) Fundamental component of many enzymes involved in protein and carbohydrate metabolism.	Decreased energy production and protein utilisation, hence growth and condition adversely affected.	Good quality grass and hay should provide much higher levels than the estimated requirements.

Table 18.2 *contd*

Name	Function	Deficiency signs	Sources
Vitamin B$_6$ (pyridoxine)	Protein and carbohydrate metabolism.	Not reported in horses.	Forages, grains, pulses.
Vitamin B$_{12}$ (cyanocobalamin)	(1) Contains cobalt, production of red blood cells. (2) Enzyme function.	Anaemia, reduced red cell number. Mature horses less affected than youngsters.	Synthesised exclusively by micro-organisms in horse's gut, presence in food is of microbial origin.
Vitamin B$_{15}$ (pangamic acid) .	Allegedly increases the supply of blood oxygen to the horse.	Not known.	Isolated from apricot pits. Not recognised by the US Food and Drugs Administration as there is no exact chemical formula.
Folic acid	Intimately linked to B$_{12}$, vital for red blood cell production.	Anaemia and poor growth.	Good quality pasture, hay etc., cereals, extracted oilseed meals. Requirement increases with exercise.
Pantothenic acid	Metabolism of fats, carbohydrates and certain proteins.	Unusual, weight loss, growth failure.	Peas, molasses, yeast, cereal grains.
Biotin	(1) Contains sulphur. (2) Fat, protein and carbohydrate metabolism. (3) Positively linked with the sulphur-containing amino acid, methionine.	Skin changes, poor hoof horn and faulty keratinisation.	Present in bran and barley but unavailable. Maize, yeast, grass are available sources.
Vitamin C (ascorbic acid)	(1) Normal collagen formation, maintenance and repair. (2) Transfer of Fe from blood to body stores.	Impaired collagen formation hence delayed wound healing, oedema and weight loss.	Horses can synthesise their own vitamin C but horses on a high grain diet may not be able to synthesise enough. Good sources include green leafy forage.
Choline	(1) Fat metabolism. (2) Nerve transmission. (3) Maintenance of cell structure.	Despite its large requirement a deficiency is not usually seen due to wide distribution in feedstuffs. It can also be made from the amino acid methionine.	Green leafy forages, yeast and cereals.

Table 18.2 *contd*

Name	Function	Deficiency signs	Sources
Vitamin A (retinol)	(1) Night vision. (2) Normal skeletal development. (3) Fat and carbohydrate metabolism.	Poor growth, weight loss, increased susceptibility to respiratory infection, lameness, infertility (especially older mares), keratinisation of skin and cornea.	Derived from the abundant beta-carotene in grass and very good quality hay.
Vitamin D (calciferol)	(1) Ca and P metabolism, thus bone development and maintenance. (2) Has two forms: D_2 (ergocalciferol) and D_3 (cholecalciferol).	Deficiency or excess results in swollen joints, skeletal abnormalities, lameness. Excess also causes bone to be laid down in soft tissue. Horses that are rugged and housed, receiving little sunlight and a cereal-based diet are most at risk.	Occurs as two provitamins which need the ultraviolet portion of sunlight acting on the skin to be converted to the vitamin. The vitamin rarely occurs in plants but colostrum, the first milk, is a rich source for the foal.
Vitamin K	Blood clotting.	Rare, as made by the bacteria of the gut. Dicumerol, a blood anti-coagulant, interferes with vitamin K, leading to extended clotting time.	Some body storage and leafy material, e.g. lucerne.
Vitamin E (tocopherol)	(1) Group name for several closely related substances, of which alpha-tocopherol is most common. (2) Non-specific biological anti-oxidant. (3) With Se as body tissue 'stabiliser'.	Wide variety of problems: pale areas of skeletal and heart muscle, red blood cell fragility, infertility.	Alfalfa, green fodder, cereal grains (although the type of tocopherol can vary, e.g. barley has mainly alpha-tocopherol but maize also has gamma-tocopherol).

Feeds can be divided into two categories: concentrates and forage. Concentrates are energy feeds and traditionally cereals have provided the principal source of energy for horses in hard work. Cereal grains contain 12–16 MJ DE per kg of dry matter compared to about 8.5 MJ/kg in average grass hay. In other words, 1 kg of cereals can replace up to 2 kg of hay in the ration – hence the name concentrate. As we demand a higher energy output from the horse we have to feed him more concentrated energy sources in order to keep the ration within his appetite. This also reduces his natural grass belly to give a trim athletic outline.

Cereals also contain proteins but these are not as nutritionally valuable as animal protein and oilseed protein because they are relatively deficient in the essential amino acids lysine and methionine. All cereal grains are very low in calcium, containing less than 1.5 g/kg, but they contain three to five times as much phosphorus. The phosphorus is principally in the form of phytate salts which reduce the availability of calcium and zinc, further increasing the horse's need for a calcium supplement.

The 'heating' effect of grain

Grain is often said to be 'heating', meaning that it results in a horse being overexcited and difficult to control. This heating effect stems from two sources:

(1) Overfeeding energy. Many 'hot' horses are simply getting too much energy for the job that they are doing and a reduction in the concentrate ration and an increase in the roughage should solve many problems. The behavioural problems are made worse by confining the horse to its stable 23 hours a day and then working the horse to increase its fitness – a veritable time bomb!

(2) Fermentation. Any grain passing through into the large intestine is rapidly fermented by the intestinal micro-organisms. Consequently there is an increase in the acidity of the caecum which may lead to discomfort, and the products of digestion pass very quickly into the bloodstream. The resulting rise in the levels of glucose and volatile fatty acids in the blood stimulates the

Table 18.3 Nutrient values of commonly fed concentrate feeds.

	Crude protein %	Oil %	*MAD fibre g/kg	Ca g/kg	P g/kg	Lysine g/kg	DE MJ/kg
Oats	9.6	4.5	17	0.7	3.0	3.2	11–12
Naked oats	13.5	9.7	3.2	0.2	0.4	5	16
Barley	9.5	1.8	7	0.6	3.3	3.1	13
Maize	8.5	3.8	3	0.2	3.0	2.6	14
Linseed	22	32	7.6	2.4	5.2	7.7	18.5
Extracted soyabean meal	44	1.0	10	2.4	6.3	26	13.3
Wheatbran	15.5	3	12	1.0	12	6	11
Sugarbeet pulp	7	1.0	34	10	11	2.8	10.5

* MAD = Modified acid detergent

metabolic rate, thus 'heating' the horse both literally and mentally.

Processing cereals increases the amount of digestion in the small intestine, reduces caecal fermentation and keep the horse's metabolism more stable.

Rationing

When deciding on the feed for a horse, it is wise to bear in mind the theory of rationing. Horses are fed for maintenance, i.e. to maintain them in their present state. Their food provides energy for the muscles of the internal organs and for grazing, maintains body temperature and continuously replaces cells to keep the body in good order. Horses are also fed for production. This can be broken into different categories:

(a) Growth from the day the horse is born until it stops growing at 4 to 7 years old
(b) Lactation of the brood mare from the day her foal is born until the day it is weaned
(c) Growth of the embryo into a foal within its mother (most of this growth occurs in the final third of the pregnancy)
(d) Body repair, regrowth after major injury or disease
(e) Fattening
(f) Work (this can be broken down into light work, medium work, heavy work or fast work)
(g) Build up muscle for performance

To feed for maintenance, the main criterion is the size of the animal: bigger animals need more food. In practice, maintenance for the horse in the field is produced by grass supplemented with hay or straw and possibly some hard feed in winter. Maintenance for the stabled horse comes from hay or other forms of conserved grass. If the horse requires a large quantity of food for production, the hay must be of high quality and therefore less bulk is required. There is a limit to the gut capacity of a horse, and if a performance horse is filled up with large quantities of low-quality maintenance food, it will have neither room for adequate production rations nor zest for its job.

To feed for production, the main criterion is the amount of production required. Thus, with the pregnant mare, the extra feed is

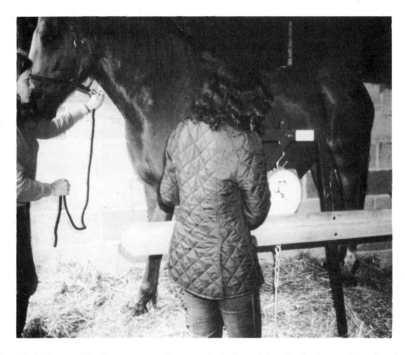

Fig. 18.1 Horses, like humans, need to watch their weight. Rationing and medication can be used more accurately if the horse's weight is known.

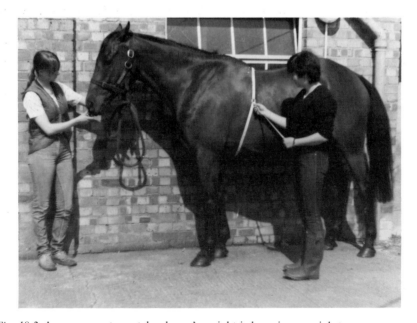

Fig. 18.2 An easy way to watch a horse's weight is by using a weigh-tape.

increased gradually through the last third of the pregnancy. With the competition horse, the feed is increased as the horse becomes fitter and is able to work harder. Production rations are mostly based on cereals. Good grass or very high-quality hay will produce a little above maintenance and therefore provide some production.

The horse can eat, each day, hay and concentrates weighing about 2½% of its body weight (2% for ponies and up to 3% for young stock).

The ratio of forage to concentrates

The relationship of forage to concentrates in the horse's diet has a clear bearing on the energy in the diet. More concentrates means more energy. Therefore the horse's diet is related to its work. A horse that is not working should be able to thrive on hay alone. A working horse, burning up energy, will need to have concentrates added to the ration.

This means that a 500 kg (1100 lb) horse in medium work has an appetite of 12.5 kg (28 lb) and is fed 40% concentrates and 60% forage, resulting in a ration of 5 kg (11 lb) of concentrates and 7.5 kg (16½ lb) hay.

It is best to feed a horse slightly below appetite so that he is always eager for his next concentrate feed and has always finished his haynet when you come to fill it again. Beware of the *ad lib* feeding system; often the hay rack is constantly topped up so that the hay at the bottom becomes mouldy, and the horse becomes over-fussy and wasteful. If you feed a weighed ration of hay and concentrates, within the horse's appetite, he should always eat up. If he does not eat all his hay and concentrates it may indicate that the quality of the feed is not up to scratch or that the horse is off-colour.

In order to design a practical ration that supplies the energy and protein requirements of an individual horse and fits within its appetite

Table 18.4 Ratios of forage to concentrates.

Work level	Hay (%)	Concentrates (%)
Resting	100	0
Light	75	25
Medium	60	40
Hard	40	60
Fast	30	70

we can follow the eight steps involved in the rules of rationing. Taken for our example is a 16.0 hh, middleweight Novice event horse.

The rules of rationing

Step one: Estimation of bodyweight
Several methods are available:

- Table of weights
- Calculation
- Weightape (Fig. 18.2)
- Weighbridge (Fig. 18.1)

Our 16hh, three-quarterbred Novice event horse will weigh 500 kg.

Table 18.5   Approximate bodyweights.

Height (hands)	Bodyweight	
	(kg)	(lb)
11	120–260	264–572
12	230–290	506–638
13	290–350	638–770
14	350–420	770–924
15	420–520	924–1144
16	500–600	1100–1320
17	600–725	1320–1595

N.B. The values in this table are averages and only approximate.

Step two: The horse's appetite
An adult working horse's appetite is about 2.5% of his bodyweight. Foals and lactating broodmares may compensate for their high nutrient requirements by eating more than this.

$$\text{Appetite (kg)} = \frac{\text{bodyweight}}{100} \times 2.5$$

$$\textit{Appetite of 500 kg horse} = \frac{500}{100} \times 2.5 = 12.5 \textit{ kg (28 lb)}$$

A 500 kg horse can eat up to 12.5 kg of dry matter per day. Remember that different feeds have different amounts of dry matter in them, so a horse will eat much more than 12.5 kg of grass a day because of its high moisture content.

Step three: Calculating the energy for maintenance
The horse requires a minimum amount of energy a day just to stay alive, this is related to the bodyweight of the horse – bigger horses need more feed than smaller ones.

$$\text{Energy required for maintenance (MJ DE/day)} = 18 + \frac{\text{bodyweight}}{10}$$

Energy required for a 500 kg horse to maintain its bodyweight
$$(MJ\ DE/day) = 18 + \frac{500}{10} = 18 + 50 = 68\ MJ\ DE/day$$

A 500 kg horse will require 68 MJ DE per day to stay alive and to keep its bodyweight constant. (The above formula and this system of ration calculation were devised by Jeremy Houghton Brown, based on comparison of feed trials around the world.)

Step four: Calculating the energy for work
The amount of energy the horse needs to carry out the work we demand of it depends on the intensity and duration of the work and the horse's bodyweight. The variation in the trainer or rider's perception of how much work the horse does has been minimised by giving the work a 'work score' of from one to eight. Examples of types of work have been outlined, but these are not rigid and you should adjust to fit your horse's individual work load.

Table 18.6 Work scoring.

Type of work	Work score (MJ DE)
One hour walking	+1
One hour walking including some trotting	+2
One hour including trotting and cantering	+3
Schooling, dressage and/or jumping	+4
Novice ODE or hunting one day/week	+5
Intermediate ODE, hunting 3 days a fortnight, Novice 3-day event	+6
Advanced ODE, Intermediate 3-day events, hunting 2 days a week	+7
Racing	+8

For each 50 kg of bodyweight, add the work score to calculate the horse's energy requirement for work.

A 500 kg Novice one-day event horse will have a work score of 5. The extra energy needed to carry out that work will be:

$$work\ score \times \frac{bodyweight}{50} = 5 \times \frac{500}{50} = 50\ MJ\ DE/day$$

The energy requirement for work is then added to the maintenance requirement to give the total daily energy requirement per day.

Maintenance requirement for a 500 kg horse = 68 MJ DE/day

Work requirement for a 500 kg Novice eventer = 50 MJ DE/day

Total energy requirement = 118 MJ DE/day

Step five: The forage to concentrate ratio

The horse's work level will determine the amount of energy to come from the forage part of the ration and the amount to come from the concentrate part. Using the table of forage to concentrate ratios we can calculate how the energy is going to be partitioned.

Table 18.7 Forage to concentrate energy partition.

Work score	Energy from hay	Energy from concentrates
Maintenance – resting	100	0
1–2 – light	75	25
3–5 – Medium	60	40
6–7 – Hard	40	60
8 – Fast	30	70

Of the total energy requirement (118 MJ DE/day) for our eventer in medium work (work score 5), 60% will come from hay and 40% will come from concentrates.

$$Energy\ from\ hay = \frac{118 \times 60}{100} = 71\ MJ\ DE$$

$$Energy\ from\ concentrates = \frac{118 \times 40}{100} = 47\ MJ\ DE$$

71 MJ DE per day are to be supplied by hay and 47 MJ DE per day by concentrates.

Step six: Making the ration

The next step is to convert these figures into a sensible ration, using the table of nutrient values. The energy value of food will be matched with the energy requirements of the feeds.

Table 18.8 Typical nutrient values of common feeds.

	Crude protein (%)	Digestible energy (MJ DE/kg)
Hay		
Average	4.5–8	7–8
Good	9–10	9
Poor	3.5–6	7
Haylage		
	9–12	9–11.5
Concentrates		
Oats	10	11–12
Barley	9.5	13
Maize	8.5	14
Extr. soyabean meal	44	13.3
Peas	23	14
Wheatbran	15.5	11
Sugarbeet pulp	7	10.5
Vegetable oil	0	35
Cubes		
Horse & Pony	10	9
Performance	13	13
Stud	15	11

The 500 kg event horse is to receive 71 MJ DE per day from average quality hay containing 8 MJ DE per kg.

$$Weight \ of \ hay \ to \ be \ fed/day = \frac{71}{8} = 9 \ kg \ (20 \ lb)$$

The horse is to receive the remaining 47 MJ DE as concentrates. This can be done by feeding a performance horse cube with an energy content of 13 MJ DE/kg.

$$Weight \ of \ cubes \ to \ be \ fed/day = \frac{47}{13} = 3.5 \ kg \ (8 \ lb)$$

This simple ration is perfectly adequate but could be enhanced with fresh apples or vegetables, etc. For those who like to make their own mix, the ration could be as shown in Table 18.9.

Along with his 9 kg (20 lb) of hay our event horse is going either to be fed 3.5 kg (8 lb) of performance cubes or 2 kg oats, 1 kg cubes, 0.5 kg bran and 0.5 kg beet pulp.

The first ration falls within his appetite of 12.5 kg. However, the second ration over-faces him by 0.5 kg, because lower energy feeds are being used. In most cases this small amount may not be of consequence, but a fussy feeder may let you know that the ration is rather too much for him.

Table 18.9   The final ration.

Feed	Quantity	Megajoules provided
Oats	2 kg (4.4 lb)	24
Sugarbeet pulp	0.5 kg (1 lb) dry weight	5
Bran	0.5 kg (1 lb)	5.5
Performance cubes	1 kg (2.2 lb)	13
Total		47.5

Step seven: Checking the protein level

Energy is the most important aspect of a performance horse's diet, and if good quality feed is being used the protein requirements are likely to be satisfied. However, growing youngstock and broodmares will have a high protein requirement and it is important to check the protein level in any ration that you have formulated.

Table 18.10   Protein requirements of horses.

Type of activity	Crude protein in the ration (%)
Light work	7.5–8.5
Medium work	7.5–8.5
Hard work	9.5–10
Fast work	9.5–10
Pregnant mare – first 8 months	7.5–8.5
Pregnant mare – last 3 months	10
Lactating mare – first 3 months	12.5
Lactating mare – last 3 months	11
Stallion	9.5–10
Weanling	16
Yearling	13.5
Two-year old	10

A horse in medium work requires 7.5–8.5% crude protein. The protein content of the ration can be worked out using the table of nutrient values.

Table 18.11 Protein in ration A.

Feed	Quantity (kg)	Protein content (%)	Protein in ration
Hay	9	6	54
Performance cubes	3.5	13	45.5
	12.5 kg		99.5

The percentage protein in the ration is therefore $\dfrac{99.5}{12.5} = 8\%$

If the oat-based ration is used the calculation would look like this:

Table 18.12 Protein in ration B.

Feed	Quantity (kg)	Protein content (%)	Protein in ration (g)
Hay	9	6.0	54
Oats	2	10	20
Cubes	1	13	13
Bran	0.5	15.5	7.75
Beet pulp	0.5	7	3.5
	13		98.25

The percentage protein in the ration is therefore $\dfrac{98.25}{13} = 7.6\%$.

This is adequate for a horse in medium work.

If the hay had been low in protein, say at 4.5% then these rations would be too low in protein and would need revising by using a high protein feed like soya or a performance cube.

Step eight: Check and adjust the ration
All horses are individuals and must be treated as such. Once a ration has been calculated and is being fed, the horse must be monitored to ensure that the ration is suitable.

- A supply of fresh clean water must be available to the horse at all times.

- The foods must be of good quality and acceptable to the horse – is the horse enjoying its food?
- Not only must the foods satisfy the horse's nutritional requirements, the horse must also be psychologically satisfied; it must not be bored and suffer a craving for roughage.
- The horse's condition must be checked by eye, tape or weighbridge. The horse may be gaining or losing weight. Is this what is wanted? If not, alter the ration accordingly. Horses have an optimum performance weight and should be kept as close as possible to this weight.
- The horse's temperament and behaviour may affect the ration fed. Part-bred horses may need more concentrates and less bulk as they are better doers and (usually) more placid. Routine and a quiet yard may save feed as horses are not fretting in their boxes.
- The horse's environment must be monitored. In a cold spell, more food and an extra blanket may be needed. A clipped horse may need more food to maintain its condition if it is not adequately rugged up. In hot weather horses may go off their concentrate ration, because their maintenance requirement has fallen; do not worry unless they start to lose condition.
- Horses must be regularly wormed and have their teeth checked for sharp edges.
- Some horses are poor doers, perhaps due to a gut damaged by worms early in life, and will always need extra attention to their feeding.

19 Practical Feeding and Watering

The 'rules of feeding'

To help us feed the horse several rules of good feeding have evolved. These include:

- Water before feeding.
- Feed little and often.
- Make any changes gradually.
- Feed only good quality, dust-free feed.
- Feed plenty of fibre and succulents.
- Keep feed utensils clean.
- Keep to regular feeding times.
- Feed according to work done, condition and temperament.
- Anticipate feeding requirements, e.g. reduce the amount of feed the day before a rest day.

Behaviour at feeding time

Like all animals horses can become protective at feeding time; this is particularly true in the field where the horse may feel in competition with others and may lash out or bite in an attempt to guard the feed. The feeder must be very aware and safety-conscious when feeding horses both in the stable and in the field.

Horses are individuals and have different feeding habits; some are always greedy, knocking over feed buckets in their enthusiasm while others are more cautious, eating only when the yard is quiet. It is important that the handler is aware of these habits so that any change from normal behaviour can be reported and acted upon immediately; a change in the horse's eating and drinking habits is often the first sign of illness. Once a horse has settled into a feeding routine it is unwise to change the type, time and method of feeding suddenly.

Feeding horses at grass

Hayracks must be of a safe design. The design often used for cattle
with a feeding trough underneath can allow seeds to drop into the
horse's eyes and may have sharp corners on which a horse can hurt
himself (Fig. 19.1). Some round cattle feeders are useful but must be of
a type where a horse cannot hit his head or become trapped. The rack
must be heavy enough not to be easily pushed over when empty.
Racks should be placed in a well-drained spot, away from the fence,
with good clearance all round. They should be moved regularly to
prevent poaching.

Haynets must be tied securely to a solid fence post or tree (Fig. 19.2)
and so that they hang just over the top of the horse's leg when empty,
or the horse may get a foot tangled in them. Obviously this is tricky if
you are feeding groups of horses as they will be different sizes; in this
case, hay is best fed on the floor – wastage is better than an accident.
One extra haynet or heap of hay should be put out than there are
horses and the nets or heaps should be well spaced so that kicking and
bullying is minimised.

Concentrate feeding should be supervised as it is a time when horses
can be very aggressive and accidents can happen. Always feed all the
horses at the same time or take the horse to be fed out of the field and
feed it out of sight of the others. There are a variety of buckets and
troughs that can be hung over a post-and-rail fence (Fig. 19.3)
although these can be knocked off and the contents spilt. Non-spill
feeders for feeding from the ground can be purchased including those
dropped into a close-fitting tyre. If feeding horses in yards, tethering
each horse before feeding ensures safety and that each horse has its
share of food.

Worming is covered in detail in Chapter 8.

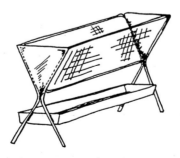

Fig. 19.1 Hayrack and feeder not suitable for horses.

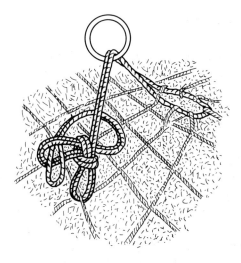

Fig. 19.2 A securely tied haynet.

Feeding the stabled horse

Most yards have a feed room containing secure, rodent-proof feed containers with a feed board stating how much and what type of feed each horse should receive in each feed. The quantity of feed may be expressed in 'scoops' in which case the amount of each different feed that a scoop holds should be known – horses should be fed by weight not volume. Some yards use a spring balance and the feed is weighed out for each horse. It is important that everybody understands the feed board and is able to make up feeds.

Horses may be fed in mangers built into the stable, plastic mangers over the door or in buckets on the floor. All utensils used in the preparation of feed, as well as mangers and buckets, must be washed

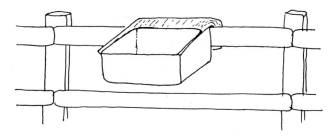

Fig. 19.3 A portable clip-on manger which can be hooked over a fence or the stable door.

out daily. Hygiene is part of good stable management; it helps in the prevention of disease and ensures that feeds are not tainted which may deter a fussy feeder.

Hay may be fed in haynets, hayracks or loose on the floor. Haynets allow a weighed amount to be fed easily. It is good practice to weight the amount of feed a horse receives – there is less wastage and the hay used can be accounted for. Hayracks are easy to use but can be difficult to empty if the horse does not eat all the hay; this sometimes means that rejected hay builds up, becoming less and less palatable. Feeding from the floor is more natural and allows the horse to sort through the hay, but tends to be wasteful with horses treading hay into the bed. A bale of hay weighs between 20 kg (44 lb) and 25 kg (55 lb) and usually falls into slices when the bale is opened, the slices varying in weight but often about 2 kg (4.4 lb).

If a mouldy and dusty bale is opened it should not be fed, nor should it be soaked in an attempt to make it more palatable. Dusty hay and feed can permanently damage the horse's lungs and handling dusty hay can cause illness in humans.

Simple rationing

The amount of feed a horse needs depends on many factors including:

- size
- condition
- age
- health
- breed
- appetite
- work done
- reproductive status
- environment
- temperament

In practice when a new horse arrives at the yard one has to decide what to put on the feed board immediately; there is no time to get out the calculator! The first thing to do is to decide the size and weight of the horse – large horses eat more than smaller ones. A weigh tape placed around the horse's girth (Fig. 19.4) will give an estimate of the horse's weight and Table 19.1 gives an approximate guide to the relationship of height to weight and the appetites of different weights of horses.

A horse will eat about 2.5% of his bodyweight each day, as seen in Chapter 18. Although in theory this is for the dry matter in food, hay and concentrates are about 80% dry matter, so the calculation works

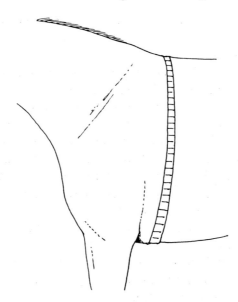

Fig. 19.4 Using a weigh tape. The tape is placed just behind the withers and in front of the girth groove.

well enough as a guide. Thus a 500 kg (1100 lb) horse will eat 12.5 kg (28 lb) of feed every day.

As discussed in Chapter 18 a rule of thumb that has been used for many years relates the intensity of the horse's work to the ratio of hay to concentrates fed (Table 18.4). The horse in light work will need more hay and less energy feed, while the horse in hard work will need less hay and a greater proportion of high energy feed.

Table 19.1   The relationship between height, girth, bodyweight and appetite.

Height (hands)	(cm)	Girth (cm)	(in)	Bodyweight (kg)	(lb)	Appetite (dry matter/day) (kg)	(lb)
11	111.7	135–145	54–58	200–260	440–572	4.5–6	10–13.5
12	121.9	140–150	56–60	230–290	506–638	5–7	11–15.5
13	132.0	150–160	60–64	290–350	638–770	6.5–8	14.5–18
14	142.2	160–170	64–68	350–420	770–924	8–9.5	18–21
15	152.4	170–185	68–74	420–520	924–1144	10–12.5	22.5–28
16	162.5	185–195	74–78	500–600	1100–1320	12–14	27–31.5
17	172.7	195–210	78–84	600–725	1320–1595	13–18	29–40

Table 18.4 showed the following guide figures for percentage hay to concentrate, at various work levels:

Resting   100/0
Light work   75/25
Medium work   60/40
Hard work   40/60
Racing   30/70

It is important to note that the low hay to high concentrate ration is the limit, and is only to be attempted by experienced trainers.

So we have agreed the likely weight of the horse, the amount of food it can cope with, the level of work it is doing and the division between hay and concentrates. For example:

● Our 16 hh riding horse weighs about 500 kg (1100 lb)
● He needs just over 12.5 kg (28 lb) of food per day (2.5% body weight)
● As he is in medium work he needs a maximum of 40% concentrates and 60% hay
● This gives 5 kg (11 lb) concentrates and 7.5 kg (16½ lb) hay

The next step is to decide what to feed.

Types of feed

Concentrates
Concentrates provide the horse with energy and protein in a less bulky form than hay or grass. Traditionally the horse has been fed cereal grains such as oats, barley and maize; these are high in energy and are suitable for the horse in medium and hard work. However, if fed in excess to horses in light work cereals have a 'heating' effect, making horses too boisterous and difficult to ride. This makes the low energy or 'non-heating' cube or coarse mix ideal for feeding to ponies and horses in light work. Cubes and coarse mixes are compound feeds containing a balanced mixture of energy, fibre, protein, fat, minerals and vitamins. They are formulated to be fed with hay or grass to meet all the nutritional requirements of the horse.

Oats
Oats are the traditional grain for feeding to horses. They can make up

all of the concentrate ration of a horse in hard work, but as they are high in phosphorus, limestone flour should be added to the ration. Oats are fed rolled or crimped, but once rolled they begin to lose their nutritional value and should be fed as soon as possible. A good sample of oats consists of plump, golden grains which are free from mould and dust.

Barley

Barley can be fed rolled but is often processed by steaming, micronisation or extrusion. Micronisation and extrusion are methods of cooking cereals to make them more digestible. Micronisation results in large rolled flakes similar to those found in the muesli we eat for breakfast, while extruded barley is reshaped into nuggets by passing it through metal dyes. Barley has a higher energy content than oats and is thus known as a fattening feed. When feeding rolled barley remember that a 'scoop' of barley is heavier and more rich in energy than a scoop of oats.

Maize

Maize is a high energy, low protein and low fibre cereal. It is generally fed steamed and rolled. Traditionally it is only fed as a small proportion of the diet of horses that are not 'good doers' or that lack condition.

Wheatbran

Traditionally bran was fed to bulk out the feed to stop the horse bolting his ration, or as a bran mash. Bran can hold much more than its own weight in water; thus a bran mash has a laxative effect on the gut and is useful if the horse suddenly has to be rested and there is a risk of azoturia. Azoturia is a metabolic disease which may occur when horses in full work and on full rations are rested. When the horse is brought back into work the muscles are said to 'tie-up'. Thus the ration must always be reduced when the horse's work load is reduced. A bran mash is also a palatable vehicle for oral medicines. Bran is deficient in calcium and very high in phosphorus and must be supplemented with limestone flour.

Sugar beet pulp

Sugar beet pulp is the dried remains of sugar beet once the sugar has been extracted. Most horses find it very palatable and it has a fair energy content and a high fibre content. The sugar is digested easily in the small intestine giving 'instant energy', while the fibrous part is fermented in the large intestine, releasing nutrients more slowly. Sugar beet pulp should be soaked before feeding. Shreds are soaked overnight for use the following day and just covered with water. Soak pellets for 12–24 hours using 1 kg (2.2 lb) of pellets in 2 l (3$\frac{1}{2}$ pt) of water. Horses can be fed up to 1 kg (2.2 lb) in dry weight of beet pulp per day; this results in about three scoops of wet sugar beet pulp.

Compound feeds

Compound feeds are convenience feeds for horses and have several advantages:

- convenience
- standardised diets for specific purposes
- constant quality
- good shelf life
- dust-free
- palatable
- uniform weight and size, making the feeding routine more convenient
- economy of labour, transportation and storage
- no wastage

However, there are some disadvantages:

- It is impossible to tell good quality from poor quality ingredients.
- The horse may find them boring to eat (or humans may assume they do).

The first problem can be overcome by always using products from reputable compounders and seeking advice from their nutritionists. The label on the bag has to declare, by law, certain ingredients, and this can be a useful reference; some manufacturers now include digestible energy and digestible crude protein, which is very useful. Remember that although straight feeds such as oats may look the same, you cannot see the protein and energy in them any more than you can in a cube. The bag that a cube comes out of states its feed value, a bag of oats does not have to do this. Oats can vary in their protein content by up to 8% from one season to the next or one farm to the next, so in order to meet the legally declared analysis the compounder must analyse the oats and then add a suitable protein supplement to balance a compound horse feed.

Feeding compounds

If we are honest few of us feed compounds as intended – we add oats or barley to them, believing that horses find them 'boring'. We must be careful not to make our horses fussy: why should cubes, properly fed, be any more boring than grass? To combat this coarse mixes were produced, muesli for horses! We think that these look nice and are good enough to eat and we can see what is in them, enough to induce us to pay extra for them. However, we continue to add grain to the mix, which unbalances the compound and defeats one of the reasons for feeding a compound – a convenient balanced ration in one bag. If you feel your horse needs more energy than the present cube is giving him, then buy a higher energy performance mix – there are plenty available.

If you are in any doubt, ring the manufacturer and ask for help. Any reputable company will have a technical adviser who should be able to answer your questions.

Chaff

Chaff is chopped hay and/or straw, usually with added molasses which is added to the feed to stop the horse eating too quickly. It is also useful for ponies on a low concentrate ration. Chaff and horse and pony cubes make a simple ration which can be fed safely by the most inexperienced feeder.

Forage

The design of the horse's digestive system means that he has a high requirement for roughage or fibre – it is his natural diet. The forage part of a horse's diet consists of grass – fresh or conserved as hay, haylage or silage.

All hay contains fungal spores. Soaking hay causes the spores to swell so they are eaten rather than inhaled; inhaling the spores can damage the horse's respiratory system. Evening hay should be soaked first thing in the morning and morning hay should be soaked at evening stables. Alternatively, haylage or silage can be fed. Mouldy or dusty hay should *never* be fed, or soaked in an effort to make it more palatable.

Silage is grass 'pickled in its own juice'. It has a high nutrient value in terms of energy and protein so the concentrate ration will have to be reduced. It can be fed to horses, but once exposed to air it needs eating within two or three days. It is not practical for many yards that lack specialist equipment to move it. Care should be taken to only feed quality silage, as horses have died after contracting botulism from earth-contaminated big bale silage.

Haylage is a compromise between hay and silage; the grass is packed in plastic bales varying in weight from 25 kg (55 lb) to 500 kg (1100 lb). The product is essentially fungal-spore-free and usually highly palatable. It too has a higher nutrient content than hay and may require the concentrate ration to be cut.

Additives and supplements

Additives, for example probiotics and enzymes, are added to an already balanced ration. They may have an indirect effect on the horse's health but they are not fed for their nutritional value.

Supplements are substances added to the horse's diet to balance it by satisfying deficiencies in certain nutrients, most often minerals, vitamins and amino acids.

However, both additives and supplements are not a recipe for success. Horses likely to require a supplement are stabled performance horses, growing youngsters, brood mares in late pregnancy and early lactation, old horses and those receiving poor-quality hay especially in winter. A traditional mixture of corn and hay provides inadequate amounts of calcium for young horses and lactating mares; they will need a supplement.

Supplements vary in complexity; one of the most simple supplements fed to horses is salt (sodium chloride), while at the other end of the scale there are broad-spectrum supplements containing many nutrients. Broad-spectrum supplements are formulated on the basis of the average horse being fed an average ration, making up for likely deficiencies. Some simple supplements cater for specific problems, e.g. biotin for hoof growth.

Guidelines for feeding supplements

- Never mix or overdose supplements.
- Remember that compound feeds are already supplemented; if being fed the amount of cubes recommended by the manufacturers, the horse should not need another supplement.
- Split the supplement between all the feeds.
- If feeding a hot feed like a mash, wait for it to cool down before

adding the supplement; otherwise nutrients may be denatured. If feeding a bran mash, be sure to add some limestone flour to compensate for the low calcium level in bran.

- As with any new feed, introduce supplements gradually, taking about a week to build up to the full dose.
- Mix the supplement thoroughly into the feed.

Salt

Whatever diet you are feeding you will need to add salt. The performance horse should have at least 40 g ($1\frac{1}{2}$ oz) per day of common salt added to his feeds, with a salt lick in the manger for insurance. Horses and ponies that are not working so hard could rely on a salt lick either in their manger or out in the field. Grazing horses that eat soil and bark are almost certainly seeking salt.

Calcium and phosphorus

On a grass/hay and cereal diet you will need to add calcium; 25–30 g ($\frac{3}{4}$–1 oz) per day of limestone flour is a minimum requirement. Most broad-spectrum supplements contain some calcium and phosphorus but not enough to balance the ration. Requirements will vary depending on the horse's diet, age and reproductive status.

Minerals and vitamins

A stabled horse is likely to require vitamins A, D and E, plus folic acid. A selection of B vitamins may be necessary for performance horses receiving more than 50% of their diet as concentrates. Of all the trace elements, inadequate intakes of copper, selenium, manganese, iodine and zinc are most frequently detected and should be included in a supplement. The form in which the mineral is fed can affect its availability to the horse as well as how it interacts with other nutrients, for instance iron affects the uptake of vitamin E. Unless you are feeding a high quality protein diet, you may have to feed supplements containing lysine and methionine.

Monitoring condition (Fig. 19.5)

Once a ration has been decided upon for a horse and written on the feed board it is vital to monitor that horse's reaction: Does he eat up?

Condition score	Back	Pelvis	Comment
4	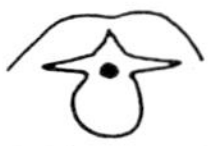	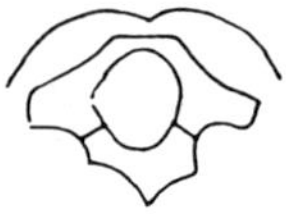	*Obese:* Large masses of fat carried on neck quarters and back. Can only feel ribs on pressure.
3	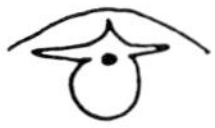	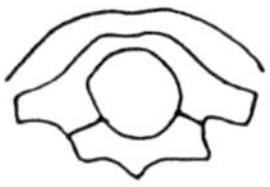	*Getting fat:* Bones becoming more difficult to feel. *Show horses.*
2	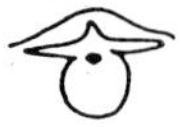	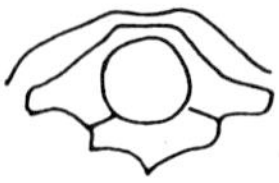	*Approaching normal:* Hip bones and vertebrae of back defined but not prominent. *Hunters & eventers.*
1	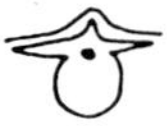	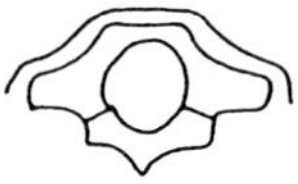	*Thin:* Bones still prominent but a little more muscle definition.
0	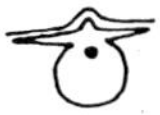	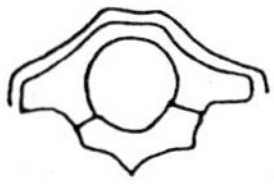	*Starvation:* Croup and hip bones sharp and prominent. Cut-up behind. Rib cage prominent.

Fig. 19.5 Monitoring condition.

Are temperament and performance affected? Is he gaining, losing or maintaining condition? A diet too high in energy may make the horse 'fizzy' and he will grow fatter, while too little energy will result in loss of condition and possibly a lethargic temperament. Some horses are naturally energetic no matter how little they are fed and it must be remembered that training, fitness and discipline will affect temperament. Remember too that a horse must be regularly wormed and have his teeth checked twice a year and rasped if necessary.

Preparation of feeds

Bran mash
Add the required amount of bran to a clean bucket. This is usually about 1.5 kg (3.3 lb), plus a teaspoon of salt and a sprinkling of oats if

the horse needs to be tempted to eat the mash. Pour on as much boiling water as the bran will absorb and stir well. Cover to retain the steam and leave to stand until cool. Before feeding stir in a heaped teaspoon of limestone flour. Correctly made the mash should have a crumbly texture. Molasses or cooked linseed can be added to make the mash more appetizing. A bran mash can be fed to tired horses the night before a rest day or after hard work.

Linseed jelly
Cover linseed with cold water and soak for 24 hours. Allow 0.5 kg (1 lb) linseed per horse. After soaking add more water and bring to the boil. Boil for 1–2 hours until the linseed is soft, taking care that it does not stick and burn. (Soaked linseed that has not been well boiled is poisonous.) Allow the linseed to cool and add the resulting jelly to the horse's feed. To make a linseed mash, add 1 kg (2.2 lb) of bran to soak up the fluid, cover and cool.

Boiled barley
Soak the barley for 12 hours. Then boil gently until the grains are just beginning to split and the water has been absorbed. Boiled barley can be added to every feed if the horse is lacking condition or added to a small feed for a tired horse.

Sugar beet pulp
Sugar beet shreds should be covered with water and soaked for 12 hours. Cubes or pellets should be covered in two-to-three times as much water and soaked for 24 hours. Sugar beet should be freshly made every day as it can ferment, especially in warm weather. Sugar beet pulp is a useful source of both fibre and energy for all horses; it helps the horse put on condition.

The nutrient requirements of elderly horses

Elderly horses need frequent attention to their teeth, as the loss of a tooth or the formation of sharp edges and hooks can cause considerable discomfort, leading to loss of condition. Consequently old horses may need food that is easy to chew; stemmy hay and whole oats would not be suitable as the horse's teeth would not be able to process the food sufficiently to allow adequate digestion.

Nutrition of the sick horse

Providing the horse with a balanced ration plays an important part in the horse's ability to fight illness, and correct nutrition provides one of the body's defence mechanisms. Proper feeding of the sick horse should always be considered as an integral part of the nursing and therapeutic regime.

The task of feeding a sick horse can be difficult and tiresome; the horse's appetite is likely to be depressed, swallowing may be difficult and the function of the gut may be disturbed. Any upset in gut function may lead to dehydration and a disturbance of the electrolyte balance (the ratio of salts in the body), all of which may occur just when the horse's metabolic requirements may be substantially greater. This means that there is often marked weight loss during illness, with a resultant decrease in the horse's defence capacity and prolonged illness and convalescence.

The sick horse's diet must have several special characteristics:

- palatability
- good quality protein
- fibre
- minerals and vitamins

Palatability

The sick horse must be provided with the most palatable feed possible to encourage eating. Barn-dried hay is ideal if the horse has previously been fed poor quality hay. Maize can be gradually introduced into the diet; it is acceptable and has a high energy content. Molasses, mashes and succulents can all be fed providing that the food is fresh. If swallowing is difficult the feeds should be soft and any carrots cut into very small pieces. If chewing is a problem the horse may need a liquid diet.

Feeding little and often is vital for the sick horse with up to eight feeds a day, including first thing in the morning and last thing at night. Any rejected food should be removed immediately. Soaking or damping the hay may help and will also mean that the horse is taking in water. A smear of vapour rub in the false nostril may mask the smell of medicines in the feed. Plenty of fresh clean water must always be available, and it should be changed frequently. If the horse is using an automatic drinking system, close it off and give the water by bucket so that you can monitor the amount the horse drinks.

Good quality protein

The protein content of the sick horse's diet is more important than the amount of energy the food is providing because the horse is not active, but protein is needed for the repair of body tissue. Good quality grass nuts, milk pellets, stud cubes and soyabean meal are all high in good quality protein; milk pellets have the advantage of being highly palatable. Care must be taken not to overfeed the horse as he recovers.

Fibre

Fibre is important in maintaining normal gut function, but as the fibre content of the diet increases so its digestibility falls and a compromise has to be reached. Molassed sugar beet pulp and bran are useful palatable sources of fibre and can be fed as mashes.

Minerals and vitamins

The sick horse may become severely dehydrated and it is important to supply a suitable source of electrolytes to help restore the fluid balance of the body. A supplement of minerals, vitamins and/or amino acids may be recommended by the vet, depending on the horse's blood profile; an anaemic horse would require iron, folic acid and vitamin B_{12} as well as his normal broad-spectrum supplement. As always calcium and salt are important.

Watering horses

Water makes up 65–75% of an adult horse's bodyweight and 75–80% of a foal's. Water is vital for life; it acts as a fluid medium for digestion and for the movement of food through the gut. It is necessary for growth and milk production and is needed to make good the losses through the lungs, skin, faeces and urine. Restricted water intake will depress the horse's appetite and reduce feed intake, resulting in loss of condition. Under most circumstances the horse should have free access to fresh, clean water at all times. After hard, fast work during which the horse has been denied water, care should be taken to cool the horse before allowing him substantial amounts of water. Excessive consumption of cold water by hot horses can cause colic or laminitis.

The 'rules of watering'

- A constant supply of fresh clean water should always be available.
- If this is not possible, water at least three times a day in winter and six times a day in summer. In this situation always water before feeding.
- Water a hot or tired horse with water which has had the chill taken off it. (This is sometimes confusingly called 'chilled water'.)
- If a bucket of water is left constantly with the horse, swill out the bucket and change the water at least twice a day, topping it up as necessary throughout the day. Standing water becomes unpalatable.
- Horses that have been deprived of water should be given small quantities frequently until their thirst is quenched. They must not be allowed to gorge themselves on water.
- During continuous work, water the horse as often as possible, at least every two hours. Hunters should be allowed to drink on the way home.
- If horses have a constant supply of fresh clean water there should be no need to deprive the horse of water before racing or fast work. However, the horse's water can be removed from the stable two hours before the race or competition, if thought necessary.

The horse at grass

Access to rivers and streams can be a good way of watering horses at grass provided that the river contains running water with a gravel bottom and a good approach. Shallow water and a sandy bottom may result in small quantities of sand being ingested, collecting in the stomach and eventually causing sand colic.

Ponds tend to be stagnant and are rarely suitable; usually it is best to fence them off and provide alternative watering arrangements.

Filled from a piped water supply, field troughs provide the best method of watering horses at grass. Troughs should be from 1 to 2 m (3 to 6 ft) in length and about 0.5 m (18 in) deep. There must be an outlet at the bottom so that they can be emptied and scrubbed regularly. The trough should be on well drained land, clear of trees so that the ground around the trough does not get poached and the trough does not fill up with leaves. During freezing weather troughs should be checked twice a day and the ice broken if necessary. They must be free from sharp edges or projections, such as a tap, which might injure a horse.

If the trough is tap-filled, the tap should be at ground level and the pipe from the tap to the trough fitted close to the side and edge of the trough. The best method is to have a self-filling ball cock arrangement in an enclosed compartment at one end of the trough. Ideally the trough should be sited along a fence or recessed into it (Fig. 20.2), rather than at right angles to it or in front of it. If not in the fence line the trough should be at least three to four horse's lengths into the field so that there is free access all round and horses cannot be trapped behind it.

The stabled horse
Stabled horses are usually offered water in buckets or automatic drinkers, both of which have advantages and disadvantages.

Buckets
Buckets can be placed on the floor, in the manger, hung in brackets or suspended from a hook or ring at breast height. They should be placed in a corner away from the manger, hayrack and door, but should still be visible from the door for checking. Providing water in buckets is time-consuming, heavy work and wasteful on water; they must be emptied, swilled out and refilled at least twice a day, and topped up three or four times a day. Horses frequently knock buckets over and may damage themselves by getting a leg caught between the bucket and the metal handle. However, they have three advantages: you can monitor how much the horse is drinking – a change in a horse's drinking habits may be the first sign of illness; buckets are a very simple method of providing water which cannot go wrong; they are cheap – though the cheapest buckets will not last long.

Automatic drinkers
Although expensive to install, automatic drinkers (Fig. 19.6) are an asset in a large yard, saving time and effort. They should be fairly deep

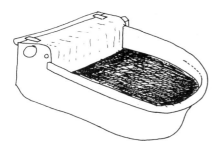

Fig. 19.6 Automatic drinker.

so that the horse can take a full drink, they should be cleaned out regularly, sited away from the manger and hayrack, and well-insulated to stop the pipes freezing in winter. Some horses are reluctant to drink from the small noisy automatic drinkers and water intake cannot be easily monitored. Each drinker should have its own tap so that if it malfunctions, or one needs to monitor the horse's water intake using buckets, it can be switched off.

20   The Horse at Grass

The horse's natural environment is at grass; it evolved as a nomadic grazer, roaming freely over an extensive area which provided it with food, exercise, shelter when needed. As the horse grazed it left its droppings behind it, so avoiding the build-up of a worm problem. However, man has enclosed the horse in intensively grazed paddocks, effectively putting the dining room and the loo in the same area – hardly an ideal situation!

At one time, horses in England were only turned out to grass during their rest season. This is still the case with most hunters, which are kept at grass during the summer thus giving them a rest from work. However, many horses are kept wholly at grass throughout the year. This is a method practised by many private owners. Another possibility is the combined system, whereby the stabled horse spends part of each day at grass and the remainder in its stable.

Requirements of a paddock

Horses need daily attention even when turned out at grass. From the owner's point of view easy access at all times of the year is important. A paddock near the house is ideal but not always possible. Adjacent activities should also be considered: a railway line may be tolerable but not, perhaps, a go-kart track.

Owners should also consider how the land lies: a level field is to be preferred to a steep one. Steep fields can create stress for exuberant Thoroughbreds and youngsters. They also limit the possibilities of ridden exercise within the field.

The aspect of the paddock is also significant. A field is warmer if it faces south, and the grass will grow earlier in the spring. Trees and hedges are a great asset, as they provide natural shelter from wind and rain as well as shade from the sun in the summer. If there is no natural shelter, an artificial field shelter or wind-break should be provided (see Fig. 20.1).

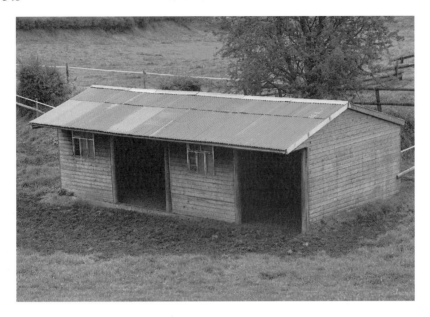

Fig. 20.1 A field shelter.

In winter-time, horses will tend to eat from the bark of trees, so ideally trees within reach should be protectively fenced.

Adequate fencing of the field boundaries is essential. Hazard areas, such as rabbit holes and obstructions, must also be fenced. Large stones and rubbish such as old corrugated iron sheeting should be removed. The use of barbed wire should be avoided.

Soil type is of great significance. Light sandy soils stay dry all year round, but they grow poor grass, particularly in midsummer. However, they are best for riding on, and this may well be an important consideration. Heavy clay soils (even with drains) get deep and muddy in winter. They are slow to start grass growth in spring, but they are productive. A serious disadvantage is the tendency of such soils to go so hard in midsummer that they are a hazard to ride on. Loam, a mixture of sand, silt and clay, is a good compromise between the two extremes.

Paddocks should be properly drained. Good drainage is essential to avoid 'poaching' or treading of the ground. Also, a cold waterlogged soil will not warm up and start growing grass as quickly in the spring. Drains are expensive to install and should be kept in good order. Ditches should be tended regularly and, if there is a drainage problem, expert advice should be sought.

The paddock must have an adequate water supply. This may be either natural or artificial. Stagnant ponds are best fenced off, and the ideal natural supply is an unpolluted running stream, preferably with a good stone bed. Sand or mud is easily stirred up by horses and can result in colic when swallowed over a long period.

Water troughs must be properly sited and adequately protected (Fig. 20.2). They should be of good construction and preferably purpose made. A trough which has a sharp edge at knee height, such as an old bath, can injure horses, and any ball-cock or other projections should be well protected from inquisitive horses. Pipes rising from the ground should be protected against frost.

A trough sticking out from a fence is not really ideal. The ground around the trough will tend to get poached in winter, and hence it is best to excavate the top soil, lay a builder's permeable membrane, and then cover the area with stone topped with sand. The same procedure should be followed in gateways and in front of field shelters if the field is to be used during the winter months.

Good fencing is pleasing to the eye and a good investment, both financially and otherwise. It reduces worry about stock getting hurt or straying. Fencing must be safe and tidy, must stand up to pressure, must be easily maintained and not easily chewed, and must be fairly

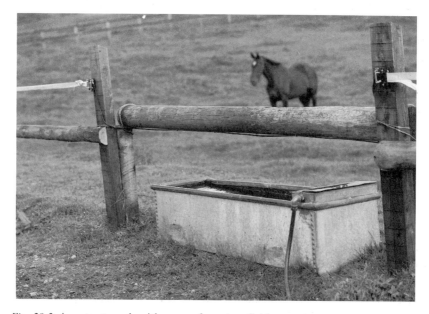

Fig. 20.2 A water trough with access from two fields.

inexpensive. A good fence is plain high-tensile wire with strong straining posts, with the bottom strand of wire 0.3 m (1 ft) from ground level. The traditional post-and-rail fencing is excellent, though on the costly side. Well-creosoted rails are not usually chewed but tanalised ones are.

A possible compromise fence is to have a strand of taut plain wire along the top of the fence about 2.5 cm (1 in) above the top rail to prevent chewing, with a rail or two below it and a plain wire at the bottom. If cattle are also to be fenced against, the lower strand should run through insulators and be electrified. If this precaution is not taken, cattle may graze under the wire and tend to push the fence over.

Where sheep are a problem, a different type of fencing is needed: special sheep wire is available. An alternative is to have two lower strands of wire which must be kept taut for safety.

Several substitutes for wooden rails are now available in both metal and rubberised webbing. They are strong, durable and maintenance free, but must be erected with considerable tension to stay stock-proof and smart.

Where it is necessary to create a temporary partition in a field, as for strip grazing or to prevent horses coming right up to the permanent fence, an electric fence can be used. This should be of the type specially designed for horses, with a broad and easy-to-see band.

Paddock management

The owner's aim is to provide nourishing food for as long as possible during the year. This requires a sward of good nutritious grasses and a base that will stand up to the wear and tear imposed by stock. A further consideration is to try to reduce reliance on drugs for controlling parasites. This can be achieved in three main ways: (a) the use of mixed grazing; (b) rotational grazing; and (c) good grass husbandry. In small paddocks near to home it is important to keep the field as free as possible of droppings, by collecting them on a regular basis before they have time to cause trouble.

The division of land so that good management can be practised raises problems of stocking rates and size of paddocks. The question of size includes so many variables that it is difficult to be specific. Any clear-cut answer is open to misinterpretion. However, assuming 16-hand horses weighing about 500 kg each, with well-managed paddocks on loam soil about one horse per acre (which is just over two per hectare) is about right. This stocking rate allows for some poaching of the ground in winter, with its inevitable effect on grass production in summer. Even without the use of fertilisers, there will be too much grass in summer unless some is conserved. If the best use is to be made of land, large fields will be split into paddocks. Hopefully, only one paddock will then become poached in winter.

During the summer the horses should be moved from paddock to paddock in rotation, with each paddock having at least three weeks' rest. When a paddock has been grazed and the horses have been moved on, fertiliser should be broadcast on it and the paddock should be rested. Horses should not be allowed to graze on a fertilised paddock where the granules can still be seen, as this would risk colic or poisoning through ingestion of the chemical.

Grass for horses should not be very lush or high in nitrogen content. If a high-N compound fertiliser is used, it should be at a lower dosage than that advised for cattle. A typical pattern might be a 20 : 10 : 10 analysis at 200 kg per hectare when the grass starts to grow in spring. Thereafter, just 100 kg per hectare of straight nitrogen fertiliser should be applied after each grazing, although considerably more should be applied before a hay cut. After a conservation cut, a fertiliser with extra potash is often used to make good the nutrients taken from the land.

Excess grass in summer calls either for extra stock (horses, cattle or sheep) or conservation. It can be sold to a farmer to take for hay or silage. There are problems in taking hay for one's own use unless the acreage is sufficient to justify owning the equipment. Agricultural contractors can be employed to take hay, but horse-owners are often their smallest and least important customers. Thus, the hay is not turned often enough or will be baled wet or old and the hay will be poor. Good hay can be made by hand, using old-fashioned tripods, if one has the time and energy.

The advantage of cattle and sheep is that they tidy up the pasture and consume the worms that damage horses but not themselves (Fig. 20.3). Cattle and sheep need especially strong fencing to restrain them. If the extra stock are one's own, when winter comes some of them must be housed or sold; however, sheep do not poach land to the extent that horses or cattle do.

Where land is poached after the winter, a good harrowing aerates the soil and levels the surface for grazing. If a good riding surface is required, the harrowing should be followed by a ring- or flat-roll. The timing of this treatment is critical to the day.

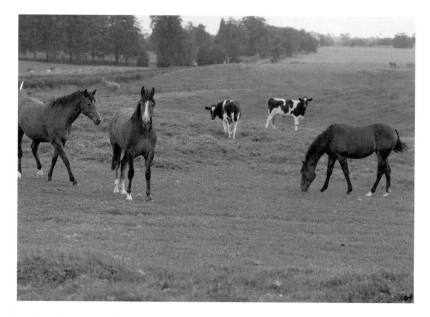

Fig. 20.3 Mixed stocking can be financially beneficial and is good for the pasture.

As the summer progresses, the pasture should be mowed to top weeds and rejected grasses. This is especially desirable if only horses are kept. Mowing is important, because without it all the wrong plants will prosper. On very hot days, the field may be chain-harrowed to scatter horse droppings in the hope that the sun will dry out and kill both worm eggs and larvae.

Pasture improvement

Poor pasture can always be improved. Pasture improvement is an aspect of horse management that is ignored by many people. The foundation of good pasture is the soil, and just as the gardener can improve his vegetable patch, so can the paddock-owner improve his soil. A sandy soil will benefit from organic manure; this helps to hold both nutrients and moisture. A clay soil will benefit most from drainage.

The acidity of the soil is important and should be considered every five years or so. The local lime company's representative will take soil samples and analyse them. Acidity is measured on a pH scale, with 7 being neutral. Lower numbers are acid and higher numbers alkaline.

For grass a pH of 6.5 is about right. If the soil is too acid, the wrong plants prosper, and if it is too alkaline, the grass cannot take up certain minerals from the soil. This is bad for the nutrition of growing stock. If the soil is very alkaline, a good dressing of farmyard manure will tip the balance towards acidity. If possible, horse manure should be avoided as it may contain worm eggs.

Acid soil (pH 6 or lower) needs different treatment, and a good dressing of lime or ground chalk should be applied.

Apart from calcium (which is in lime and generally freely available in the soil) the main nutrients to consider are nitrogen (N), phosphorus (P_2O_5 is phosphate) and potassium (K_2O is potash). Nitrogen is leached out of the soil by rain and so is only used during the growing season. Phosphates and potash are needed for plant efficiency. Local agricultural merchants can put paddock owners in touch with a fertiliser representative who knows the soil types in the locality. If there are likely to be phosphate or potash deficiencies, he will advise the appropriate compound fertiliser to use.

However, too much quick-acting phosphate will upset the horse's calcium : phosphorus balance. Some people are anxious about the use of 'chemical fertilisers' and prefer to use those with an organic base. These are generally slower acting and more expensive, but they provide some minor nutrients which the soil might lack and they may well be free of fluoride which is often found in compound fertilisers. Owners of breeding stock will be anxious that their mares cycle regularly and produce healthy foals every year. They should, therefore, consider soil nutrition as it affects horse nutrition.

Phosphate encourages clover which produces free nitrogen from nodules on its roots. A little clover is desirable in the sward; one plant of wild white clover for each square metre is sufficient. An excess of clover makes the herbage too rich for horses.

The bulk of the sward should come mainly from a late-flowering perennial ryegrass of prostrate growth. A grass called S23 meets this need. Creeping red fescue is productive and gives a good turf; crested dog's-tail also resists treading. In dryer areas, a little smooth-stalked meadow grass may be added to the mixture, and in wetter areas rough- stalked meadow grass is good. Cocksfoot is hard-wearing but grows into clumps. Timothy is persistent, and most horses prefer tall fescue.

The main ingredients in the grass mixture should be represented by two similar varieties. A suitable seed mixture for a hard-wearing, palatable and productive paddock might be as follows:

Species	kg/ha
Perennial ryegrass (two varieties)	18
Creeping red fescue	5
Crested dog's-tail	1
Rough- or smooth-stalked meadow grass	2
Cocksfoot, timothy, tall fescue (two of each)	6
Wild white clover	1
	33 (30 lb/acre)

This mixture is mainly for grazing, but an occasional cut of hay may be taken from the sward. It is best not to put herbs into the mixture as they make it harder to use weedkillers (called herbicides!) and for hay to dry out. However, horses like herbs, the deep roots of which bring up minerals from the soil. A compromise can be achieved by hand-sowing a strip of herbs along the fence. These herbs should include chicory, ribwort, yarrow and burnet.

Horse pasture is rarely ploughed up, but the mixture suggested can be used to renovate old pastures as well as to create new ones. If a paddock is thin, renovate by mixing the seed with fertiliser, applying by means of a spinner or by hand-broadcasting. Seeding must be done in spring or autumn. Chain-harrow before seeding and ring-roll afterwards.

Topping and selective scything will control weeds. Ragwort needs pulling and burning, and docks, thistles and bracken can be spot-treated using a knapsack sprayer. Major infestations need specialist herbicides, and if necessary expert advice should be sought. Excess clover is reduced by taking a hay crop or by spraying with a herbicide that contains MCPA and is designed to kill broad-leaved plants.

Many fields are badly neglected but can be renovated without too much difficulty. A suggested programme might be: make good the fencing, water, drainage and lime. Put in a herd of cattle to eat it bare, harrow hard, fertilise, seed and roll. Make the early grazings light using sheep and avoid using cattle until the grass is well established. The routine then is horses, cattle, top if necessary, fertilise and rest. This cycle is then repeated. Grazing too tight (5 cm; 2 in) should be avoided, as should letting the grass get so long that treading wastes good food.

Working from grass

Many advantages are claimed for grass-kept horses. It is a natural system, and has much to recommend it. Less straw and hay are used and less time is spent on routine management. The horses need not be ridden because they exercise themselves.

This system has corresponding disadvantages. The horse is often too fat in summer, and in winter it is often wet and muddy. Where a horse is kept at grass, it should be caught up and handled daily if possible. Supplementary feeding will be necessary in wintertime, and where there is insufficient grass during the summer as well.

It is easier to operate on the 'combined system' where the horse spends part of each day at grass and part in its stable. Thus, in summer the horse, or more particularly the pony, is shut in for part of the day to limit its food intake and also to protect it from flies. In winter the horse may be stabled at night or else shut in well in advance of being ridden so that it can be dried off. This is an ideal method for keeping hunters.

Horses working from grass in winter will usually be given a trace or blanket clip. This makes grooming easier and the horse can gallop about without undue sweating. A clipped horse will need a good New Zealand rug. The best designs have two straps at the front, a well-fitted back and good leg straps so that the rug will stay in place even when the horse rolls.

The unclipped horse can stay out without a rug, but its long coat means that there is the problem of drying its back in wet weather before saddling up. The best method is to put it in the stable with a thatch of straw, lightly covered with a cut-open lightweight sack held in place with a loosely fastened surcingle. After half an hour or so, the worst of the mud may be brushed off. It is undesirable to remove the natural protective grease from an unclipped horse living at grass, and so only a dandy brush should be used. If the back is not cleaned before saddling up, mud will be ground into both the saddle and the horse's back, which could cause sores.

A wet horse must not be left in the stable after riding. If it is to remain stabled, it should be thatched. If the horse is to be turned out, this should be done straightaway so that the horse can roll and keep on the move. A cold, draughty stable and a wet horse will soon lead to a chill.

A variant of the traditional system which, although expensive in initial outlay, offers many advantages of the paddock without the mess, is that of the shelter/stable with a free-draining sand yard attached (see Fig. 20.4). The ever-increasing cost of bedding and labour means that this system will become more important.

Whether in field, yard or stable, there is always the problem of how best to feed hay and concentrates. In the field, concentrates may be fed in bowls. Those set in car tyres are good as they tip less easily and have fewer sharp edges. Bowls should be spaced out and it is a good idea to have one more bowl than the number of horses as there will be plenty of swapping when the greedy see off the timid. Hay can be fed on the ground along the fence line to reduce treading. On clay fields, the fence line soon becomes poached. Nets are laborious and a slight hazard, and hay racks tend to be wasteful. Feeding hay in a shed may induce

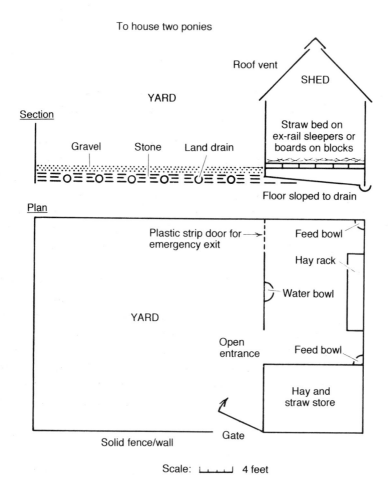

Fig. 20.4 Accommodation with exercise area.

kicking or biting. If available, cheap plastic pods set along the fence are the best answer. Hay is pushed in at one end of a tube, which is like a flute, and the horses pull it out through the holes.

Management routine

When horses are kept solely at grass, a daily visit is essential. The experienced eye will spot small details that may give a clue to more significant events.

Is the horse always standing away from hedges bordering roads because children throw stones at it? Is the good summer weather going to produce a heavy crop of acorns, which will fall and be of sufficient quantity to poison the horse if eaten? Is the coat 'staring', indicating an increased worm burden? These are the sort of questions to ask. Changes are sometimes so slight that only a visit with someone who has not seen the horse for several weeks may draw attention to subtle changes.

The daily check of the horse at grass is usually made entirely by eye. The horse should be looked over for injuries. Particular attention should be paid to the feet. A hand run under the belly, down the legs and over the back may detect something which the eye has missed. This last check may need two people for safety and convenience: it may be carried out weekly. It is a good plan to have a hoof pick and to lift, inspect and pick out the feet at least once a week.

The daily check must include the water supply and the general state of the field, including the grass. By October, for example, grass has less feed value, and hay or concentrates may need to be started or increased.

The field boundary should be walked regularly and any fencing defects noted and made good. Areas by footpaths, public roads or people's gardens all need regular checks for items thrown away, particularly wire, tin, glass or rubber. Like litter collecting, weed removal needs constant attention: poisonous plants such as woody nightshade, foxglove and so on should be uprooted and removed. Ragwort repays pulling up. Docks and thistles do not spread if the field walker carries a sharp billhook or light scythe and constantly tops them.

Horse people have a bad name because of fields that are a mess of mud and weeds, fallen-down jumps, botched-up fencing and tatty buildings. This reputation should be scotched by careful appraisal by the field-owner, and by good husbandry and constant vigilance.

21   Travelling Horses

Travelling is an important aspect of horse care today. Loading, unloading and travelling are hazardous procedures and it is vital to be well prepared and well practised to minimise the risk of accidents; once a horse has had a bad experience or has travelled badly he can become very reluctant to load and can panic when on the move.

Clothing for travelling

Horses wear rugs and protective clothing during travelling; what they wear depends on several factors including:

- time of year
- weather
- length of journey
- whether the horse is alone or in company
- how well the horse travels
- type of vehicle

The equipment needed includes the following (see also Fig. 21.1):

- headcollar, rope and poll guard
- sweat rug or thermal travelling rug
- surcingle or roller
- in winter the horse should wear the equivalent of his normal day rugs
- travelling boots or bandages with knee boots, hock boots and coronet boots
- tail bandage and tail guard

Spare rugs should be available in case the rugs get wet or the horse sweats profusely.

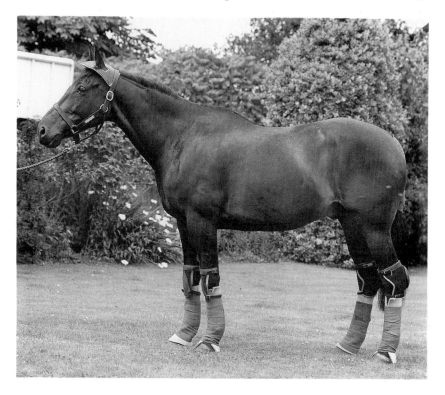

Fig. 21.1 Horse partially dressed for travelling.

Procedure before travelling

Vehicles and trailers must be regularly serviced and checked thoroughly before any journey. Checks should include: the floor and tyres of the trailer including tyre pressure; oil; water; petrol; battery; and lights.

Once the trailer has been hitched up check:

- the coupling hitch and safety chain
- indicators, side lights, brake lights and the internal light
- the jockey wheel and cables are clear of the ground

It is useful to carry insurance and registration documents as well as your driver's licence. Up-to-date maps and small first-aid kits for both horses and humans are essential. After travelling, the vehicle should be skipped out, the floor swept and left to dry. It is advisable to do this immediately so that the floor is protected from the rotting effect of urine and wet patches. If the weather is suitable the floor may be scrubbed and hosed. Remember to lift the rubber matting regularly so that the floor underneath can be cleaned and left to dry out.

Loading a horse into a vehicle

Loading a fractious horse into a vehicle can be dangerous for both horse and handler and it is wise to think ahead if you do not know how the horse is going to behave. The procedure is as follows:

(1) Position the vehicle alongside a wall so that the horse can only escape one side. Make sure that the gap is very small so that the horse is not tempted to run between the wall and the vehicle.

(2) Avoid slippery surfaces – concrete and tarmac tend to be slippery. If the horse is going to be awkward it may be better to park on grass.

(3) Bed down the floor with straw or shavings so that it looks inviting and is less noisy and slippery.

(4) Swing back and secure the partitions so that the horse is not having to enter a narrow space. It may be better to remove the partitions completely if possible.

(5) Open the jockey door or the front of front-unload trailers so that it is light inside the vehicle and the horse can see a way out.

(6) Make sure the ramp is level and firm so that it does not shift under the horse's weight.

(7) It is very important to have enough experienced help if you suspect that the horse will be difficult; even with well behaved horses it is useful to have an assistant standing by the side of the ramp. The assistant should not stare at the horse as he approaches – nothing stops a horse going forward more quickly (Fig. 21.2).

(8) The handler standing at the horse's shoulder should lead the horse forward and straight up the ramp (Fig. 21.3). It is important not to pull on the horse's head. If he stops, give him a pat, look ahead and walk forward. If he pulls back, do not get into a fight but move back with him until he is happy to move forward.

(9) Once the horse is inside the vehicle, do not duck under the breast bar but stand by his shoulder until the back is secured by

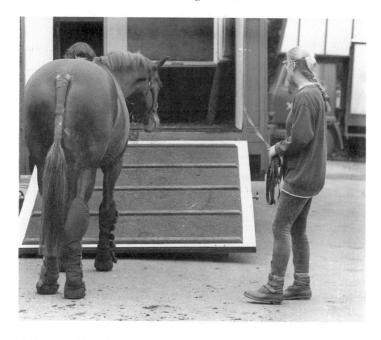

Fig. 21.2 Approaching the horsebox.

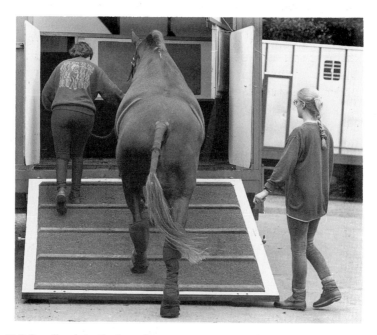

Fig. 21.3 Loading into the horsebox.

the assistant. The assistant should stand to one side when lifting the ramp so that if the horse does rush backwards the ramp will not fall on them.

(10)   Once the ramp has been lifted and secured tie the horse to a loop of string so that he cannot swing round but not so tight that he cannot balance himself. The string should be breakable string so that if the horse panics and goes down the string will release him.

If you are on your own then the horse should be loaded in exactly the same way but using a lunge line instead of a lead rope; once the horse is loaded, the lunge line can be threaded through the tie-ring and the tension on the horse's head maintained as the handler backs down the ramp and lifts it. It is important that the horse does not learn that he can rush back down the ramp so never load on your own until the horse is reliable.

Coping with a shy loader

Horses can become difficult to load for many reasons including:

- Reluctance to leave the other horses – position the vehicle out of sight and earshot of other horses.
- Fear of the enclosed space or steep ramp.
- Habit – some horses are 'trained' not to load by inexperienced handlers.
- Memories of a bad journey or forceful loading.

Loading difficult horses should not be undertaken lightly; all handlers should be suitably dressed, including gloves, suitable shoes and a hard hat. The equipment needed includes a lunge whip and two lunge lines, food in a bucket, a snaffle bridle for control or a lunge cavesson.

The horse should be quietly led to the ramp and allowed to look where he is going. If he has a quiet temperament, first one front leg and then the other can be lifted and placed on the ramp, making much of him at each step. If the horse moves back, follow him and start again. This way his confidence can be gradually built up until he is happy to enter the trailer. If a quiet or stubborn horse is not liable to kick, two people can link fingers behind the horse's hindquarters and push him up once his front feet are on the ramp.

Alternatively a lunge line can be buckled to each side of the vehicle, the lines held by two assistants and crossed behind the horse's hindquarters to encourage him forwards. Some horses give in as soon as they realise there is no means of escape while others can lash out or rear against the lunge lines so care must be taken.

Young horses or horses that are reluctant to leave their companions may load more readily if a companion is loaded first. They can gain confidence from the fact that the other horse is not worried by the ramp or the enclosed space. Once the 'problem' horse is loaded, the companion can be unloaded, but take care that the horse does not panic once his friend has gone. Young horses may benefit from the company of an experienced traveller during their first few journeys.

Transporting horses

Many horses become reluctant to load, especially into trailers, after they have experienced a bad journey or forceful loading. Prevention is better than cure:

- Avoid sudden braking, rapid acceleration and fast cornering.
- Use the gears with brakes to decelerate gently into a corner or to a halt.
- Pull away from a standstill or out of a bend steadily.
- Pay attention when travelling over a rough or uneven surface.
- Remember that horses can become frightened if they have previously had a bad experience travelling.
- Overhanging branches and uncut hedges along narrow lanes can be very frightening.
- Trailers towed too fast can start to sway and become so unstable that they jacknife or turn over.
- A speed of 30–35 mph (48–56 km) on normal roads is suitable for most vehicles.

Unloading a horse from a vehicle

The vehicle should be parked in a safe, suitable place with enough room around it. The horse must be untied before the partition, front bar or breeching strap is undone. Many horses can become quite

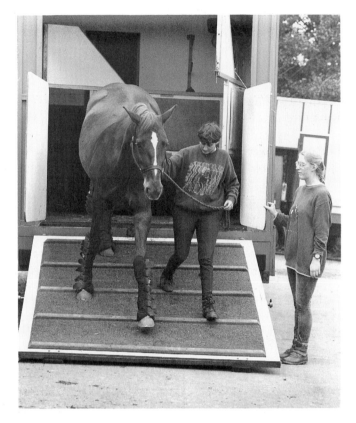

Fig. 21.4 Unloading.

excited in anticipation of being unloaded; they must not be allowed to rush or jump off the ramp (Fig. 21.4).

Care of the horse when travelling

The horse should be kept warm in winter and cool in summer, but remember that the vehicle and the number of horses will influence the temperature and the air available. A single horse in a trailer may get cold, even in summer, while a lorry with three or four horses may become very warm even in winter.

There must be adequate fresh air but no draughts; many lorries are very poorly ventilated. It is better to put an extra rug on the horse and have more air than a warm stuffy environment.

A non-slip floor which makes minimum noise and hence disturbance to the horse will help the horse travel more calmly as will ensuring that horses have adequate space and that the vehicle has suitable suspension.

Travelling mares and foals, inexperienced travellers and stallions

Some horses have special requirements during travelling. A mare and foal will require about twice as much room as normal; the mare should be tied up while the foal travels loose. The partitions may need to be adapted so that the foal cannot pass under them.

Inexperienced or very poor travellers may prefer to travel loose in a large area so that they can find a position that suits them. Studies have shown that travel stress is reduced when horses travel backwards.

Stallions need special partitions to prevent them biting the horse next to them. Alternatively they can be muzzled.

Feeding and watering on journeys

One of the major problems horses experience when travelling long distances is dehydration; it is very important to offer the horse water at frequent intervals. If the horse is sweating it is wise to include some electrolytes. Some horses are more fussy about water than they are about food so take some water from home in a couple of containers so that the taste of unfamiliar water does not put the horse off drinking. If he refuses to drink try adding a little molasses to the water at home so that you can do the same at your destination and disguise the different taste. Fortunately most horses will drink when they are thirsty, no matter what the water tastes like!

The horse will spend a long time standing still during the journey so to avoid swollen legs or any other metabolic upsets the concentrate ration must be reduced. However, in order to avoid loss of condition, allow the horse plenty of good quality hay during the journey so that the gut is kept moving and partially full the whole time; this will reduce the risk of colic. Concentrate feeds should be small, easily digested and given at regular intervals. The horse may be given a bran mash the evening before the journey and only hay or a very small feed, including bran, the morning before setting off.

22 Lungeing

Why lunge?

Lungeing is carried out for many reasons:

- to train the young horse
- to retrain or improve the older horse
- to train the rider
- to exercise the horse
- to warm a horse up prior to ridden work
- for the pleasure of working a horse from the ground

Some people only lunge mature horses when the roads are too icy to ride on or some other reason prevents their normal riding routine. However, lungeing is a pleasant and useful part of the gymnastic preparation of every equine athlete; the hunter, dressage horse, show jumper, eventer, racehorse, carriage horse and so on will all benefit from lungeing if done well. Similarly it is a pleasing skill in which the lunger gains satisfaction from the quality of the performance. Good lungeing improves a horse's obedience and can be used to build up muscle in the horse as well as developing his rhythm, balance, suppleness and willingness to go forward.

The lungeing equipment

- Bridle – if the horse is being lunged for exercise a snaffle bridle with the noseband and reins removed may be used. If the horse is being warmed up prior to work the horse's normal bridle should be used.
- Lungeing cavesson – this has a padded noseband with three metal rings attached at the front. The lunge rein is fitted to the central ring (Fig. 22.1).

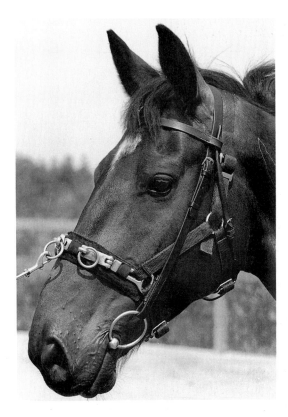

Fig. 22.1 Lungeing cavesson and snaffle bridle.

- Lunge rein, about 10 m (33 ft) long with a large loop at one end and a swivel joint attached to a buckle or clip at the other.
- Side reins.
- Saddle or roller adequately padded with a numnah or pad.
- Breastplate – this may be necessary to stop the roller or saddle slipping backwards.
- Brushing boots.
- Lunge whip.
- Gloves.

Fitting lungeing equipment

The lungeing cavesson has a thick padded noseband which has to be fastened tightly. To achieve this the cavesson noseband of the bridle must either be removed or lie just below the protruding cheekbones. The lungeing cavesson can then be fastened immediately below the noseband of the bridle. Some lunge cavessons fasten below the bit like a drop noseband. The throatlash of the cavesson, if fitted, should not be tight and, as with a bridle, should allow four fingers to be inserted inside the slack.

Further down the cheekpiece, another strap called the cheek or jowl strap should be pulled tight as it helps to stop the cavesson twisting. Care must be taken with a strong horse in case the cavesson pulls round and the cheek strap moves close to the eye. The lunge cavesson should be set over the bridle but the noseband of the cavesson normally goes under the cheekpieces of the bridle to avoid interference with the action of the bit. However, this is not possible with some nylon cavessons. If the bridle has reins attached for riding later, the reins should be twisted under the throat and then passed over the head and secured by passing the throatlash through the loop thus formed.

The lunge line should be clipped or buckled to the centre ring on the front of the lunge cavesson. This ring and the lunge line may be fitted with a swivel; one or other is essential to stop the lunge line twisting as it comes off the coils from the lunger's hands. The lunge line should be soft, strong and long; sharp-edged nylon lines should never be used.

The side reins should be about 2 m (6 ft 6 in) long with a clip at one end and a buckle at the other. The horse should be fitted with a suitable roller with a 'D' ring on each side to which the side reins can be attached. Alternatively, the side reins can be attached to the girth straps on a saddle; this arrangement is normal practice when a horse is being lunged as a warm-up prior to ridden work. The side reins should be passed under the first girth strap in use and secured round the second (Fig. 22.2). The stirrups should be run up the leathers and the loop of the leather passed round the tread of the stirrup and then back under itself towards the rear (Fig. 22.3).

Some people like side reins to have elastic in them and some do not; such discussion calls for a long evening and a drink or two! The side reins should act parallel to the ground, with the horse's head and neck in a posture similar to that when ridden, i.e. the side reins must not be set too low or allowed to slip downwards. The side reins should not be fastened to the bit rings when the horse is first tacked up; they should be clipped to the roller or saddle (Fig. 22.3). This arrangement should be adopted until the horse has relaxed on the lunge and again at the end of the lunge work.

For lungeing, the horse must wear brushing boots on all four legs;

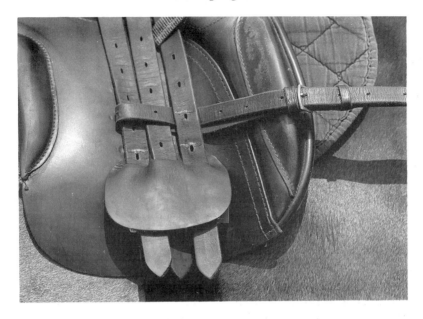

Fig. 22.2 Side rein attached to the girth straps.

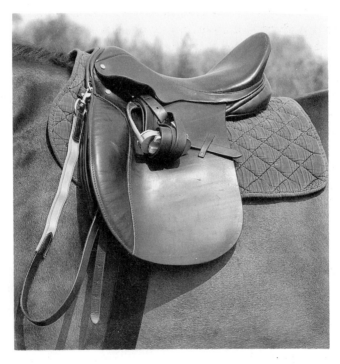

Fig. 22.3 Stirrup leathers secured and side reins clipped up out of the way.

even with sympathetic and disciplined lungeing on a large circle the horse may knock himself, so protection is essential (Fig. 22.4).

Lungers must wear stout footwear in case their toes are trodden on. The footwear should also have a good heel as a smooth under-surface gives poor grip. Properly fitting gloves are essential when lungeing to protect the hands and enhance grip. Those breaking horses on the lunge must wear a hat for obvious reasons; for all others a hat is a matter of preference or exam board protocol (Fig. 22.5). Spurs are best not worn when lungeing.

The aids

The main aid to control when lungeing is the voice. Instead of the horse being between the leg and the hand he is between the lunge whip and the rein; the lunge rein is used to keep a light consistent contact with the horse and if the horse becomes strong the tension on the rein is relaxed and retaken consecutively until the horse stops resisting. The horse should be accustomed to the whip.

Lungeing a horse for exercise

The horse is led to the lunge area with the side reins clipped back to the roller. There are two schools of thought about sending the horse forward from the halt. One method is as follows: the horse is stood on the circle facing for instance to the left. The lunger has the lunge line leading from their left hand to the horse. The spare coils of lunge line may be held in the left hand or, if preferred, in the right hand. This latter style is better for a frisky horse. The lunge whip is tucked under the left elbow, pointing to the rear. The horse should stand still as the lunger takes a few steps back towards the centre of the circle. Not all horses will stand still but such discipline and good practice should be instilled in every horse; it is a matter of patient, calm insistence and consistency.

When well clear of the horse the lunge whip can be brought quietly round behind the lunger's back into the right hand to point a metre (yard) or two to the rear of the horse and towards the ground. The command is 'walk on' but it may be prefixed with either 'and' or the name of the horse; either prefix warns the horse that, whatever else the lunger may have been saying, they are now about to issue a command.

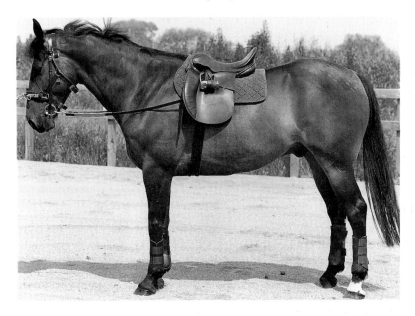

Fig. 22.4 Horse tacked up ready for lungeing.

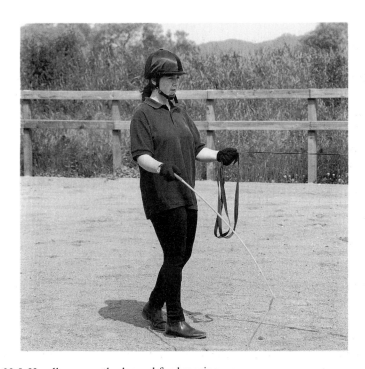

Fig. 22.5 Handler correctly dressed for lungeing.

The 'and walk on' is enforced by raising the whip to buttock height with a little shake that curls out the thong of the whip so it can be seen by the horse. As the walk proceeds the lunger moves on an inner circle, but by gradually letting out the lunge line makes spiral progress to the centre of the circle. This method establishes the horse on the outer track from the outset.

The second and more common method of sending a horse forward in walk is for the lunger to step just clear of the horse before sending him forward using the whip quietly to encourage the horse to go forwards and outwards. Thus the horse spirals outwards. The thinking behind this method is twofold: firstly, it encourages the horse to go away from the lunger rather than the lunger drawing back towards the centre of the circle; secondly, it does not require the horse to be obedient enough to stand still on the circle – many horses will turn in because they have not been taught good behaviour in this respect. Thus this method copes with strange horses and those lunged by many different people, as at a riding establishment. With this method of sending the horse out particular vigilance is required with a fresh or cheeky horse which might plunge forwards and kick out at the lunger.

The walk should be purposeful, long and unhurried with the hind feet overtracking the print left by the front feet. A walk of this quality may not be achieved in the first few minutes, particularly if the horse has just come from the stable.

Control of the horse is subtle and requires both concentration and anticipation. Lungeing is a great skill and, like riding, there is great pleasure in doing it well. If the lunger stands in the centre of the circle they are in a neutral position with the horse balanced between the whip pointing towards him and the taut lunge line; that is to say, equally between the lunger's two hands (Fig. 22.6). If the horse is on the left rein and the lunger wishes to increase the pace, the lunger takes one step to the right. They are now slightly behind the horse and raising the lunge whip a little and clicking the tongue can send the horse forward more purposefully. On the other hand, if the horse is rather too forward, the lunger steps a pace to the left and lowers the whip point towards the ground. Now they are slightly ahead of the horse and with a gentle command of 'steady' can adopt a quieter pace.

Typically the horse appears to find that the entrance gate to the lunge area has a 'magnetic' effect! Thus the horse hurries round that part of the circle which heads towards the gate and then dawdles when heading away from the gate. A good lunger will quickly notice such things and by quiet movement will anticipate and counteract them

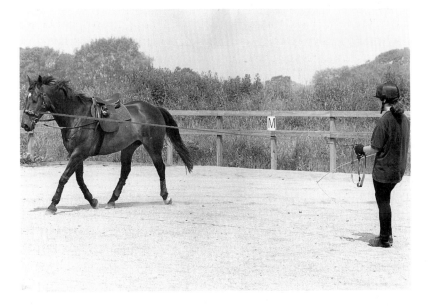

Fig. 22.6 Handler in the neutral position.

though this may not be apparent to an observer. If the horse pulls outwards, which may happen if the horse is over-fresh or badly trained, then it is helpful to lunge in an enclosed place. This may be the corner of the field or at the end of a school. In severe cases the open side can be enclosed with some jump poles on large oil drums or other temporary fencing. Such provisions should soon become unnecessary as the horse's manners improve.

On the other hand some horses charge inwards; the procedure is to stand your ground or even advance towards the horse with the lash of the whip looping towards the horse's barrel. If the lunger backs away then the horse has taken control and started to train the lunger. Commonly the horse will cut corners or fall in on the circle; in this case the whip should be pointed and, if necessary, flicked in the direction of the horse's shoulder. Sometimes a horse behaves like a hooligan and then it is necessary to attach the side reins straight away as clearly the horse is neither going to stretch down or relax, and the side reins will aid control.

When the horse has walked calmly for a few minutes on the left rein (anticlockwise), he should be sent round on the right rein (clockwise). The procedure is first to halt the horse out on the circle. He must not turn in and if he does he should be made to walk on again in the original direction. The command is a low and drawn out 'and whoa' accompanied by gentle vibration on the lunge line. If the horse does not halt, shorten the rein and bring him to a standstill. Firmly and consistently repeat this until he is obedient to the voice. When the horse is halted the lunger tucks the whip under their elbow, pointing to the rear, and walks towards the horse taking in the coils of line so that it does not hang slack or, worse still, touch the floor. Then, taking the horse on a short line, he is led round or across the circle to face the other way. Proceeding as before, the horse is sent round at a relaxed walk.

The time spent on the lunge will depend on the horse's stage of training, fitness and the type of work on the lunge; some purists like to see a horse walking for 20 minutes before trotting, but at least five minutes is a good aim. Having walked well on both reins, the horse can be given the sharp, quick command 'and trot'. If he does not respond at once a touch of the whip will serve to remind him. A crack of the whip takes only a flick of the wrist and can be useful and effective; however, care must be taken if other horses are close lest they too respond. The point is that the command should be said clearly and sharply but only once and the horse must obey instantly. Good lungeing makes the horse a better ride by enhancing obedience.

After the horse has trotted on both reins he can be halted and have the side reins fitted; initially these should be fairly long. The light pressure of the side reins on the bit may tend to shorten the horse's stride and so a little click of the tongue, a flick of the whip plus a sideways step to put the lunger a little behind the horse may be used selectively to maintain the quality of the movement. In trot the horse should put his hind feet into the prints left by the forefeet (Fig. 22.7). The trot circle should be at least 15 m (16 yd) in diameter.

Most lungeing for exercise is carried out at the working trot; this is a purposeful gait, not rushed but with a spring in the step. The side reins are shortened after a while as the horse is asked to accept a contact with the bit. In order to do this he must relax the jaw and flex the neck at the poll. He should also engage the hindquarters so that the hind legs step more actively under the body. However, he must not drop the contact with the bit by ducking the nose towards the chest so that the face makes a line behind the vertical. From time to time it is a good idea for the trainer or an experienced person to come and watch the lungeing so that bad practices do not creep in. When turning the horse round while he is still wearing side reins, lead the horse forwards in a small half circle; do not turn him on the spot.

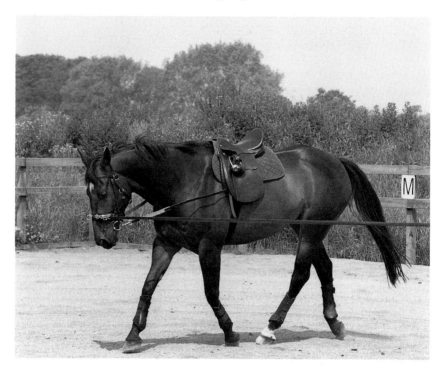

Fig. 22.7 A horse working happily on the lunge in trot.

Within the trot it is useful sometimes to ask the horse to do a few lengthened strides. The easiest way to achieve this is to select a point of the circle where there is a straight fence on the outside. Then with the lunger running just a few steps parallel to the horse, he can be encouraged to lengthen his stride before turning away from the fence back onto the circle. Later it may be possible to produce lengthened strides on the circle, but it is not an essential requirement to be able to do so.

When the horse has worked calmly yet with good activity at the trot on both reins he can be asked to canter. Experience will show the best length of side reins in order to allow the horse to move freely forward yet assist control and produce the round outline of the well-engaged horse (one that is using his hindquarters to propel himself forward actively). Sometimes, particularly in canter, the horse goes faster than intended; in such cases the lunger should never resort to roughness. The lunge line attached to the horse's nose has considerable leverage and so a hefty yank could cause damage to the horse. The procedure if the horse refuses to obey the voice commands of 'steady' or 'trot' is to reduce the length of line fairly swiftly and bring the horse to a halt. Then impose discipline with walk to halt to walk transitions before proceeding to faster paces again.

In the canter it is particularly important that the circle is large enough; 20 m (22 yd) across is ideal so a lunge line of 10 m (11 yd) is required and for a fresh horse it should be longer. If the horse is to be cantered on the lunge the ground should not be deep or slippery as a poor surface can result in the horse knocking himself, losing confidence or losing the quality of the action. As in all lungeing, it is important that there is always a light, even tension on the lunge line. You should not have a tug-of-war or a slack line. Control of the spare coils of line is a skill needing practice and lack of good line discipline will result in the lunger either tripping over spare line or having line wound round the hand which could result in a nasty accident.

Practice for lungers

Lunge beginners can practice with the line attached to a fence post, letting it out, gathering it in, passing it into the other hand and so on; it is essential that the lunger never fails to have all the line under control and available as necessary. Even in practice, gloves must always be worn so that it is only natural to handle a lunge line when wearing gloves.

Similarly beginners must practise handling the lunge whip. Typically the whip is about 2 m (6 ft 6 in) long and the thong with lash an additional 3 m (9 ft 8 in). With the thong twisted round the whip it must be carried pointing behind the lunger; it must be brought quietly into the usable position and then tucked out of the way, pointing to the rear again when adjusting the side reins or turning the horse onto the other rein. The whip must not be laid on the floor in case it is trodden on; also, the lunger is in a vulnerable position and not in control when bending to pick it up. In use the whip rarely has to touch the horse, but such a delicate flick needs to be practised.

More advanced work

Trainers schooling horses on the lunge may sometimes shorten the inside side rein, but this is not usual when lungeing horses for exercise.

Similarly, trainers may usefully jump horses on the lunge; this is done without side reins and is an advanced skill.

In some cases an ill-disciplined or exuberant horse will go too fast or its hindquarters will keep flying outwards; in such a case a second lunge line is taken from the cavesson, round the hindquarters and so to the lunger's other hand. Great care has to be taken to prevent this line riding up under the horse's tail or slipping to the ground; this too is a form of exercise which is only suitable for those who are more experienced.

In long-reining there is a line to each bit ring and the lines either run through terrets on a roller or pad, or through rings on either side of a roller, and back to the lunger. Long-reining can be carried out using circles (Fig. 22.8) or straight lines (Fig. 22.9). Unless done with great care and skill the horse may tend to come behind the bit, that is drop the bit by bending the neck too much, tucking the nose into the chest, so that the face makes a line behind the vertical, and not go forwards with sufficient impulsion. Long-reining is a useful and enjoyable advanced skill.

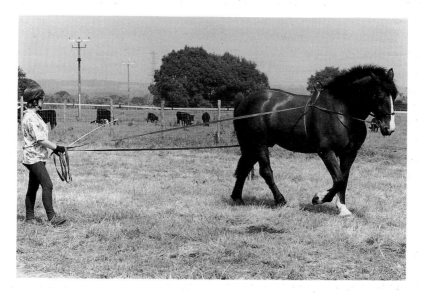

Fig. 22.8 Long reining on a circle.

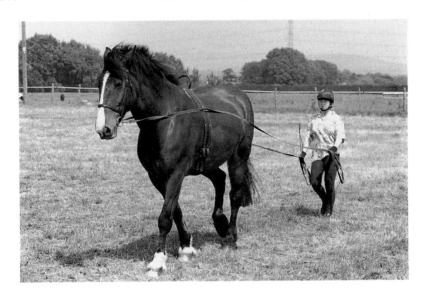

Fig. 22.9 Long reining on a straight line.

Part V
Horse Care in Action

23 Care of the Hunter

Getting the hunter fit

A fit horse is one that can do the work that is required of it without becoming overtired or overstressed. Getting a horse fit requires a mixture of correct work, feeding and health care. Regardless of the type of horse, the idea of the fitness programme is to improve the horse's ability to tolerate work by gradually increasing his workload and energy intake in a slow, steady progression.

The traditional methods of getting horses fit have developed from getting hunters fit from grass. Traditionally, hunters are brought up from grass at the beginning of August, allowing three months to get them hunting fit – equivalent to one-day-event fitness or 20-mile-distance ride fitness – before the Opening Meet in November. This three month period can be split into three four-week blocks: preliminary walking and trotting work, development work and fast work.

Bringing the hunter up from grass
After the hunting season the hunter will be roughed off and have a complete rest to allow him to unwind mentally and physically. The event horse has his break in the winter. The routine for bringing an unfit horse up from grass follows the same basic pattern, although there may be differences from yard to yard.

- *Vaccinations* – if the horse did not have the annual vaccination boosters before his holiday they should be given before starting any work. The horse will need seven days with no more than light work after vaccination to minimise the risk of any adverse reaction.
- *Teeth* – the vet or horse dentist should check the horse's teeth for sharp edges before the horse comes back into work and again six months later.
- *Worming* – a worming programme should be planned, with horses

being wormed when they are first brought in, and then every four-to-six weeks.

- *Shoeing* – horses must be shod all round once road work starts; a heavier set of shoes will last longer during this initial fittening period. The horse should be shod every four-to-six weeks.

- *Equipment* – the tack should have been stored in good condition at the end of last season. Check the stitching and restuff the saddle if necessary. Hunters can get very fat and soft during their summer break and so a thick numnah and a girth sleeve are a good idea to prevent rubbing and absorb sweat. The numnah and girth sleeve must be washed regularly. Salt water or methylated spirit can be applied to vulnerable areas on the horse to harden up the skin. Many people exercise horses in front boots plus knee boots when on the road; back boots can also be used if the horse's action makes them necessary.

- *Turning out* – the horse will benefit from being turned out for a few hours every day; this will help him unwind and stay sane. He has been accustomed to being out for most of the day and if part of the routine is a daily turn-out he is unlikely to have too wild a fling and gallop about. In the summer, horses should be protected from flies; otherwise they may become very frustrated and actually start to lose condition. Some people turn the horses out at night, exercise them early in the morning and keep them in during the day to avoid flies. This 'half and half' system is much better both physically and mentally for the horse than suddenly bringing him into work and stabling him full-time.

- *Feeding* – if the horse has not been receiving any concentrate feed, a small feed of a low energy food such as horse and pony cubes may be fed in the field the week before he is brought up. This will help his digestive system adjust to the feed he will be getting once stabled.

- *Trimming and bathing* – the horse will have his mane, tail, heels and whiskers trimmed, depending on individual preference. If the weather is mild he can be washed to help rid the coat of parasites, grease and scurf.

- *Preparation of the stable* – prior to the horse being brought back into work the stable should have been cleared of bedding, well scrubbed and then disinfected. Every so often the walls may need painting or treating with wood preservative. Hay and feed should be ordered and equipment such as buckets, clippers, etc., checked to ensure they are in sound working order.

Preliminary work

The preliminary work exercises the horse slowly for increasing lengths of time to tone up the muscles, tendons and ligaments and to harden the soft horse's skin. The initial walking and trotting work is very important.

Weeks 1 and 2: walking

The hunter is likely to have spent about four months in the field and may be rather fat and very unfit. This means that the work must progress slowly and steadily, starting with 20–30 minutes walking a day, building up to an hour by the end of the first week and two hours by the end of the second week. A horse walker can be used to do some of the walking work, or the horse can be led from another horse. Remember that this does not accustom the back muscles to carrying a rider and the girth region stays soft. Ideally the horse should be walked on the roads for up to two hours a day for four weeks and never less than two weeks – the longer the holiday the more road work is needed.

The horse must be carefully checked every day for rubs, galls and injuries. Girths and numnahs must be brushed after use and washed regularly to prevent them irritating the horse's skin.

Weeks 3 and 4: trotting

After at least two weeks walking work, trotting can be introduced; initially the trot should only be for a couple of minutes at a time, building up over the next few weeks to 15 minutes in total.

Development work

The next four weeks involve development work – the introduction of canter work so that the heart and lungs become accustomed to exercise. This builds up the horse's stamina while the muscles continue to strengthen and adapt to the work the horse is being given. The ground chosen for the first canter should be flat and not soft or dotted with potholes. The fresh horse may want to buck and gallop so be prepared for this – ask for canter quietly and keep the horse's head up. If the horse is known to be strong make sure that he is in suitable tack.

Canter work should be slow and steady initially and gradually increased so that by the end of the sixth week (mid-September) three or four periods of steady cantering a day can be included in the work. The horse should now be ready to go autumn hunting one or two mornings a week. Initially the horse should not stay out too long; it is very easy to start early and then stay out until lunch-time and find you have been out for four or five hours. Although you may not have been galloping and jumping, remember that just carrying a rider for a long time will be tiring to the semi-fit horse.

Fast work

The horse will need clipping as soon as his winter coat has grown adequately.

The hunter is rarely given any fast work during his exercise programme as October hunting usually provides enough cantering and the occasional short gallop (or 'pipe-opener') to prepare the horse for the Opening Meet. It is wise to school the hunter over cross-country fences once or twice before taking him hunting. It has been five or six months since he last jumped and it is a good idea to remind him about jumping. If you do not hunt in the autumn the horse will need to follow the programme outlined in Chapter 24 for the Novice event horse.

During the season

Throughout the hunting season days of sport will be interspersed with days of exercise. The exercise will vary depending on how hard the horse is working. A Hunt horse may do one or two hard days hunting a week. This will keep the horse fit and no more than 60–90 minutes walking with a little trotting will be needed on exercise days. Sunday is likely to be a rest day but rather than stand in his box the horse should be walked out in hand and allowed to graze for 10–15 minutes. This will help reduce the risk of azoturia.

A subscriber's (Hunt member's) horse may only hunt one day a week, that day being considerably less arduous than the Hunt horse's day. The subscriber's horse should have a short walk the day after hunting (usually a Sunday) and possibly a day off midweek when he should be turned out or walked in hand for 10–15 minutes. The remaining four days the horse should have 60–90 minutes of exercise including trotting and cantering. This horse may also benefit from a short gallop the day before hunting to clear his wind and prepare for the next day's galloping.

All horses vary in the amount of exercise they need to keep them in peak condition depending on how much hunting they are doing, their temperament and type. A hunter correctly worked and fed should stay in tiptop condition for the whole of the hunting season.

Roughing off

At the end of the season (March–April) the hunter is usually roughed off and turned out to grass for the long summer's rest. A clipped, corn-fed horse should not suddenly be turned out at this time of the year when the weather is cold, wet and unpredictable; the horse should be gradually 'let down'. Exercise should be reduced and at the same time the concentrate ration should be decreased and the amount of hay increased. As the weather gets warmer the number or weight of rugs should be reduced and the horse turned out for a greater length of time every day. Once the paddocks have dried up sufficiently to allow the horse to stay out all day he can stop being exercised and have his shoes removed. If the feet are likely to crack and spilt it may be necessary to leave the front shoes on. By the end of April or beginning of May the horse should be able to stay out day and night. A horse roughed off rapidly and turned out too soon tends to lose condition which may take a long time to recover.

During June and July flies can bother the horse, so any field should have adequate shelter. Alternatively the horse can be brought in during the heat of the day. The horse's feet must be regularly trimmed, he should be wormed every four-to-six weeks and checked daily for injury. The field must also be regularly checked for hazards that may injure the horse.

Feeding the hunter

As with feeding any horse it is a mistake to generalise and each horse must be fed as an individual and according to the amount of work done. A horse hunting two long days a week has widely differing requirements from a horse doing a short day once a week. However, the following points should be remembered:

- The horse must be fed to maintain condition for a long season. Traditionally boiled barley and linseed are fed; they are palatable feeds which help maintain the condition of horses that are working hard.
- The hours the horse spends out of the stable with a rider on his back are just as tiring as galloping and jumping.
- The hunter does not need to be as disciplined as the eventer or dressage horse; it does not matter too much if he starts the day a little fresh so long as he is still going at the end of the day – providing that the rider can cope!

- Feed should be reduced the day before a rest day. Traditionally the hunter receives a bran mash on the evening before his day off, its laxative effect helping to prevent azoturia.
- Tired horses tend to lose their appetite so it is better to feed smaller amounts of a high energy feed (performance cubes or cereals) rather than large amounts of a lower energy feed (horse and pony cubes).
- Succulents will tempt the shy feeder.

Care of the horse during the hunting season

The day before hunting

It is essential to be properly organised; equipment should be gathered together, cleaned and made ready for the morning. The following list covers the majority of equipment needed for hunting:

- Plaiting kit
- Grooming kit
- Tack – check the stitching for wear and polish bit rings and stirrups if necessary
- Brushing boots and over-reach boots if worn
- Headcollar and rope
- Travelling equipment for the horse
- Haynet for the return journey
- Sweat rug for the return journey
- Full water carrier and bucket
- Human first-aid kit
- Equine first-aid kit to include a small bowl, scissors, cottonwool, crepe bandages, gamgee, salt, wound dressings and sprays, and ready-to-use poultice

The horse should be thoroughly groomed and have his mane, tail, feet and any white socks washed. If the whiskers and bridle path (parts of the head where the bridle rests) are trimmed they should be tidied up.

The hunting morning

Work backwards from the time of the Meet to calculate the time you should arrive and thus the time you must leave home, start plaiting and doing all the rest of the morning routine tasks and finally the time you must set the alarm clock. The horse must be fed at least an hour before the expected loading up time.

Before leaving, the horse should be groomed, the feet oiled and a tail bandage put on. Any small cuts should be dressed with antiseptic cream to protect them during the day. In countries where mud fever is a problem the horse's legs and belly are sometimes wiped over with oil to stop mud getting into the pores of the skin.

Hunters often travel tacked up with the headcollar on over the bridle and a rug and roller or surcingle over the saddle. If the journey to the Meet is short the horse may not wear any protective travelling gear except for a tail bandage. For longer journeys it is preferable for the horse to be adequately protected and tacked up on arrival.

The vehicle should be parked about a mile from the Meet – the hack helps settle the horse. Ensure that all equipment is safely put away and the vehicle locked up before leaving it.

Care after hunting

On a dry day the horse should be walked the last mile back to the vehicle so that he is cool and dry on arrival. However, if it is raining it may be better to keep trotting so that he arrives ready to be loaded warm and wet rather than cold and wet.

The bridle can be replaced with a headcollar and the horse either loaded immediately or tied to a string loop on the side of the vehicle. If the vehicle is parked on a busy road, it is wet or the horse excited it is probably better to load him immediately. The saddle will have been on for a long time so either the girth can be loosened, the sweat rug and top rug placed on top and the horse travelled home with the saddle on, or the saddle can be removed and the area under the saddle patted briskly to help the circulation in the blood vessels under the saddle to return; sudden removal can cause scalded backs and pressure lumps. The horse can then be rugged up.

The horse can be offered a small drink of water (no more than a quarter of a bucket) and any obvious injuries attended to. Travelling gear can then be put on the horse and he can have another small drink before travelling home with his haynet.

On returning home

The routine followed varies between yards but the following guide-lines may prove useful.

(1) Once the horse has been unloaded he can be taken to the stable, tied up beside a haynet, have the saddle and travelling gear removed and the rugs thrown back over him.

(2) He can be offered water at regular intervals. If he drank a couple of times before being loaded he can have half a bucket of water, followed 15 minutes later by as much as he wants to drink. However, if he has not drunk all day he should be restricted to a quarter of a bucket every 15 minutes until his thirst is quenched. Very tired horses may appreciate water that has had the chill taken off it. Dehydrated horses can either be offered electrolytes in the feed or in a separate bucket of water. It is important that the horse drinks but does not gorge himself on water, risking colic.

(3) Meanwhile the horse can have his feet picked out, shoes checked for soundness and legs checked for injuries such as thorns and cuts. He can then be cleaned. If he is dry the mud can be brushed off and sticky sweat marks sponged off with warm water. If the mud is wet some people prefer to leave it to dry and to brush it off in the morning while others wash it off immediately, either with a hose or sponge and warm water. If the horse is washed he should be towelled dry before being rugged up with dry rugs. Stable bandages will help support tired legs and dry wet ones. The tail should be washed and the plaits taken out. If the horse is very tired just make him clean enough to be comfortable and leave him to rest. Keep offering the horse water until his thirst is quenched.

(4) The horse can now be left in peace with his haynet and a small feed.

(5) The tack can be cleaned. Some yards wash the mud off now, leave the tack to dry and soap it the next day, while others clean it completely the same evening.

(6) The horse may break out in a sweat. Check him every 15 minutes for cold, sweaty patches, restless behaviour, disturbed bedding or a reluctance to eat. If the signs are mild keep the horse warm by rubbing his ears until they are warm and walk him (if the weather is suitable) until he is dry and comfortable. If the horse does not respond or looks very distressed then veterinary help should be called.

(7) Before leaving the horse, top up the water buckets. The horse should be checked later in the evening, given more water and hay as well as a late night feed.

The day after hunting

Providing that the horse has eaten up and looks well he can be fed and given hay as normal. Depending on the routine followed the previous night the horse may be clean or dirty. Any stable bandages should be removed and the legs carefully checked for heat, pain or swelling from cuts, thorns, knocks or strains. The rugs can be thrown back and the saddle and girth area checked for lumps or rubs. The horse can then be unrugged and trotted up in hand to check that he is sound; he may seem stiff initially but this should soon wear off. The rugs can then be thrown back over the horse while he is thoroughly cleaned, making sure that awkward areas such as between the hind legs and elbows are attended to. Once the horse is clean he can be exercised. The amount of exercise will depend on how hard he worked the day before; it is likely that 15–30 minutes' walk will be enough. The horse can then be returned to the stable and left in peace to recover from his exertions.

24 Care of the Competition Horse

Getting the competition horse fit

Bringing the competition or event horse up from grass and then getting him fit varies very little from the programme outlined in Chapter 23 for the hunter. The main differences are that, firstly, the event horse is being got fit in the winter prior to competing in the summer and, secondly, he needs to follow a more formal fast work plan in order to reach the desired level of fitness.

Bringing the competition horse up from grass
The event horse usually has a rest in the winter and is brought back into work in December or January ready for the first event in March or April. This means that he is generally stabled at night and is already being fed concentrates so that unlike the hunter his system does not need to become accustomed to a completely different regime. He will also need clipping as soon as he comes into work; a blanket clip keeps his back warm during the preliminary work. He can have a hunter clip when he starts to do faster work.

Interval training
Interval training has become popular for training competition horses. It consists of giving a horse a period of canter followed by a brief interval of walk during which the horse is allowed to partially recover before being asked to work again. Interval training increases the horse's capacity for using oxygen to create energy; the point at which the horse runs up an oxygen debt is delayed as much as possible. This results in the horse being able to work for longer before fatigue sets in. The interval training workouts are fitted into the total training programme of the horse. (See also Appendix II: Interval Training to Novice One-day-event Fitness: a Detailed 12-week Schedule.)

An essential part of the interval training regime is monitoring the horse's temperature, pulse and respiration (TPR) to gauge the horse's reaction to the work. Interval training cannot cut corners and the following factors must be considered before starting such a programme:

- The horse should be capable of 90 minutes walk and trot over rolling terrain without distress. The horse conditioned slowly and carefully will stay in peak condition longer than one pushed too fast in the early stages.
- It is essential to keep a notebook with a running record of the horse's response to the workout, allowing the programme to be adjusted accordingly.
- As in any form of training the rider must be alert to any change in the horse's attitude, appetite, coat, droppings, appearance, muscle tone, etc.

During interval training the horse is cantered at a predetermined speed for a certain time. After this the horse is pulled up and the pulse and/or respiration rates are recorded immediately. The horse is then walked for a set time and the rates recorded again. The difference between the two readings is the 'recovery rate' of the horse. This fast then slow work is repeated two or three times.

These workouts are repeated, usually every four days, and the pulse and respiration rates recorded at the same points; as the horse gets fitter he will recover faster from the work. Fitness is gradually built up by slowly increasing the total amount of work the horse is asked to do and by increasing the speed and/or length of the workout or using more demanding terrain. If the recovery rate is not good enough after a workout, the work should be adjusted so that the horse is never overstressed.

Points to remember

- Interval training must be monitored by pulse and respiration rate, not by time alone. It is the pulse rate immediately after the workout that shows how much stress the horse has been subjected to, and the recovery rate that shows how fit he is.
- If the pulse and respiration have not returned to normal within 20 minutes of completing the workout the horse has been overworked and the programme should be adapted accordingly.

- The respiration rate should not exceed the pulse rate; if it does stop work.
- Never complete the day's planned programme if the horse becomes distressed.
- On the other hand the horse must be stressed enough to stimulate the body systems to become better adapted to exercise. The heart rate must be raised above 100 beats per minute after work.
- The interval training programme should be planned backwards from the proposed date of the competition(s) so that workout days fall appropriately.
- Always warm up and cool down thoroughly before cantering, particularly if the horse has to travel in a lorry or trailer to the work area.

Preliminary work
The preliminary work is no different for the competition horse than for the hunter – they both need plenty of slow work at the beginning of the programme.

Weeks 1 and 2: walking
Not all riders allow their horses to become completely unfit; they may only give their horses a short holiday of two-to-four weeks, after which they are walked two or three times a week for up to an hour each time. This helps to maintain a basic level of fitness and to keep the tendons and bones strong. The risk of girth galls and sore backs is also lessened.

During preliminary work, ideally the horse should be walked on the roads for up to two hours a day for four weeks and never less than two weeks – the longer the holiday the more road work is needed. If the horse has been walked two or three times a week from the field, another two weeks on top should suffice once the horse has come in to be stabled. This work strengthens the horse and prepares him for the next stage. The walk should never be sloppy; it should be purposeful and with a good rein contact.

Weeks 3 and 4: trotting
After at least two weeks' walking work, trotting can be introduced; initially the trot should only be for a couple of minutes at a time, building up over the next couple of weeks to 15 minutes in total. If the trotting is done in an arena sharp turns and small circles must be avoided at this stage. Flat work or lungeing can be incorporated into

the routine towards the end of the fourth week; this should be no more than 30 minutes before or after an hour's road work.

It is far better to underfeed than overfeed the horse with concentrates at this stage, but a good amount of hay (or a dust-free equivalent such as haylage) must be fed to prevent the stabled horse becoming bored.

Development work (weeks 5–7)

Development work involves the introduction of canter work and suppling exercises so that the heart and lungs become accustomed to stronger exercise, building up the horse's stamina while the muscles continue to strengthen and adapt to the work the horse is being given.

The initial canter work may be done in a schooling environment where horses often respect their riders more than in an open space. The horse should be cantered for two-to-three minutes at 400 m per minute to start with, bringing the horse back to walk through trot. These little bouts of canter should be built up so that by the end of two weeks the horse is cantering for a total of nine-to-ten minutes split into three or four sessions. The horse should always be walked for two-to-five minutes after each canter.

During week 5 or 6, jumping can be introduced into the programme starting with pole work, grid work and small jumps in the school. This can be incorporated into the schooling programme so that by the end of the second month the novice horse should have done a small local show jumping class or two.

Discipline work (weeks 8–12)

The third period of the fitness programme is even more specialised; the power and athleticism of the dressage horse (Fig. 24.1) and show jumper (Fig. 24.2) are developed further, while the racehorse and the event horse are given fast work. Some horses, for example ridden show horses, do not need speed, power or athleticism but should continue to build up body, skin and coat condition and become more highly trained.

Now interval training can start in earnest. Canter work is repeated every fourth day, building the sessions up minute by minute. The day after a canter session should be less stressful with a hack or some gentle schooling. Over the next two weeks the sessions are built up so that the horse can do three lots of five minute canters at 400 mpm, with 3 minutes' walking in between.

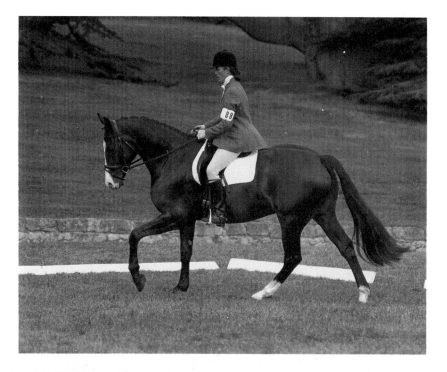

Fig. 24.1 The dressage horse.

By now the horse will have been stabled about ten weeks. Road work continues each day; it can form a useful warming up and/or cooling down period. Show jumping, cross-country and dressage schooling all continue in a balanced programme.

The final two weeks (weeks 11 and 12)

The first horse trial can be planned for week 12; on a couple of occasions, the last minute of the last canter can be increased to a speed of 500 mpm.

Table 24.1 shows a sample workout. The heart rate after the third canter should drop below 100 beats per minute after ten minutes walking. All horses are individuals and must be treated as such. Tables are merely a guideline and do not allow for lost shoes, heavy-going or lazy horses. The real skill in training lies in the ability to design programmes for individual horses and to recognise the need to adapt the programme without hindering the horse's progress. The same programme may take up to two weeks longer with a different horse.

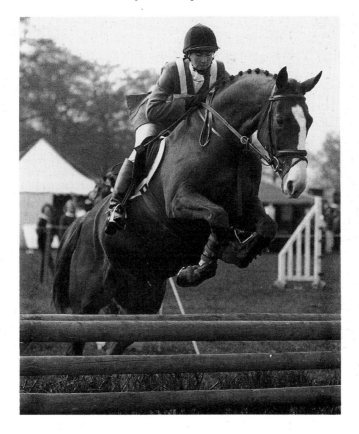

Fig. 24.2 The show jumper.

Table 24.1 Interval training to novice one-day-event fitness.

20 minutes warm-up

Canter 1: 5 minutes @ 400 mpm
trot 30 seconds
walk 3 minutes

Canter 2: 4 minutes @ 400 mpm
1 minute @ 500 mpm
trot 30 seconds–1 minute
walk 3 minutes

Canter 3: 4 minutes @ 400 mpm
1 minute @ 500 mpm building up to 550 mpm
trot 1–2 minutes
walk at least 20 minutes

Roughing off

Once the competition season has finished the horse may be roughed off and turned out to grass for a holiday. The horse's work is cut down or stopped and he is turned out in the field for an increasing amount of time during the day, regardless of the weather. Gradually the number of rugs worn is reduced and the ratio of forage to concentrates increased. The shoes may be removed or left on according to the state of the horse's feet. Hind shoes may be removed if there is a danger of horses kicking each other. The horses should have their feet checked regularly while at grass and also should be wormed.

Feeding the competition horse

The competition or event horse has to be fit enough to gallop and jump at speed and yet disciplined enough to perform dressage and show jumping; this has led to many event riders trying to keep their horses happy both mentally and physically by feeding as few concentrates as possible and turning their horses out in the field every day. The three-day-event horse may have a very rigorous training programme and yet only compete in a few events on the run up to the main competition before being turned away, while the lower level horse may compete once a week throughout the long event season. These horses have widely differing feed requirements.

Prior to the event do not be tempted to change the horse's ration. Some people reduce or omit the sugar beet pulp from the feed before the event, while others would only do this on the morning of a cross-country event. If the horse frets away from home, reduce the quantity of concentrate food and use high energy palatable ingredients such as milk pellets and flaked maize. Generally speaking, however, it is better not to alter the horse's feed too much; you may just cause problems.

A three-day-event horse should have a concentrate feed no less than four hours before the start time of the first phase of the cross country day. If competing in the afternoon he could also be given a small haynet. If the horse has had free access to fresh water there is no reason why he should have his water bucket taken away before competing – why should he suddenly decide to have a huge drink?

A novice event horse could munch on a haynet while being plaited on the morning of the competition. If he is competing early he should not receive any bulk feed while travelling until after his cross-country event. If he is competing later he could have a small haynet while travelling. Depending on your competing times, he may be able to have a concentrate feed between the dressage and the show jumping, providing that there is at least two hours digestion time. He should be offered water frequently throughout the day and allowed to wash his mouth out between the show jumping and the cross-country, even if they are very close together.

The fluid and electrolyte balance is very important and the horse must be watched for signs of dehydration. If a pinch of skin on the neck or shoulder lingers after it has been released and the horse has a gaunt tucked-up appearance he may well be dehydrated – this can limit the next day's performance severely. Ensure that the horse drinks and provide electrolytes in the food or water.

Colic can be a problem after severe exertion, and the intestines must be kept moving. Once the horse is cool and his thirst has been quenched he may appreciate a small bran mash, with his normal feed later on. Tired horses are easily overfaced by a large feed, but dividing the normal feed in two and feeding it at intervals may overcome this.

After the competition the horse's appetite will indicate how tired he is. Until he is eating normally, he has not really recovered from his exertions and should be allowed plenty of rest. Hacks and grazing in hand will help the horse relax and recover.

Care of the horse during the competition season

The week before the competition
This is the time for those finishing touches. The mane and tail should be tidied up and the horse clipped if necessary. All tack and equipment must be examined thoroughly and repaired or replaced; any items missing from your checklist must be purchased and ensure that any medications are not out-of-date. The horse should be shod with stud holes as necessary and the farrier asked to check that the horse's spare set of shoes still fit correctly. The numnahs, boots and rugs, etc., that are being taken to the competition should be clean and in good repair.

The day before the competition
If staying overnight before or after the competition it is essential to be properly organised; clean equipment should be gathered together and

packed. The following list gives the general requirements for most situations:

- Stable tools, muck skip and muck sack
- Shavings or paper bedding
- Two haynets
- Two water buckets and full water carrier
- Feed bowl
- Pre-packed concentrate feeds clearly labelled, for example, 'Monday lunch'
- Soaked sugar beet pulp if fed
- Hay or haylage
- Supplements, for example, electrolytes
- Grooming kit including extra sponges, towels, sweat scraper and hoof oil
- Fly spray
- Plaiting kit
- Spare set of shoes, studs and stud fitting kit
- Tack cleaning kit
- Spare rugs and blankets
- Sweat sheets or coolers
- Waterproof rugs
- Stable bandages and gamgee or wraps
- Passport/vaccination certificate
- Rule book and details of entry
- Equipment for all those going on the trip (food, clothing, toiletries, money, etc.)

Other essential items include:

- Tack – depending on the horse and competition
- Bandages, brushing boots, over-reach boots plus spares
- Spare girth, leathers, irons and reins
- Spare headcollar and rope
- Hole punch
- Lungeing equipment
- Travelling equipment for the horse
- Human first-aid kit
- Equine first-aid kit to include a small bowl, scissors, cottonwool, crepe bandages, gamgee, salt, wound dressings and sprays, ready-to-use poultice and leg coolant

The horse should be thoroughly groomed; if the weather permits it may be possible to bathe him, and you will need to wash the mane, tail and any white socks. If the whiskers and bridle path are trimmed a last trim will prevent a designer-stubble look.

Packing the vehicle

Equipment should be listed and ticked off as loaded; this will avoid vital items being overlooked. Containers as simple as plastic washing baskets will make loading and unloading easier, but they should not be too large or too heavy as this makes handling tricky. Containers should have an easily-read list of contents so that items can be located quickly. Filled water containers and buckets should be packed so that they are easy to get at during the journey for watering the horse.

At the competition

Find out when the class starts or your specific start times so that you know in advance the time your horse is expected to compete. Work backwards from this time to calculate the time you should arrive at the showground and thus the time you must leave home, start plaiting and doing all the rest of the morning routine tasks, and finally the time you must set the alarm clock.

The horse must be fed at least an hour before the expected loading up time. Allow extra time for delays in the journey and about 45 minutes-to-an-hour to get yourself organised and the horse settled and tacked up before he needs to be ridden. If you have a cross-country course to walk allow yourself an hour to do this plus 10 minutes to walk the show-jumping course.

Once at the competition ground, park where the ground is as level as possible, and if the weather is warm try to find some shade. If you have help and the horse has had a long journey he should be quietly unloaded and walked in hand; letting him graze will help relax him. Meanwhile you can go and declare for the class, pick up your number and find out where everything is. The next step is to brush the horse over; he will have been thoroughly groomed at home and should only need the finishing touches such as hoof oil, quarter marks and the last shaving taking out of his tail. If the competition is on grass the horse may be fitted with studs to give him more grip. The type of stud used will depend on the state of the going with pointed studs being used on hard ground and square studs on soft ground. The horse is now ready to be tacked up, mounted and warmed up.

Overnight stays

If staying overnight at a showground or racecourse all the horse's vaccination papers should be up-to-date and ready to show the officials. Before putting the horse into the stable, which may be temporary or permanent, carry out a few checks:

- Clean out contaminated or mouldy bedding.
- Wash out the manger, disinfect and then wash it again.
- Clean out the automatic drinker if present.
- Check that the lights work and are out of reach of the horse.
- Check that glass-covered windows are safe and out of reach of the horse.
- Ensure that there are no sharp edges or projections which may cut the horse.
- The door must be strong with secure latches and bolts.

Once the horse has been unloaded and has had a walk to stretch his legs he can go into the stable for a roll. After being offered a drink, he will benefit from a small haynet to munch on so that by the time he is offered a feed he is relaxed enough to eat it. Even if the horse does not have a late night feed he should be checked last thing to see that he has settled in this strange environment and is not too warm or too cold.

Care after the competition

After the horse has finished an arduous competition he will have a higher temperature, pulse and respiration rates and it is important to bring these body systems back to normal as quickly as possible.

(1) Immediately after the horse has stopped the rider should dismount and loosen the girth; it is important to keep the horse moving so that the circulating blood cools the muscles. After 5 minutes walking, the horse can have the tack removed and a cooler or sweat rug put on and walking continued. If the saddle has been on for a long time, it should be left in place for about 10 minutes to allow the circulation in the blood vessels under the saddle to return; sudden removal can cause scalded backs and pressure lumps.

(2) As soon as the horse stops blowing hard he can have a few sips of water. Until the horse is cool and his thirst quenched he should be given water little and often; as a guide allow five swallows of water for every 50 m walked.

(3)   The pulse and respiration rates of a fit horse that has not been over stressed should return to comfortable levels within 15 minutes and the horse should be checked every 15 minutes thereafter until the values return to normal, which should be within an hour of completing exercise.

(4)   Once the pulse and respiration are within comfortable levels the horse should be stood in a sheltered place, out of the sun on a hot day and out of the wind on a cool day, and washed down. The lower legs, inside the legs, the head and belly should be sponged.

(5)   During untacking and sponging, the horse must be checked for injury; once he has recovered, these areas can be cleaned and dressed. The horse should also be jogged for a few yards to check for soundness while he is recovering.

(6)   Once the horse has cooled completely he can have a nibble of grass or a small haynet while you attend to his legs. The leg treatment will vary according to personal preference, but after strenuous effort it is a good idea to apply a cold dressing to constrict the blood vessels and soothe any bruising and inflammation that may be present. A clay or cooling gel dressing can be used and applied thickly down the back of the leg from the knee to below the fetlock joint, and then covered in dampened newspaper, tinfoil, clingfilm or plastic with gamgee and a stable bandage applied over the top.

(7)   Although the skin and surface muscles are now cool, the horse may break out in a sweat. Check the horse every 15 minutes for cold, sweaty patches, restless behaviour, disturbed bedding or a reluctance to eat. If the signs are mild keep the horse warm and walk him until he is dry and comfortable. If the horse does not respond or looks very distressed then veterinary help should be called.

Welfare of the competition horse

Whatever type of equestrian sport is being followed it is vital that the competition horse is looked after in the best way possible. The following points are included in a Code of Conduct which has been drawn up by the Federation Equestre Internationale (FEI) in conjunction with The International League for the Protection of Horses (ILPH) and the British Equestrian Federation (BEF).

- In all equestrian sports the welfare of the horse must be considered paramount.
- The well-being of the horse is more important than performance in a competition; horses must not be exploited to satisfy a sponsor or team.
- The pressure to compete must not result in the misuse of medication.
- The highest standards of feeding, health and stable management must be maintained.
- The horse must be travelled with adequate ventilation, feeding, watering and rest periods.
- The horse's rider or driver must be fit and competent.
- No training method should cause pain, injury or distress.

25 Care of the Leisure Horse

A large number of horses are kept by riding schools or private owners as leisure animals. They are not kept to take part in a specific equestrian sport, but provide enjoyment to their riders hacking and taking part in a variety of competitions and club activities. These horses may compete in dressage, hunter trials, show jumping and showing classes as well as doing the odd day's hunting and the occasional sponsored ride or team chase.

The majority of texts are written for the professional full-time horse person. However, many horse owners are in other full-time work; indeed, they need to work in order to pay the bills associated with keeping a horse! Fitting a horse in around your life and commitments is not easy and must be planned so that neither the horse nor the family are neglected.

The right horse for the job

Selecting the right horse is the first step on the way to a happy partnership. Owning a leisure horse is supposed to be fun; unfortunately it can turn out to be a nightmare if the horse is unsuitable. The ideal horse is a 'can't go wrong' character; he should be rugged, amenable and a pleasure to own and look after. There are guidelines that will help in choosing the right horse:

- A cob or pony cross is likely to be sensible and easy to feed.
- The horse does not need to be much higher than 15.2 hh. Providing that he is sturdy and has plenty of bone, that is the circumference of the leg below the knee is adequate for the size of horse, he should be able to carry any person's weight. Ability is not related to size and a 15.2 can do anything that a 16.2 can do.
- Smaller horses tend to be more sound and easier to look after. Large often means trouble.

- Avoid Thoroughbreds as they tend to need plenty of work every day and are not suited to being amenable at the weekend having done little all week.
- Avoid buying a young horse unless you have enough time and expertise to train the horse.
- When choosing a horse take a knowledgeable friend with you.
- Before buying the horse have it vetted; the expense is well justified.

Keeping the horse in the stable

The horse is not designed to be kept in a stable; he does not have enough space to move around in, there is very little air space, the air only changes slowly resulting in a stuffy atmosphere and he has no real physical contact with other horses. All in all it is a totally artificial lifestyle. However, stabling horses is very convenient for us: we can feed and exercise them, keep them warm and dry, prevent them being kicked or bitten by other horses and keep more animals on a small piece of land. After all, most people cannot afford to buy a paddock but we can afford to rent a stable.

It is important that the stable is an adequate size: for example, 3.5 m^2 (12 ft^2) is a minimum size for a 16 h horse. Further details regarding the size of stables can be found in Chapter 11. The stable should also be well ventilated; in most ready-made boxes the window and door are on the same side and as a result the open top half of the door often blocks the window and there is no movement of air through the stable. While the horse must not stand in a draught it is useful to have a window or gap below the eaves on the opposite side from the door to ensure that the air within the box changes regularly, creating a healthy environment. There should also be an exit for air in the ridge of the roof; this allows the warm air to escape from the stable as it rises and effectively 'sucks' air in through the open top half of the door.

Keeping the horse at grass

There are many advantages in keeping the horse at grass: it is a natural system; less straw and hay are used; less time is spent on routine management; and the horse need not be ridden because it will exercise itself. However, there are disadvantages: the horse may become too fat in the summer; he may be wet and muddy in the winter; he still needs to be caught and checked over every day; supplementary feeding will be necessary in the winter and in the summer where there is insufficient grass.

It is easier to operate a 'combined system' where the horse spends part of the day at grass and the rest of the time in the stable. In the summer the horse can be stabled during the day to protect him from the flies. In the winter the horse may be stabled at night or brought in well in advance of being ridden to give him time to dry.

A variation of the traditional system of in at night, out by day which, although expensive initially, offers many advantages of the paddock without the mess, is that of the shelter/stable with a free-draining sand yard attached. The horse can be shut in the stable at night and then allowed access to the yard during the day. This way the horse has a little more exercise, plenty of fresh air and a more natural environment.

Horses working from grass in the winter can be given a trace or blanket clip. This makes grooming easier and allows the horse to work without undue sweating. A clipped horse will need a New Zealand rug. An unclipped horse can be turned out without a rug, but the heavy winter coat will take a long time to dry before the horse can be tacked up. The horse will dry quite quickly if put in the stable with a thatch of straw on his back, lightly covered with a cut-open light-weight hessian sack held in place with a loosely-fastened surcingle. After half-an-hour or so the worst of the mud can be brushed off with a dandy brush. If the horse's girth and saddle area are not free of mud there is a risk that the horse's skin will be rubbed and sore after riding.

After work the wet horse should not be left in the stable. If he is to remain stabled, he should be thatched in order to aid drying. If the horse is to be turned out, this should be done straight away so that he can roll and keep on the move.

Keeping the leisure horse fit

The leisure horse is unlikely to undergo a formal fitness programme. The work done will vary according to the rider's ability, facilities and preference, but the horse will rarely be more than half fit, having undergone the equivalent of the preliminary and development stages outlined earlier.

If the horse is going to compete in hunter trials or to go hunting it is important that some faster work is done prior to the event. This faster work may take the form of going round a farm ride, for example, and cantering where possible. This also gives the rider the opportunity to pull their stirrups up and get themselves fit for riding short at the same time. Alternatively, the canter work could be done in the arena – the horse will not be able to go fast but there is no reason why the rider cannot shorten the stirrups, adopt a forward seat and do, say, three three-minute canters. Both horse and rider may be competent at jumping but unless they are both fit problems are likely to arise towards the end of the course.

Feeding the leisure horse

It must always be borne in mind that the domesticated horse is being given a diet that is quite different from the one he is designed to cope with. In the wild he would graze and browse a high fibre diet for up to 16 hours a day. In an effort to keep the horse slim and athletic we cut down the fibre, reduce the eating time and add highly digestible concentrates to the ration.

It is easy to overestimate the feed requirements of a horse that is working for an hour a day, hacking or doing school work. Just because we have worked hard riding the horse does not mean that the horse has worked equally hard. Many behavioural problems as well as health problems are caused by overfeeding. The golden rules for safe, economical and effective feeding are:

● Feed simply
● Feed plenty of roughage and as few concentrates as possible
● Buy the best quality hay you can afford

Feeding a low energy, high fibre compound feed such as horse and pony cubes along with dust- and mould-free hay should be all that the healthy leisure horse needs. If he is inclined to bolt his feed, chaff can be added to slow him down and make him chew the feed more thoroughly. There should be no need to add a supplement or 'a bit of this and a bit of that' to the feed as it will only unbalance the ration that the equine nutritionist has created. In the winter the horse will appreciate carrots in the feed. Horses that are allergic to the dust and fungal spores found in hay may need to have their hay soaked or they can be fed a dust-free alternative such as haylage.

If the horse is turned out onto reasonable grazing in the summer he may only need feed and hay if he is brought in at night. The amount of feed will depend on the quantity and quality of the grazing available. If the horse is inclined to become fat try to turn him out on sparse grazing so that he has to work hard for each mouthful of grass. Keeping him in and starving him during the day will only encourage gorging at night.

Caring for the leisure horse after exercise

Although the leisure horse may not work hard in the accepted sense he will often be hot and tired after exercise. As he is only half-fit he will find the exercise just as strenuous as the fit horse in an arduous competition. See the section 'Care after the competition season' in Chapter 24.

Selecting a system of management

The important thing with a leisure horse is to set up a system which maximises the pleasure of ownership, whether it is your own stable and paddock or a 'do-it-yourself' livery. Take good local advice to ensure that the system and facilities will meet your needs and provide you and your horse with the greatest enjoyment.

Part VI
Stud Management

26   The Stallion

The same basic rules of stable management apply to stallions as to all other horses, but even pony stallions can become aggressive in the breeding season and special attention should be paid to the safety of both stallion and handler at all times. The route to safety lies in a well thought out routine with calm, confident but firm handling and a consistent insistence on discipline. While the stallion needs to be able to express his individual personality, the correct balance between permitted high spirits or enthusiasm and stepping out of line calls for fine judgement which comes with experience.

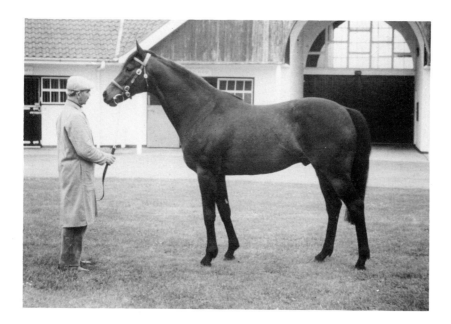

Fig. 26.1 Mutual esteem between stallion and handler is the ideal relationship.

General care

Accommodation

Like all horses, stallions are gregarious and should be kept where they can see other horses and some activity. Many competition stallions are kept very successfully in a mixed yard but most Thoroughbred studs have a separate range of stallion boxes. The stable must be sound and strong, and extra care should be taken to ensure that there are no sharp projections or edges as an excited stallion can be quite violent in his box. The bars at the window or grille over the door must be designed so that the stallion cannot get his foot caught up.

The box should be as large as possible; some Thoroughbred boxes are 6 m (20 ft) square. The lower door may be higher than average to prevent the stallion getting his forelegs over it. While some stallions are permitted to look out over the top of the stable door except when horses are being led past, many busy yards will have bars or a grille across the top door. If this is the case it is important that the box is big enough for the stallion not to feel caged in as this may make him more aggressive. A solid top door must be available so that the stallion can be shut in if he gets very excited, for example when strange mares arrive on the yard or if another stallion is covering.

Fittings within the box should be kept to a minimum but strong tie rings are important so that the stallion can be 'racked up', i.e. tied at eye level with chain, away from the door if he is likely to become excited.

Ideally the stallion box should have a second door leading directly into a stallion paddock.

Exercise

The stallion needs daily exercise. During a busy covering season, the amount of exercise may be reduced but the stallion should never be confined to his stable and brought out only to cover the mare. This would be bad both physically and psychologically.

As competition horse breeding becomes more popular, many stallions are ridden and compete throughout the covering season. Competing helps advertise a stallion and his greater fitness may actually enhance his stud performance. A stallion obviously needs a competent rider and care must always be taken, particularly when riding in mixed company. Risks should be avoided and even when leading the stallion from his box to the mounting block the route should be planned and the handler should wear gloves and carry a whip.

Many Thoroughbred stallions have a good pedigree and a successful track record so are deemed too valuable to ride and are exercised by walking in hand. For safety they are led in a bridle and wear side reins from the bit to a roller.

In addition to ordinary exercise a stallion may usefully be lunged, long-reined or loose-schooled if the facility exists. This adds a little variation to prevent him becoming bored, particularly in the late winter or early spring when he is being got fit for the approaching stud season.

All horses appreciate being turned out in a paddock, preferably every day, even if only for a short time. The stallion paddock must be safely fenced with post and rails of sufficient height to discourage him from jumping out. It is an advantage if the corners can be rounded off and it may be necessary to build a solid fence to screen the stallion so that he cannot see passing mares or adjacent stallions. While a calm stallion may not find it upsetting to see other horses, young or highly strung stallions can become overexcited and lose condition walking the fenceline.

Some stallions, particularly ponies, run in the field with their mares and may overwinter in the field with them. It is very unwise to turn a stallion out with or adjacent to geldings as the stallion will become very aggressive, particularly if there are mares in the vicinity.

Ideally, the stallion should have plenty of human contact. The stallion needs consistency of treatment with fair reward and punishment administered mostly by voice. A relationship of mutual esteem is ideal.

Diet

A popular stallion may cover up to three mares a day throughout the covering season and so he must start the season muscularly fit and in good condition. Some stallions lose condition dramatically and will need careful feeding with good quality hay or haylage and a concentrate ration similar to that of a competition horse. If he is competing he will obviously need to be fed for the work that he is doing. Other stallions keep their condition well and should not be overfed concentrates as they may become more difficult to handle. The horse's psychological wellbeing will be enhanced by allowing him as much good quality forage as he wants. If a stallion is overweight, decrease his concentrate ration and increase his exercise.

Fresh water should be available at all times and the total ration should include about 10% protein. A high protein stud cube need only be fed if the hay is of poor quality. A traditional ration of oats and bran should be supplemented with salt, limestone and a mineral and vitamin supplement.

Health
Even when the stallion is living in, routine worming is needed. It is important that parasites sapping the stallion's energy are reduced to a minimum. The stallion should also be injected against tetanus and equine influenza. Teeth need checking regularly, and the stallion's feet must be kept in good order. If the stallion is doing much roadwork, he will have to be shod.

Proper strapping will promote good condition as well as making the horse feel good and look more attractive to the owners of mares.

The stallion's penis will need swab testing by the veterinary surgeon at the beginning of the stud season to ensure that the stallion is free from any venereal disease that could be transmitted to a mare during covering. The vet wipes a sterile cotton wool swab on the penis, the swab is cultured in the laboratory and any bacteria found identified and appropriate treatment given to the stallion.

Some studs take a semen sample from the stallion before and during the covering season to ensure that the stallion is producing adequate amounts of viable sperm.

Choosing a stallion

Types of stud management
The first step in breeding a foal is to choose the stallion that the mare is going to be covered by. For most mare owners choosing the stud is equally important as it is essential to be happy with the environment in which you have left your mare.

The majority of horse stallions standing at stud are segregated from other horses and cover mares 'in hand', i.e. both mare and stallion are restrained during the covering procedure. However, many pony stallions run with their mares at grass, covering the mare when his instinct determines, not when a human being lets him. While this method is more natural it is obviously not practical for valuable Thoroughbreds and competition horses.

The Thoroughbred stud season runs from 15 February to 15 July in an effort to have foals born as early in the year as possible so that they have an advantage when racing as two-year-olds. The non-

Thoroughbred season tends to finish later than this as early born foals are not as important if the horse is not working and competing until it is four or five years old. Occasionally, mares that are very difficult to get in foal may run with the stallion during the autumn.

Maiden mares and mares with foals at foot are normally covered in hand and turned out in separate fields; mares with foals can be very aggressive to mares without foals.

In an ideal world, the young colt would run with mares to learn to live in the company of others as he would in the wild. Boisterous behaviour would be punished with a hefty kick, teaching him to approach a mare with discretion, from the side and enquiring before mounting her. Understandably, the owners of colts which have the potential to be good stallions are rarely willing to take the risks associated with this education.

How to choose a stallion

Stallions are no longer licensed by the Ministry of Agriculture and it is left to the Breed Societies to make their own arrangements for validating the use of a horse at stud. This validation may involve an inspection to observe conformation, soundness and freedom from hereditary defects.

If you wish to breed from a particular breed of stallion it is wise to get in touch with the Breed Society, otherwise you can browse through Stallion Directories or rely on word of mouth to make your choice. Bear in mind the location of the stud, the breeding record of the stallion, what his progeny look like, what they have done and how much the stud fee is, as these are all important factors.

Viewing the stallion

The next step is to send for the stallion's stud card which will tell you more about him and the stud, and then to make an appointment to go to the stud. As you arrive your first impressions are important – remember that you are going to leave your mare here for several weeks. First view the stallion in the stable to assess his temperament, taking a note of the standard of stable management. He will then be brought out and trotted up – depending on the type of stallion he may also be ridden. Observe his conformation, movement, action and attitude – he should look like a stallion without being aggressive and unruly.

It is important to see some of his progeny as this will give you some idea of the type of foal he tends to breed, although the conformation and type of mare you are using will obviously affect this.

You may also need to look at the stabling and foaling facilities available.

Stud fees and terms

Remember that the stud fee is often the least of your worries. You must also budget for grass keep or stabling, vet's bills, a groom's fee, a foaling fee, a swabbing, worming, the farrier, transport to and from the stud and VAT. Producing a foal is expensive and it is false economy to try and save on the stud fee – use the best stallion that you can afford.

The amount charged as a stud fee is a matter for the discretion of the stallion owner, but he must ensure that the price is competitive, especially if the stallion is not well known or there are others of the same breed in the area. The stallion must not be undervalued or he may be perceived as 'cheap', receiving poor quality mares and thus breeding poor quality stock – this will not enhance his reputation.

There are several arrangements for payment:

(1) A straight covering fee payable when the mare is collected from stud. This is generally used for less expensive stallions as there is no refund if the mare is not in foal.

(2) 'No foal, no fee (1 October terms)': the fee and keep fees, etc., are paid when the mare leaves the stud but if she is tested not in foal on or before the 1 October, the stud fee only is returned to the mare owner.

(3) 'No foal, free return': the fee is paid as before but if the mare does not hold that year, she will be covered without further fee the next year. Keep fees, etc., will still be payable.

(4) Live foal terms: if the foal does not live 24 or 48 hours, the stud fee is refunded.

(5) Part payment or split fee: part of the fee is paid when the mare is covered and the balance is payable under an arrangement such as (2) or (4).

The stud fee tends to get higher as the risk to the mare owner decreases. Thus a straight fee is likely to be less than a live foal fee. Concessions may be offered to the owners of approved mares with a good breeding record, particularly if the stallion is young and unproven. The more selective the stallion owner can be about the mares visiting his stallion the better will be the stallion's performance figures, both in terms of the percentage of mares in foal and the quality of foals born.

Thoroughbred stallions are often owned by a syndicate of owners. In a typical case, the stallion's value might be divided into 40 shares, with the owner of each share getting a free nomination, which may or may not be transferable.

Promotion

The stallion must be advertised. This could be in the local press, in special stallion numbers of weekly and monthly magazines and in breed society publications. The stallion may also be paraded at shows or else he may compete himself. On such occasions stud cards will be available to give more information about the stallion and the stud. Where there are several stallions at a stud, an annual open day and stallion parade are effective ways of advertising.

The young stallion

Colts may reach sexual maturity when two years old. It is all too easy to think that he is only a youngster and fail to take precautions against his popping over the fence and covering a mare. The three-year-old may be permitted a few experienced mares. The four-year-old may be advertised and take up to 20 mares while the mature five-year-old should be able to cope with twice that number.

Getting a mare in foal

Teasing or trying the mare

If mares are being covered in hand and the stallion has many mares, it is best that he should cover a mare as rarely as possible. Covering is time- and energy-consuming. The object is to cover the mare just before she ovulates so that the sperm going up meets the egg coming down. The difficulty is to know the precise moment. In the field the stallion repeatedly covers the in-season mare as long as she will receive him and he has the energy.

In a Thoroughbred stud the vet will put his hand in the rectum and feel the ovary through the gut wall. On some studs, the stud groom may observe the cervix through a sterile speculum.

On most studs, past experience of the particular mare will give a clue as to how long she will be in season. She will ovulate in the last two days of being in season, so, if the mare is going to be in season for five days, there would be little point in covering her before the third day. The semen of most stallions will still be viable in the mare 24 hours later and so to cover her again on the fifth day would be merely a safety measure.

However, even if the mare worked to such a typical pattern, the success of the plan depends on knowing exactly when the mare comes into season. This knowledge is essential and is gained by keeping accurate records and by observation. These two procedures are backed up by letting the mare know that the stallion is about. Although some well-mannered stallions are taken into the mare's field, the normal pattern is to walk the stallion in a bridle past the field where the mare is.

When the mare is in season she can be tried by the stallion. However, trying a mare will involve the stallion in some slight risk and so very expensive stallions will not be used. This job will be done for them by a rig or a low-value stallion called the teaser. Trying the mare is much easier with an experienced stallion and such a horse will sometimes show very clearly by his behaviour whether the mare is ready or not. If the stallion trying the mare is well mannered, life is less fraught for the handlers. Some stallions are over-enthusiastic and do not make the best teasers. The actual process of trying or teasing the mare may induce her to come into season.

A stud where the stallion runs with the mares will need no special facilities. However, on most studs there is a 'teasing' or 'trying board' where the stallion can tease or try the mares to see if they are in season. Although some owners will tease a mare at the stallion's door, there is then a danger that the mare will strike out and hurt herself on the door catches.

An alternative is a hatch where the stallion can put its head out and the mare stands, possibly in a crush or race which confines her. The wall below the hatch should be well padded, and similar protection should be affixed to the opposite wall towards the rear of the crush. An alternative arrangement is a free-standing padded wall (Fig. 26.2), well secured into the ground. This should be set on a free-draining and non-slippery ground surface. If protected from the worst of the wind and rain, this is an advantage. The area should be free from disturbance and out of public view.

In some studs, an indoor teasing board is used. This is often hinged out from the wall of a barn. Indoor facilities are a particular advantage for Thoroughbred studs which operate earlier in the spring

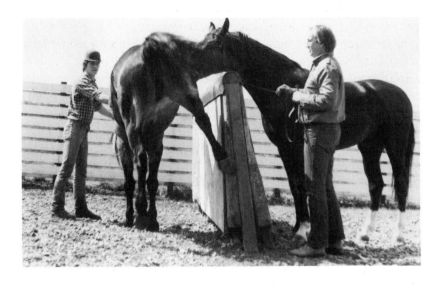

Fig. 26.2 A stallion at the trying, or teasing, board and a mare who is not in season.

because of the need to produce well-grown yearlings by the January following the foal's birth. In a stud barn, the floor will be a 'tan' mixture such as is used in a riding school, and the surface must be kept rolled level and watered so that it is firm and dust-free.

The board itself should be very robust and of a height such that it is level with the dip in the back of the average mare. The board must be longer than the mare so that she cannot kick the stallion or strike out in front of him. Some studs have a small pen at the front, offset from the line of a teasing crush. The purpose of this pen is to enable a groom to hold the mare's foal safely near her head. Some mares may be distracted if their foal is left away from them.

Another feature of a crush may be a bar at the front. This stops the mare running forwards. There may be a second bar at the back for use when the mare is being prepared for service or is undergoing veterinary examination.

In addition to teasing mares in the stud yard, it may well be necessary not only to walk the stallion past the mare's field but also to try mares over the fence. For this purpose, a plain close-boarded teasing board is set in the fence. At one time, protection on the top of the board took the form of a large wooden roller in case the stallion got a foreleg over the top, but anything safe and smooth will suffice as protection, and heavy duty rubber is commonly used.

Where the mares are to be tried at a trying board in the field fence-line, the stallion or teaser is taken to the board. He will probably call to his mares. The stallion handler notes which mares come to the stallion and how they react. An assistant will fend off protective or over-attentive mares. Some mares are shy about coming to the stallion and the assistant should put a head collar on these and bring them up to the board to be quietly teased.

Trying procedure

Each yard has its own procedure but the following is typical. The mare is led up in a bridle and stood behind the trying board with the handler standing by her left shoulder in the conventional manner. The stallion is then led up to the trying board in a bridle and lead rein. The handler carries a whip or stick and should wear gloves for safety. Some yards also insist on the handler wearing a hat: any hat gives some protection but a hard hat with chin harness is clearly the safest.

The stallion may make first contact with the mare nose to nose and the assistant must be on guard in case the mare strikes out. If the signs look hopeful, the assistant turns the mare parallel to the board so that the stallion can first nuzzle her right shoulder and then work his way back to the vulva.

Reactions that indicate a mare is in season include interest in the stallion, clear discharge from the vulva, slight squatting as she micturates and 'winking'. The vulva may be a little more filled with blood and look smoother and longer than normal. Although a mare may be coming into season and show some of the symptoms, she may not be ready to receive the stallion and will show this by kicking out, squealing, tail-swishing and laying back her ears.

Some shy mares will resist initially but, with patience, they will come round to the idea that they are ready to be mounted by a stallion. The stallion or teaser must therefore be willing to remain both enthusiastic and patient as he tries the mares. An over-noisy or aggressive stallion could prove off-putting to some mares but, on the other hand, a placid slow stallion might not be sufficiently stimulating.

Covering

When the mare is covered in hand, there are two styles common at studs. The main difference between the styles is accounted for by the conflicting requirements of being natural and being safe. To be totally safe, the mare may have hobbles put on her hind legs and these are attached by very strong cord to a neck strap. Other safety precautions include blindfolds, holding up a front leg, and twitching the mare. At the other end of the scale, the two horses on long lead reins are allowed to meet and mate in their own time and own way.

Procedure

A reasonable compromise is as follows. The upper hindquarters of the mare are groomed so they are free from dust and dirt and then they are washed with mild disinfectant, paying special attention to cleaning the dock, vulva and anus. Several swabs are used so that a dirty swab is never put back into the clean liquid. The tail is bandaged with a freshly laundered tail bandage. The long hair may be plaited and turned back into the bandage. The important point is that a tail hair should not lie across the vulva as the stallion's penis is inserted.

Felt overboots are then strapped on to the mare's hind feet to lessen the risk of her kicking the stallion. She is then held in a bridle and a long twitch is left ready in case it is needed. The stallion in his covering bridle with its lead rein is brought into the covering yard (Fig. 26.3). He should be brought to the mare's left flank where he can nuzzle the mare quietly and gain her confidence. If the stallion were to approach from behind, he might get kicked.

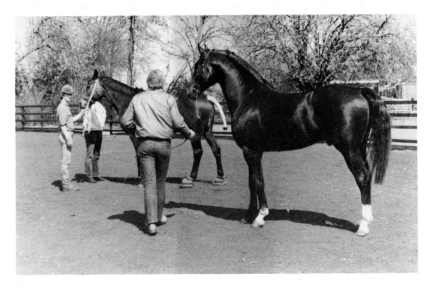

Fig. 26.3 A well grown three-year-old stallion showing good manners.

As the mare gets well aroused, the stallion will be similarly aroused although each stallion has his own speed of operation. If the mare is inclined to kick, a twitch can be applied for extra safety. In general, it is not necessary to twitch a mare, but with high-value stallions, twitching may be used as routine.

The smell of the mare causes the stallion to draw back his upper lip with his head held high in the Flehman posture. By the time the stallion has worked his way to the mare's rear, he should be fully drawn, i.e. he should have a fully erect penis. He may then mount. At this point some handlers like an extra assistant to hold the mare's tail out of the way and even to put the penis into the vulva. However, most stallions and mares can cope quite well.

As the penis goes up into the vagina, the mare may step forward a pace to balance herself. She must be kept straight. In the rare cases where the stallion is over vigorous with his front feet on her shoulders or his teeth on her withers, a protective leather may be put on the mare. A drop noseband is useful for stallions that are inclined to bite their mares.

Once into the mare the stallion will 'flag' his tail, which shows he is ejaculating. In his own time, he will quietly get down off the mare.

As soon as the penis is withdrawn, the stallion handler signals to the

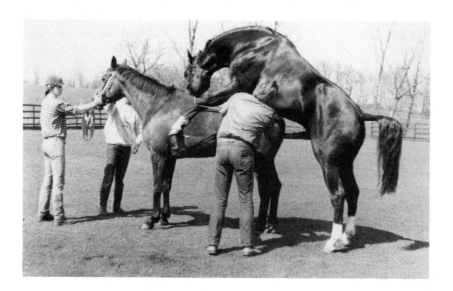

Fig. 26.4 The mare is kept straight and the stallion mounts her confidently.

mare's attendant who pulls the mare's head and leads her left and forwards. This move automatically turns the mare's quarters away from both the stallion and his handler so that they do not get kicked. The second assistant steps forward quickly with a jug of warm water to wash the stallion's penis. This must be done in the few seconds before the penis is taken back into the sheath. The use of a mild disinfectant is now discouraged as it kills harmless natural bacteria, allowing harmful ones to grow.

As the stallion withdraws, a little semen may be lost from the mare. The kicking boots must be unbuckled at once and the mare is then walked on for some while until she is settled, because some mares wish to urinate after service and it is considered that the mare might thus expel further semen. The semen should be in the uterus but some may be at the top of the vagina by the open cervix. The stallion, too, may like to be walked round while he cools off.

Young, inexperienced stallions need quiet experienced mares of the right height, who will stand steady. If the young stallion mounts at the side, the mare must be walked and repositioned for him to try again. Patience and time may be needed. A very enthusiastic youngster may require a second line to help restrain him. The second handler on the other side may become at risk if the stallion or mare turn out of line.

Where there are significant height differences between the mare and the stallion, it may be possible to use a slope or bank to help the stallion or even to stand a big mare in a hollow such as the water jump.

The young stallion will cover a mare a day; the older stallion will cover a mare in the morning and another in the afternoon. However, even covering mares only on alternate days, it may be that several mares will need to be covered in a single day and then the stallion must cope with these demands. The stallion who was got really fit before the stud season begins, and who is kept fit and strong through the season, will be better able to cope and is more likely to get a higher percentage of his mares in foal.

It is important to remember that as a stallion is used more often he may not be able to produce enough sperm to keep up adequate levels in the ejaculate – demand is greater than supply. This means that each subsequent ejaculate will become less and less fertile, thus overuse of a stallion will contribute to poor conception rates. If a stallion is so popular that he is covering two or three times a day, using artificial insemination (if he is not a Thoroughbred) may provide a successful alternative, one ejaculate being split to inseminate all the mares which are in season that day.

Getting all the mares in foal

Keeping a mare is expensive. There will be a period of at least 18 months from the day the mare was swabbed prior to covering until the foal is weaned. In addition to the costs of keeping mare and foal, there will have been the stud fee and related charges, and possibly some veterinary expenses. Producing a foal is therefore an expensive business and during the 18-month period the mare's value may have decreased. If, instead of producing a foal each year, the mare produces only two foals in three years, most of the costs are increased by 50%. It is, therefore, very important to ensure that each mare going to a stallion should be got in foal.

The first step is to spot the mare coming into season so that she can be swabbed by the vet. It is also important to identify when the mare next comes into season so that she can be tried at the right time. The mare should normally be covered on the second day of the season and thereafter on every second day until she 'goes off'. Some mares only stay in season for a few days, and they must be tried and covered daily. Other mares, particularly older ones, appear to have rather acid conditions within the genital tract and the sperm seems to fail to survive; these mares also need serving daily and artificial insemination may be of use here.

The problem mare is one who comes into and stays in season but fails to ovulate. An injection of luteinising hormone will cause the egg to be released from the ovary. A mare that fails to come into season can be helped by having the genital tract irrigated with saline solution. This should be done by the vet. Some mares will need a prostaglandin injection if a blood sample shows progesterone in the blood. Others will need progestogen, which can be given in the food for 10 days. Progestogen acts like progesterone, and when the treatment is stopped the mare will come into season some five days later. Usually she will ovulate on the fourth day of her season.

Once a mare has been covered and has gone out of season, it is important to ensure that she holds. She will therefore be checked to see if she comes into season again. A mare that has been properly covered but has failed to hold will need veterinary palpation of the ovaries to ensure that they are in a normal condition.

Pregnancy diagnosis

Rectal examination
Six weeks from the last service the vet can test the mare by manual examination to see if she is in foal.

Ultrasound scanning
Ultrasound scanning is the most up to date method of determining if a mare is in foal. The principle of the scanner is based on the echoing of sound waves such as used by a ship's sonar navigating in shallow water. High frequency sound waves are emitted from the scanner head or probe, directed through the tissues of the uterus and reflected back – echoing – to be picked up by the probe and converted to electrical impulses, which are displayed as a picture on the scanner television screen. The echo is proportional to the density of the surface of the tissue – the greater the density, the higher the rate of echo and the whiter the picture on the screen.

The scanner probe and cable are introduced through the anus into the mare's rectum (cleared of faeces) and manipulated forwards over the vagina, cervix and uterus. The sound waves are directed downwards through the floor of the rectum which contacts the upper wall of the uterus and reflects back from the uterine wall and its contents. Solid tissues of the uterus shows light-grey to white; fluids show black (non-echogenic) or flecked grey and black from pus, blood or urine.

The foetus in very early pregnancy diagnosis is too small to pick up but it lies within its yolk sac which is non-echogenic and shows as a black hole on the screen within the grey white uterus. The uterus appears like a slice of cucumber or orange and the fetus is usually clearly visible within it.

The normal period for initial scanning for pregnancy diagnosis is 17 to 21 days after ovulation. The conceptus is no longer mobile and has grown to a 'hole' of 2–3 cm diameter. Usually twins can be clearly differentiated at this stage and a skilled vet can pinch one out with a 90% chance of success, without disturbing the other, providing they are well separated. Seventeen days also coincides with the mare's return to oestrus after a non-fertile season.

Blood testing

The earliest blood test is taken between 40 and 100 days and is used to look for the presence of PMSG (Pregnant Mare Serum Gonado-trophin) produced by fetal cells in the uterine wall. This test can give false positives following fetal death and occasional false negatives where PMSG production is very low.

A second blood test is for the progesterone, produced by the corpus luteum, in pregnancy. This normally rises to a high level, remaining high throughout pregnancy. Although rather variable, the levels of this hormone can give a fair indication of pregnancy from as early as 30 days. However, progesterone levels remain high following fetal death without a return to oestrus.

Blood or urine oestrogen levels

From 60 days onwards oestrogen rises and peaks at about 210 days.

Paperwork

Memory is a fallible thing and consequently proper records should be kept in respect of each mare. These should be an ongoing record of the mare's performance at the stud, with particular reference to the days the mare was tried, in season, served, and tested in foal (or not), and when she foaled. Other items noted will be farriery and veterinary treatment.

27   The Mare

Selection for breeding

There is universal agreement that the wrong reason to select a mare for breeding is because she is not fit for anything else. A good reason to select a mare is because she is an outstanding example of quality. It may be that she has proved this quality in competitions, be it in the show ring, the racetrack or elsewhere. Usually it would be wrong to go on breeding from a mare that has difficulty in holding her fetus or in foaling, or from one that is a bad mother. Only an exceptional mare would justify these extra problems.

It is also wrong to breed from a mare with poor conformation or a poor temperament. Certainly, sentiment is no justification for breeding from such a mare. It would be wrong to breed from a mare if her foals are not full of quality, and are of good conformation and

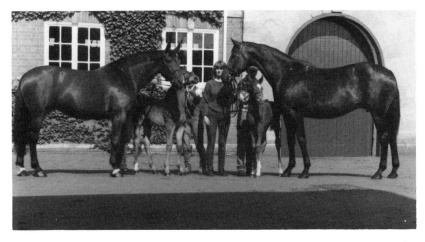

Fig. 27.1 Good brood mares. On the left a warmblood and on the right a Thoroughbred.

temperament, and robust and healthy. All too often a mare is bred from because she is there and not doing anything else. There are too many horses around and there is only room for the best.

Not all brood mares are beautiful. A mare may be a good type, but lack quality: when crossed with a suitable Thoroughbred, that mare will produce superb offspring. In Britain, in spite of originating the Thoroughbred and having superb native breeds, when it comes to sending out National Teams to compete in driving, dressage, show-jumping and eventing it is mostly imported horses that are used. The ideal is a home-bred horse with the courage of a Thoroughbred, the good temperament and strength of an Irish Draught, and a combi-nation of quality and presence. For showjumping and driving the stronger middleweight version would be used and for eventing the faster lightweight version; for dressage one would look for movement and good temperament. The British Horse Foundation Database allows the linking of breeding with performance records and will ultimately provide a national register of horses. Not only will this allow Britain to compete with the efficient breeding schemes on the continent, it will also have welfare and anti-theft applications.

The traditional English hunter is such a variable commodity that it is hard to standardise the type, even though, through the work of the National Light Horse Breeding Society (formerly the Hunter Improvement Society), most hunters are now sired by Thoroughbred stallions.

Sadly, the qualities now being sought are those that have been frittered away through lack of foresight. The Yorkshire Coachhorse was amalgamated with the Cleveland Bay, the Devon Packhorse disappeared, and so few Norfolk Roadsters survived the war that they could only point to what might have been. Even now no national effort has been made to save these blood-lines, which soon will have gone for ever. The only draught-lines remaining, other than the cobs and carthorses, are the Hackney and the Cleveland Bay. The former has been bred for action, and the latter, although it has the size and bone required, seems to lack the zest and willingness of spirit to meet with general approval for competition work. There is thus a great shortage of British stallions to cover Thoroughbred mares for cross-breeding.

Where pure breeding is proposed, the task is made easier by breeds, other than the Thoroughbred, having showing classes where skilled judges can indicate their personal preferences. Mare owners must ask themselves what type of foal they want to breed; what will its eventual use be and is the foal being bred for profit or for pleasure? It must always be remembered that the mare contributes 50% of the genetic input and it is unrealistic to expect a top class foal from an inferior mare, no matter how expensive the stallion.

Selecting a suitable stallion

There are three aspects to consider when selecting stallions to look at for a particular mare. These are genetic potential, performance and progeny.

Genetic potential

Genetically, the stallion is half of each of his parents, one quarter of each of his grandparents and one eighth of his great-parents. The information concerning his relations is generally available and is worth considering because his offspring will be half of him genetically. Within the Thoroughbred 'General Stud Book' there were 50 mares with traceable offspring in the first issue and this gives the 50 numbered families. In any breed, to breed within a line or family is called inbreeding and this will intensify both good and bad points. Inbreeding can be quite safe where the genes of the family are known to be pure, e.g. the Exmoor pony. Inbreeding can also bring a recessive and undesirable characteristic to the surface. Consideration of any pure siblings (brother and sisters) of the stallion will show the same genetic potential in a different light. Consideration of half-siblings is also relevant, as a study of a Thoroughbred sale catalogue will show.

Performance

What has that stallion done? Consideration should be given to his competitive achievements, his winnings and whether he stood up to training. If the stallion was a racehorse, what sort of distance was he best over? Has he a good reputation for temperament? Does he move well? Is he sound? Has he good fertility? These are all relevant questions.

Progeny

The stallion's progeny must also be considered to see whether he throws desirable characteristics and stamps his type. It may be that the offspring have undesirable traits or conformation faults.

Having shortlisted two or three stallions which are suitable for the mare in question, they then have to be visited. At the stud, the conformation, movement and temperament of the stallion should be studied. Another very important consideration is the standard and style of the stud. The mare owner must feel confident that the mare will be well cared for and pleasantly treated.

Sending a mare to stud

Before the mare is sent to stud there are several tasks for the mare owner to carry out. Initially a nomination form may need to be completed. This books the mare in to a particular stallion and acts as a written agreement between the stud and the mare owner. It will confirm the stud fee and set out any conditions of acceptance – for example that the mare will need swabbing before arrival at the stud.

When a mare goes to stud she must be in good condition. Her skin must be clean and free from parasites. Her feet must be in good order, recently trimmed and unshod behind. If she has not been very recently wormed, then the stud may worm her on arrival. Many studs like the mare to be vaccinated against tetanus and equine influenza and they may require documentary proof.

In terms of body weight and condition, it is difficult to breed from fat mares or very thin ones. The mare should go to stud fit and well, with a reasonable cover over her ribs and on a rising plane of nutrition. This slight increase in feeding mirrors the natural increase in spring grass which is part of the trigger mechanism to start the mare cycling regularly. Improved weather giving her sun on her back is a second trigger factor, but the most significant is the longer day.

With Thoroughbreds it is desirable to have early foals so it is necessary to start the mares cycling in February. To trigger the system, from January onwards bright lights are switched on in the mare's quarters to give at least 16 hours of light per day.

When the mare arrives at the stud she has to adjust to different feeds, different water and even different germs. Thus, when she first arrives she will regress slightly in condition, and it is therefore wise for the mare to arrive at the stud a week before she is next due in season. This aids the chance of getting her in foal. However, if it is required to cover her at the foal-heat, it is not wise to travel the mare and newborn foal so it is best for her to foal at the stud. In order to ensure that a mare is not too heavy, and to enable her to acquire immunity to the germs in her new environment (and thus pass on this immunity to the foal), she may go to stud as much as a month before foaling.

A minimum of equipment should be sent with the mare and anything left at the stud must be clearly marked. The mare should be sent to stud in the same condition as you expect to get her back – it is not the job of the stud to put condition on a thin mare, remedy neglected feet or to wash and trim manes and tails.

Swabbing

Internal and external parasites must be controlled as routine. The mare should be vaccinated against tetanus and equine influenza a month before foaling. Diseases affecting the genital tracts may interfere with the reproductive processes and be transferred from mare to stallion or vice versa.

To avoid the risk of sexually transmitted disease the stud is likely to insist that the mare has two swabs before she is covered. A swab is taken by the veterinary surgeon, wiping a sterile cotton wool swab on areas of the mare's reproductive tract. The swab is then cultured in the laboratory and examined for the presence of disease-causing micro-organisms.

The mare is swabbed for Contagious Equine Metritis (CEM) before she is sent to stud; the swab is taken from the clitoral fossa and the results take at least a week to be returned. The mare owner must take this into consideration when arranging for the mare to go to stud.

The second swab is usually taken at the stud and is taken from inside the genital tract to detect bacteria which may cause low grade infection, preventing the mare from conceiving. This cervical swab is taken when the mare is in season and her cervix is relaxed; the vet inserts a speculum into her vagina and passes the swab through the cervix. The results are available within 24 hours so that, if the mare is clean, she can still be covered that time.

Care of the in-foal mare

Management of the in-foal mare divides itself into three overlapping periods. During the first two months it is essential that the mare should not have a fall, blow or experience that might disturb the embryo. Once all is secure, there is the middle period of the pregnancy when the mare must simply be kept fit and well. Finally there is the last three months before foaling day.

The early months of pregnancy

Hopefully, when the mare does not come back in season after being covered, she is pregnant. The pregnancy can later be confirmed by the vet making a manual examination, by blood or urine samples, or by machine (see Fig. 27.2).

When a mare is not confirmed in foal, it may be that she did conceive but the embryo or fetus failed to take up a good anchorage, died and was reabsorbed. Germs infecting the mare's genital tract can be another cause of loss: there are various viruses, bacteria and fungi that may cause abortion. Unfortunately, an abortion at an early stage of pregnancy is not easy to detect. The small heap of reject material is quickly reduced by natural scavengers and will go unnoticed.

The conformation of the vulva of some mares is such that the lips are slack or incorrectly aligned. This defect can be remedied by

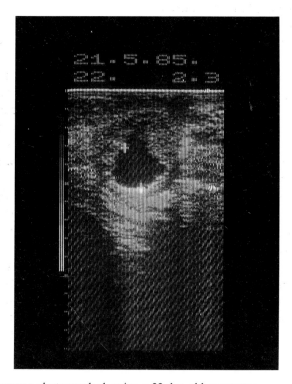

Fig. 27.2 A scanner photograph showing a 22 day old conceptus.

Caslick's operation. A mare with poor vulval conformation is prone to vaginal and uterine infections which would make it difficult for her to conceive.

A further possible cause of abortion is that the mare has conceived twins. If this happens, in the majority of cases the mare will abort. If a mare carries twins to full term, they rarely survive.

Although the use of pregnant mares is now less common, there is no reason why the mare should not continue to do ordinary light work for the first two-thirds of her pregnancy. Throughout her pregnancy it is important that the mare be kept fit. She should therefore take daily exercise. Many mares will remain out at grass and thus exercise themselves by grazing. Thoroughbreds and horses on heavy clay soils that poach may have to come in at night. Where there is no suitable field for grazing, daily controlled exercise is better than wandering around a straw yard. The 'horse-walker' machines have a useful part to play here, and twenty minutes' brisk walk would be a minimum for stabled mares. Alternatively, the exercise may be ridden or in-hand.

The middle months of pregnancy

The mare must be kept in good order. Feet, teeth, and worm control will all be of importance. Some wormers are not suitable for pregnant mares.

During this period, the mare will go into her winter routine and feeding will change accordingly. The aim is to keep the mare fit and healthy but not fat. A mare which is over-fed at this stage will lay down fat in her body which will hinder foaling and increase the strain on her legs. However, feed must be good. It must contain adequate minerals, vitamins and essential amino acids. It must be mould-free as some toxic foods will cause abortion.

As winter approaches, the mare's owner must ensure that the hay fed is clean, well made and well stored. The concentrates may be a cereal with a proprietary supplement which may include vitamins A, D, E and folic acid as well as minerals.

If the mare has a foal at foot, supplementary feed may be avoided until weaning is complete and the milk supply has dried up. At weaning, mares may be stabled for a day or two and fed only on hay or they may be turned away on to a bare, well-fenced pasture with a companion. The supply of milk should start to dry up after a few days. The udder should continue to be checked for mastitis.

The last three months of pregnancy

During this period, the main essentials are continued fitness, freedom from undue stress and a healthy diet. As the food is increased, it is best to change gradually to stud nuts. These contain the right level of protein as well as the essential amino acids. If a home mix concentrate is being used, the feed compounders produce a high protein balancer nut for adding to a home mix; it should not be used alone. Alternatively, grass meal and soya-bean meal or milk powder can all be included in the ration for the final month before foaling. This may be continued for a month or two after foaling, depending on the availability of grass. The stabled mare's diet should be kept reasonably laxative. Eighty per cent of fetal growth occurs in these last three months, and as the foal takes up more and more room in her abdomen the mare's appetite for bulk may fall. Fat mares should maintain, not lose, weight during this period and thin mares should gain condition.

In the later stages of this period it is more important than ever to be familiar with the normal habits and behaviour of the mare. A change in the pattern may be the first sign of foaling.

Foaling

Foaling is a natural process which most mares would rather cope with unaided and undisturbed. However, things can go wrong and whether it is policy to foal indoors or out, a foaling box or mare-and-foal box may be needed.

Foaling box

A foaling box must be larger than an ordinary box, and 4.6 m (15 ft) square is a good size. The reason for a big box is that when a mare goes down to foal she may lie sideways across the box, leaving inadequate room behind her. The box has to be cleaned out in advance and scrubbed clean. It should be disinfected throughout.

If a mare is going to be brought in when foaling commences, a thin layer of sawdust should be put under the bedding to prevent the mare from slipping. The box must be free of all sharp projections or obstructions. It should have a small night-light bulb for nights and be well lit for times of action: a dimmer switch is ideal. An infra-red heat bulb should be available.

An adjacent room where an attendant can sit up without disturbing the mare is desirable. On large studs, closed-circuit television is used, but regular visits, although more disturbing for the mare, will provide a reasonable chance of viewing the activity.

A plastic beer-making bucket with a close-fitting lid will provide a suitable container for the requirements. A clean working smock should be available and it is good for the mare to get used to people wearing such a garment. Fawn is more practical than white as a colour. A place is needed for thorough hand-washing and nail-scrubbing. Hot water may be required.

The equipment ready for various eventualities at foaling might include the following:

- Some clean towels to rub dry a foal if necessary
- A foal rug (or old jersey)
- An enema syringe, plus liquid paraffin
- A torch (for foaling in the field or in case of power failure)
- Some string
- Water, soap and towel
- A rug for the mare
- Head collar and tail bandage
- Cotton wool substitute
- Iodophore liquid (dairy teat dip) or antibiotic spray
- Baby's feeding bottle and calf teat
- Vet's telephone number

Signs of foaling

Mares carry their foals for about 330 to 340 days. The foal may therefore be expected eleven months from the last service, but an earlier or later delivery is not uncommon. After Christmas the mare's legs may fill after a night in the stable and she may need walking in hand, even if she is turned out during the day. About one month before foaling her udder will start to fill, known as 'bagging up', but this filling will go down on exercise. About a week before foaling she will stay bagged up all the time. When foaling is imminent a drop of 'wax' should form on the teats and milk may run. The muscles around the tailhead soften to a jelly-like consistency and sink. The quarters look slightly impoverished. The vulva normally looks firm and dry, and a hand placed across the hind quarters will not touch it. At this stage it will relax and moisten, and it may touch a hand placed across the quarters, showing that it has moved a little to the rear. Some of these signs can be seen in Fig. 27.3. Some mares will have people

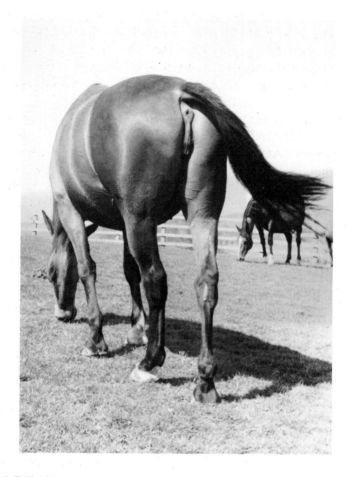

Fig. 27.3 Full udder, wax on teats, muscles round the tail-head soft, quarters looking less round, vulva relaxed and moist, and stood apart from the others – this mare did foal that night.

anxious weeks before the event; others may show only a slight change in behaviour, with increased restlessness.

Foaling

Foaling in the field is natural and is common for all native stock. A foaling box is common for Thoroughbreds. The foaling box offers convenience. Checking a field at midnight with a torch is a slow business! A modern foaling alarm is a useful but expensive piece of equipment which gives peace of mind and saves many hours. It is attached to the mare and sounds a remote alarm when foaling starts.

Mares usually lie down to foal, but at any stage they may get up, walk around and lie down again. The mare will look round anxiously, even before there is anything to see. The mare with contractions pushes the placenta membrane out through the cervix. The membrane then bursts, releasing the 'waters'. This first stage may be followed by a short rest.

The second stage occurs within ten minutes and is the appearance of the amnion surrounding the foal. This, too, will generally burst, releasing mucus. At this point many stud grooms like to enter the box quietly and check that the bulge showing at the vulva now contains a front foot, with a second front foot just behind it. Just behind and above the front feet there is the nose. This is the position for normal presentation and the attendant should leave the box quietly.

Even for this simple check, the attendant should be 'scrubbed up' or wear disposable surgical gloves. If the position is not normal or there is a delay in progress, then experienced help may be needed and the vet should be summoned. Most mares cope without help.

The front legs, head and then the shoulders emerge from the mare. The foal should be left to lie with its hind feet still in the vagina. This is important, as the mare will lie still and blood is being transferred through the umbilical cord from the mare to the foal. Possible action at this stage, if necessary, is to enter the box quietly and break the amnion covering the foal's nose, wiping it clear of mucus so that the foal can breathe. Normally, this help will not be needed as the foal breaks the membrane with its front feet. Although it is tempting to doubt the mare's and foal's ability to cope, nature generally knows best.

In due course, the mare will move, the foal's hind feet will be clear of the mother, the umbilical cord will break and seal itself, and the mare will recognise her foal. She will lick it clean and the mare–foal bond will be formed. A brief intrusion may be made to dip the naval stump of the foal into iodophore liquid, which can be obtained from the vet in advance (iodine is too strong). Dangling from the mare's vulva will be the umbilical cord and amnion. Sometimes the attendant will tie this up to itself so that it is clear of the ground.

A foaling box should not be warm at foaling time because the foal starts breathing as a result of its initial contact with the colder air. If a foal fails to start breathing, a bucket of cold water can usefully be thrown over its head and chest, followed by covering one of its nostrils and blowing up the other. When the foal is three hours old the stable may be kept a little warmer if mare and foal need to stay in.

Two things must happen within six hours. The afterbirth (placenta)

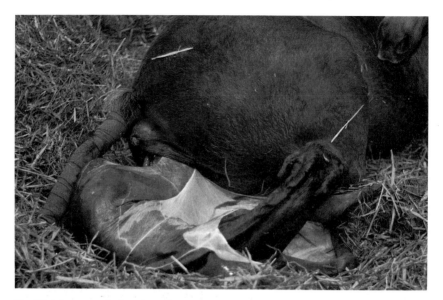

Fig. 27.4 Leave well alone!

must be passed naturally by the mare to complete the act of foaling. If this does not happen, the vet should be called. If it does occur, it should be checked to make sure the horns are intact, and put in a bucket with some cold water over it so that if there are complications within the next 24 hours the vet can check to see if all the afterbirth has come away.

The second vital happening is that the foal must suck. Assistance is often given when it is not needed. If the foal does not get to its feet after an hour or so, some assistance may be given. However, just as a foal will fail to get up several times before it succeeds, so too it will fail to find the teat at first. Interference should be avoided if possible. If it is necessary to help the foal, an assistant may be needed to hold the mare.

The mare's first milk is the colostrum and contains the antibodies necessary for the foal to survive. It is high in essential nutrients. It is vital that the foal receives this and, as a last resort the mare may have to be milked and the foal bottle-fed until it has the strength to cope on its own. If the mare was not given a tetanus booster 6 weeks before foaling, then the foal will need the vet to give it protection against tetanus.

The foal's first droppings, called the meconium, are delivered within the first 24 hours, provided the mare has been on a reasonably laxative

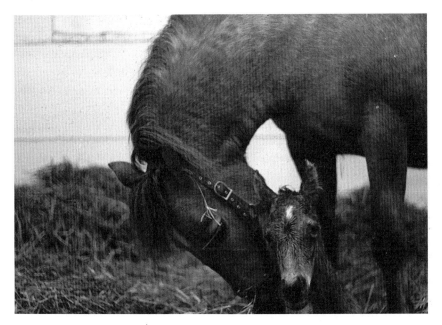

Fig. 27.5 Mare-foal bonding is important and best done without distraction.

diet prior to foaling. If the foal is unable to pass meconium, experienced attendants may try back-raking or using an enema syringe. Those with less experience will need the vet's help.

Once the mare has got rid of the afterbirth (has cleansed), her hindquarters should be cleaned with warm disinfectant. The vulva should be checked for tears. If the vulva is torn, it will need stitching by the vet. The mare should be given a bran mash with added limestone for extra calcium and then left in peace to enjoy her new foal.

Artificial insemination (AI)

With the aid of a suitable mare it is not difficult to collect semen from a stallion by means of an artificial vagina. The semen can be stored at a very low temperature. It may be diluted, or it may be used in its natural state.

There are several benefits of artificial insemination, notably disease control. If the stallion does not physically touch the mare he cannot contract any form of venereal disease. The contagious equine metritis epidemic in 1977 had a profound effect on the finances and reputation of many Newmarket studs; hence the stringent and expensive precautions now in force on most studs.

The second major benefit of artificial insemination is reduced risk of injury to the stallion. He never mounts a strange mare and this avoids his being kicked in the penis or testicles and so of being put out of use.

The third major benefit is that the semen is actually placed up through the cervix into the uterus of a mare at the right time.

These three benefits can combine to allow the stallion to cover an economically viable number of mares without the quality of the service suffering, ensuring high fertility rates. Many competition horse studs offer AI but the process is not allowed in Thoroughbreds. It is felt that AI is too open to abuse in terms of the number of foals one stallion could sire in one season and that ensuring that the right semen is inseminated into the right mare would be too difficult.

The use of chilled and frozen semen has made possible the use of stallions from the other end of the country or even abroad, so that mare owners now have a greater choice of stallion.

A further development in the competition horse world is the use of embryo transfer. A competition mare is covered and the resulting embryo flushed from her uterus after several days and collected. The pinhead-size embryo is then inserted into a recipient mare which then carries the foal to term and acts as its mother while the donor mare can continue her competition career. While this technique remains expensive it has been used successfully for several years with top class mares being able to breed foals without having to retire from competition.

Table 27.1 Stud facts and figures.

		Average	Normal range
Oestrus	In heat/in season/in use/on	Approx. 5 days	
Dioestrus	Not in season/off	Approx. 17 days	
Anoestrus	Not in season	Late autumn to early spring	
Pregnancy diagnosis			
Manual		42 days to end of pregnancy	
Blood test		45–90 days	
Urine sample		100 days onwards	
Scanning		Approx. 21 days	

Table 27.1 continues

Table 27.1 *continued*

	Average	Normal range
Length of gestation (full term)	340 days	320–360
	300–325 days described as premature	
	Before 300 days no hope of survival	
Bagging up of udder	10 days	2–30
Running milk	0 days	0–10
Waxing up	3 days	0–6
Foaling		
First stage		
(steaming up to breaking water)	30 mins	10 mins–2 days
Second stage		
(breaking water to showing amnion)	5–15 mins	
(breaking water to hips through pelvis)	30 mins	5–60 mins
Third stage		
(birth to passing afterbirth)	2 hours	20 mins–12 hours
	Get vet if longer than 8 hours	
Newborn foal		
Birth to breathing	90 secs	
Birth to breaking umbilical cord	5–15 mins	
Birth to suck reflex	up to 20 mins	
Birth to standing	20–100 mins	
Birth to suckling	60–120 mins	
Birth to passing meconium	0–2 days	
Temperature	101°F–101.5°F (38.3°C–38.6°C)	
Respiration rate	30–40 per minute	
Heart rate	80–140 per minute	

28 The Foal and Young Horse

The first few days

Foals born in the field are often brought in with their mothers so that they can be observed at three-hourly intervals for the first day so as to ensure that all is well. The mare will appreciate some cut grass while she is stabled. Providing the weather is fine, on the second day mare and foal can go out for exercise, and on some studs the foal may run loose behind the mare.

The foal will have to have a foal-slip (small head collar) put on at some point in the first week. The foal-slip is secured with an assistant holding one arm round the chest and the other arm round the quarters. If the foal is hard to catch, the mare can be so placed as to corner it. Right from the start, leading is safer than allowing the foal to run loose. For early leading, a soft web line is placed through the foal-slip and passed back to the left hand. At first, this hand steadies the foal by being placed across its chest. A second loop of similar material is dropped around the foal's quarters and is held on the loins. The mare should be led by an assistant and the foal kept by the mare's flank. Thus, the mare's leader is in front of the foal, its leader and the mare are on either side of it, and the back-strap is behind it (see Fig. 28.1).

After a week or two, if the mare and foal are coming in at night, the foal will become accustomed to being led and then one person will be able to handle both mare and foal. However, assistance may still be needed at the field gate. The fit of the foal-slip must be checked regularly: foals grow fast!

It is essential that the foal gets an adequate supply of milk. In spite of careful feeding, it may be that the mare does not produce enough. Alternatively, the mare may be tender or nervous and will not allow the foal to suck. Some mares need to be held, sometimes with a foreleg held up, while the foal is suckling. However, such measures are rarely necessary, and even nervous or tender mares will generally come

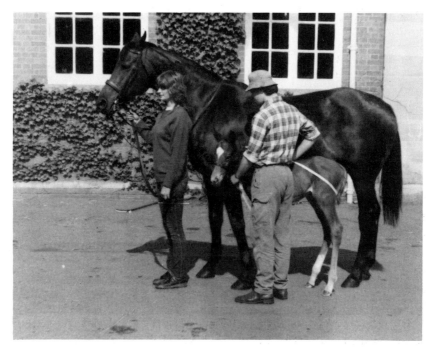

Fig. 28.1 The foal learns to be obedient and walk freely forward in its first week.

round within a few days. When suckling, the mare takes most of the hind weight on the leg next to the foal, so tilting her pelvis and making it easier for the foal to get to the teats.

Some mares are put back into work after about three weeks. It is then important that the foal should be allowed to suck every three hours. The normal pattern of sucking is a five- to ten-minute feed every two hours during the day, but less frequently at night. After taking nourishment, often the foal will relieve itself and then sleep for up to half an hour.

If either mare or foal should die or the mare have no milk, the National Foaling Bank should be consulted at once (telephone: Newport (Shropshire) 811234). This organisation has vast experience of artificial rearing and of fostering.

During the first hour of life, the foal will breathe faster than is normal, but should settle to a respiration rate of 20 to 30 per minute. This is about twice as fast as its mother's respiration rate. The pulse will be about 80 at birth but go up to 140 as it struggles to find its feet. The pulse rate will settle to nearly 100 beats per minute for a day-old foal and will be down to under 50 for a yearling. The temperature should be 38.3 to 38.6°C (101.0–101.5°F).

Diseases of the foal

Behavioural disorders
Symptoms: Excessive nervousness, muscular twitching, shivering, nodding, staggering, lack of suck reflex, convulsions, incessant chewing, etc.
Causes: May be meningitis (inflamed skin surrounding the brain) or dummy syndrome (neonatal maladjustment syndrome, NMS) caused by brain damage at birth.
Treatment: Call the vet. With good nursing under veterinary direction the foal may recover completely but it may well be lost.

Diarrhoea
Symptoms: Scouring.
Causes: A tummy upset typically caused by a chill or by a change in the mare; for example, when a mare comes into season on her foal-heat about nine days after foaling, the foal will often scour for a day or two.
Treatment: Simple treatments are available from the vet; in particular, the electrolytes (body salts) must be maintained.

Entropion
Symptoms: Ingrowing eyelid.
Cause: Congenital (born with it) imperfection.
Treatment: The vet can turn the eyelid outwards and secure it with a stitch until it settles correctly.

Haemolytic disease
Symptoms: Sleepiness, yellow (jaundiced) or pale membranes, failure to suck, listlessness, red urine.
Cause: The red blood cells in the foal are destroyed by the antibodies in the colostrum from the mare.
Treatment: The foal will need an immediate blood transfusion. Once the mare's colostrum has finished (she must be milked out regularly and the milk discarded), then the foal may use her milk again.

Thoroughbred mares and stallions are tested before covering to see if their blood types are incompatible and likely to cause haemolytic disease. Once a mare has had a haemolytic foal care should be taken to ensure that the next foal is not haemolytic. If the foal is not allowed to suckle the mare's colostrum and is given a course of antibiotics or colostrum from another mare the disease will be prevented and the foal will be able to suckle from its mother at a later stage.

Hyperflexion or weakness of lower limb

Symptoms: Pasterns and/or fetlocks hyperflexed (overbent) or weak (point of fetlock sinking so that the ergot nearly touches the ground).
Causes: Suspensory tendons and ligaments may be slightly long or short, or the muscle tension may be too weak or too strong.
Treatment: Mild cases will often right themselves. Severe cases may be aided by corrective boots carefully fitted and regularly changed. In areas of very high value foals such as Newmarket there are specialists who will provide such a service. Later on, tiny corrective shoes may be fitted with, for example, extended roll toes to sink the heel on to the ground for contracted tendon treatment.

Infectious white scour

Symptoms: Scouring (diarrhoea) within a day or two of birth, covering the foal's buttocks in yellow/grey matter which smells unpleasantly.
Cause: A bacterial infection of the gut.
Treatment: Keep the hindquarters clean by regular washing in warm soapy water. A protective cream such as udder cream for dairy cows can be used to prevent scald. Maintain scrupulous hygiene. Burn the soiled bedding. Always treat this foal last in the round. The vet must be called and treatment given to control the infection and to cope with the dehydration which is inevitable with diarrhoea.

Joint ill

Symptoms: Swelling and failure of the navel to dry up. Swollen joints and stiffness. Lack of appetite and symptoms of pain. The condition can rapidly deteriorate and cause death.
Cause: Blood poisoning by infection through navel.
Prevention: To avoid this disease or any failure of the colostrum to give early protection, it is common practice for the vet to examine a newborn foal and to give it an antibiotic injection. Also, foaling-box hygiene must be excellent and the foal's navel should be treated at birth.
Treatment: Call the vet at once.

Parrot mouth and cleft palate

Symptoms: See pages 16 and Chapter 8. The newborn foal must be examined for deformities such as these.

Cause: These are congenital abnormalities.

Treatment: As with any congenital abnormality, the vet must advise whether it will come right of its own accord, whether it may be operated on or treated, or whether the foal should be put down as not viable.

Pneumonia

Symptoms: Fast breathing, fever, coughing.

Cause: Inflamed lungs due to infection. Occurs more commonly in stuffy, poorly ventilated housing.

Treatment: Antibiotics, good nursing and warm but well-ventilated housing.

Sleepy foal disease

Symptoms: Fever, sleepiness, rapid respiration, failure to suck, loss of strength.

Cause: A specific bacterial infection.

Treatment: This disease is usually fatal.

Snotty nose (rhinopneumonitis)

Symptoms: Cold, catarrh, cough, nasal discharge.

Cause: A specific virus infection of the upper respiratory tract.

Treatment: Consult the vet.

Umbilical hernia

Symptoms: at 4–6 weeks old a soft swelling appears at the navel.

Cause: The muscular ring, through which the vessels passed to form the umbilical cord, fails to close after birth and abdominal contents protrude.

Treatment: The vet will decide if and when treatment is necessary. The condition may right itself within twelve months. If the opening is squeezing the swelling (a strangulated hernia), then it will cause pain and need prompt surgical attention.

Worms

Symptoms: Loss of condition and failure to gain weight.

Cause: Worm parasites (as discussed in Chapter 8). Adult horses may not show the effects of worms because they have a certain degree of immunity. Young stock are much more susceptible.

Treatment: (a) Rear young stock on pasture that is as clean as possible from parasite infection. (b) Keep the mare regularly treated so that she is not carrying a heavy worm burden. *Note:* some anthelminthics (anti-worm drugs) are not suitable for pregnant mares. (c) Maintain a regular monthly dosing programme from six weeks of age to cover both strongyle and ascarid worms, and bots in autumn.

Meconium retention

Symptoms: Occurs in the first three days of life – the foal rolls, strains and lies in awkward positions, refuses to suck, and the abdomen may be distended.

Cause: Inability to void the meconium easily. Meconium is the faeces stored in the rectum while the foal is in the uterus and usually only expelled once the foal is born. The brown, black or green, hard or soft pellets, with a slimy covering, are usually passed during the first three days of life.

Treatment: Call the vet who may inject pain-killing drugs, give an enema and liquid paraffin by stomach tube.

Ruptured bladder

Symptoms: Signs appear two to four days after birth and include failure to pass normal streams of urine, crouching and straining (can be confused with meconium retention). Abdomen becomes distended.

Causes: A condition of the newborn foal in which a hole or tear in the bladder wall causes continual escape of urine into the abdomen. May be due to faulty development or occur during birth.

Treatment: Treated by operation under general anaesthetic to close the tear. Most foals survive if diagnosed early enough.

Discipline

A rigid procedure is essential when several people are leading mares with foals or young stock. For example, if three mares with foals were led to a paddock, and the first handler, immediately on entering the paddock, were to release his mare and foal, the mare might well buck, kick, knock into the foal and then gallop off, thus causing problems for the other leaders, whose charges would want to join in the fun. All stud work involves care, thought, attention to detail and good discipline.

The early handling of foals is the beginning of their training and they must be taught good manners. It is important that this handling should be kindly but firm. Nothing is more confusing to animals than people who are inconsistent, or liable to be moody, or lose their tempers. A foal that rears or paws should be disciplined by slapping its chest and scolding it. A foal that bites (even in play) is best disciplined by pulling its whiskers rather than by hitting its muzzle. Violence and ill-temper must be avoided at all costs, as must over-indulgence.

When foals are two months old, they may be shown in hand with their mother. For showing it is important that the foal should be polite and lead well. The foal should be accustomed to being stood up in front of the mare and to having the mare stood up in front of it. When being shown, mare and foal will have to be separated to some degree, so that the judge can observe each move without the other masking the picture. All of this handling will help the foal to become accustomed to both humans and discipline. Foals must also learn to have their feet picked out and this will prepare them for having their feet trimmed by the farrier.

Weaning

Horses in the wild tend to live as family groups. As the colts mature, the mare will reject them, but a filly may remain with her mother for several years.

During the first winter after foaling, it is natural for the mare's milk flow to decrease markedly, and so the foal must be nutritionally independent. In stud management, it is usual to wean foals in September, when the grass loses much of its food value. However, if the mare is not again in foal, the foal need not be weaned at this stage. During weaning, the foal should be in good health and be showing independence.

In the month before weaning, the foal must get used to concentrates. Both mare and foal can be fed twice daily or, alternatively, 'a creep' can be introduced. A creep is a device for allowing the foal to feed, but not its mother. One type is a feed bowl attached to the fence, which has an adjustable narrow opening so that only the tiny muzzle of the foal can fit in to eat the food. A second type of creep is based on a narrow opening through which the youngster can pass but not the mother. However, for horses a wider opening is often used, but with an adjustable height bar across it so only the foals can pass under it. Where creeps are used, the foals must be attracted and introduced to the idea. This can be done by using highly palatable food to tempt the foal, which must also be introduced to the location of the feeder.

During weaning it is helpful if there are several mares and foals together in the field, which must be safely fenced. One of the mares is removed quietly one morning and she is placed with a companion in a far-distant well-fenced fairly bare field. Her foal is left with its friends and soon settles down. A day or so later, another mare or two may be taken. One mare should be left as long as possible as a guardian and disciplinarian.

An alternative method, which is traditional, but which tends to set back the foal due to the trauma, is to shut the foal in a stable. Probably the foal will try to climb out, and so the top door must be shut or else covered with a grille. There should be nothing in the stable that could catch up the foal, and so hay is fed on the floor. Water and concentrates are fed in safe containers that do not spill easily. When turning out, such foals may seek their mothers so they should have known company and a well-fenced field.

Colts should be separated from mares and fillies before the first spring after their birth because their natural tendency to mount the females is not to be encouraged. Colts may become fertile as two-year-olds but usually will be castrated before then.

Nutrition

When considering nutrition of young stock, the first essential is to decide on both short- and long-term aims and objectives. Is the foal to be a show winner as a foal, as a yearling, as a two-year-old, etc? Is the foal to be sold at weaning, or as a yearling, or when? Is the horse to be a competition winner? What sort of contest? All of these questions should have been considered before conception, but circumstances change and so reconsideration is necessary.

Two opposing facts must be balanced. First, the winner in the show ring or the most admired horse at a sale tends to be the most precocious animal – big, well advanced and possibly heavy-topped. To have a horse in this condition for a sale day is one thing, but to so maintain it for a show season has long-term dangers, particularly for one- to three-year-olds. Secondly, horses that have been overfed and have advanced too fast as youngsters tend not to make the best mature animals. On the other hand, it is a false economy not to feed the foal up to its growth potential. It is important that its nutrition allows it to reach full potential. The general long-term aim is good-quality food in plentiful supply so as to produce a big, strong, fit but not fat youngster.

Epiphysitis, which causes round and sometimes warm joints, is a danger to be avoided. The growing plates (epiphyses) on the long bones of the leg are just behind the bearing ends. These growing plates can get swollen by jarring. This is a particular danger with heavy-topped young stock on hard ground. The condition may also be caused by a lack of calcium, or a poor calcium : phosphorus ratio, or by bran inhibiting calcium uptake.

Young stock in winter getting a hay and cereal diet may lack some essential amino acids (e.g. lysine and methionine). To overcome this, a proprietary rearing mix may be used, or alternatively, a home mix which includes dried milk, dried grass or soya-bean meal. The home mix will also need mineral and vitamin supplements. The winter feeding should be so good that the foal moves smoothly on to spring grass on an equal plane of nutrition. An old rule of thumb for Thoroughbred foals was to feed, daily, 444 g (1 lb) of concentrates for each month of age.

Old pasture rather than new is best for young stock. Ideally, the pasture should be free from ruts or deep winter tread marks which could strain the young foal's limbs. The sward can contain up to 10% clover; a higher ratio could interfere with bone metabolism. Lush spring grass (early bite) may be high in vitamin A, and as this depresses vitamin D uptake, rickets could result. Additional vitamin D is therefore useful in spring. Slightly acid pastures are better for good mineral uptake, and so over-liming must be avoided.

Education and training

During the first three years of its life, the horse's bones are comparatively soft and are growing fast. Consequently, the horse should not be subjected to weight-carrying or strenuous work until the third year. Abnormalities are likely to occur in the bones and joints if this precaution is not taken.

Flat-race horses are subjected to earlier training, but they carry minimal weights and work on straight or gently curving tracks.

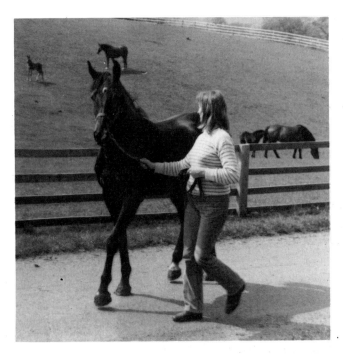

Fig. 28.2 A well-grown yearling moves pleasantly and freely forwards showing good in-hand training.

However, it should be noted that they have a very bad soundness record.

If a young horse is ruined through mismanagement, it will have to suffer for the remainder of its life through no fault of its own. Mismanagement is also costly to the owner because of all the costs that have been incurred in producing the youngster.

Probably, these costs will have been minimised by allowing the horses to live out, thus saving on labour, which inevitably reduces the amount of handling, unless they have been through a sale or have been shown. The quality of handling must be excellent even if it is minimal. A horse that has received strict but fair discipline during its most formative years will be easier to break and will therefore be set back less by the breaking process.

The procedure for breaking and initial training is outside the scope of this book. The authors' intention is to help readers to understand more about management, and the best management is *management with understanding*.

Appendixes

Appendix I: The Rationale of Feeding Horses

Rationing in six steps

Step one: *'How big is the horse or pony?'*
Estimate horse's bodyweight

Method   A   –   Table of Weights (see Table AI.1).
             B   –   Tape Measure and Table.
             C   –   Weigh-tape.
             D   –   Weigh-bridge.
             E   –   Guess.
Measure in kg (50 kg = 1 cwt)

Step two: *'How much can it eat each day?'*
Check horse's capacity

Method $\dfrac{\text{Bodyweight in (kg)}}{100} \times 2.5 = \text{capacity in kg}$

Example A 16 hh, seven-year-old riding horse weighs 500 kg

Capacity $= \dfrac{500}{100} \times 2.5 = 12.5$ kg (28 lbs) of hay and concentrates per day

Guesstimate: Horse's height in hands $\times$ 2 = capacity in lbs.

Step three: *'How much hay per day?'*
Provide energy for maintenance

Calculation 18 MJ $+ \dfrac{\text{Bodyweight (kg)}}{10} = \text{requirement}$

Provide this from fresh grazed grass or conserved grass e.g. hay, haylage, silage. (See Table AI.2.) However, don't feed too much hay, leave room for production.

455

Rough guide

	Hay (%)	Concentrates (%)
Maintenance	100	0
Light work	75	25
Medium work	60	40
Hard work	40	60
Fast work	30	70

Example Our Riding Horse.

Energy for maintenance $= 18 + \dfrac{500}{10} = 68$ MJ of digestible energy (DE).

Table AI.2 shows: average grass hay $= 9$ MJ of DE

$\therefore \dfrac{68}{9} = 7.6$ kg of hay per day (about 17 lb)

$=$ About 60% of capacity which is OK for light/medium work

Step four *'How much concentrate feed?'*
Provide energy for production

For *Work* per day, for each 50 kg bodyweight add MJ of DE:

Light work	+ 1 e.g. One hour walking.
	+ 2 e.g. Walking and trotting.
Medium work	+ 3 e.g. Some cantering.
	+ 4 e.g. Schooling, dressage and jumping.
Hard work	+ 5 e.g. Hunting 1 day/week.
	+ 6 e.g. Hunting 2 days/week.
Fast work	+ 7 e.g. 3-day eventing.
	+ 8 e.g. Racing.

For *Lactation* per day, for each 50 kg bodyweight add:

For first 3 months $+ 4\frac{1}{2}$ MJ of DE.
For next 3 months $+ 3\frac{1}{2}$ MJ of DE.

N.B. All diet changes must be gradual.

For *Pregnancy* per day, add:

$+ 12\%$ for the final $\frac{1}{3}$ of gestation or last 3 months.

For *Growth* per day, add:

Young stock over 1 year – feed at maintenance ration for their expected weight at maturity.

Up to 1 year provide 13 MJ of DE per kg of food and feed to capacity.

Example Our riding horse in light/medium work.

$$\text{Energy for production} = \frac{500 \text{ kg of bodyweight}}{50} \times 2 = 20$$

Table AI.2 shows: barley = 17 MJ of DE

$$\therefore \frac{20}{17} = 1\frac{1}{4} \text{ kg of barley per day for work (nearly 3 lbs)}$$

Step five *'Is the food suitable?'*
Provide sufficient protein

For *Maintenance* – 7.5 – 8.5% crude protein in ration

For *Production*

Light work	7.5 – 8.5%
Medium work	7.5 – 8.5%
Hard work	9.5 – 10%
Fast work	9.5 – 10%

For *Lactation*

First 3 months	12.5%
Next 3 months	11%

For *Pregnancy*

Final $\frac{1}{3}$ gestation	10%

For *Growth* – For all growth check protein quality.

Suckling foal	16 – 18%
Weaned foal	14.5 – 16% (6 months +)
Yearling	12 – 14% (12 – 18 months)
One – Two	10 – 12% (18 – 24 months)
Two – Four	8.5 – 10% (24 – 48 months)

Example Our riding horse, seven years old:

Getting: 7.6 kg of hay + 1 ¼ kg of barley per day
Table AI.2 shows the percentage of crude protein (CP) in the feed so with the feed given above the %CP per day is:

Av. grass hay 7.6 kg × 8 = 61
         barley   1.25 kg × 11 = 14

                8.85 into   75 = 8.5%CP

N.B. The nutritive values shown in Table AI.2 provide a guide based on averages, but individual food samples may show variation.

Step six *'Mixing Art with Science'*
Check and adjust

1. Check that the ration contains sufficient roughage
Supply 0.6 kg roughage per 100 kg bodyweight or more. (This is a minimum.)

Example Our riding horse weighing 500 kg.

$$\frac{500}{100} \times 0.6 = 3 \text{ kg of hay as a minimum}$$

2. Check the horse's condition
By eye and/or tape or weighbridge.
Is the horse gaining or losing weight?
Do you want it to do so?
What is its ideal performance weight?
Adjust the ration as necessary.

Example We would like our riding horse to have a bit more 'cover over his ribs'. So we will increase the concentrates. One extra kg of barley gives:

11% crude protein ⟶ Muscle
16 MJ of DE ⟶ Fat or energy

3. Check the horse's temperament
A Thoroughbred may need up to 10% extra food.
Native or draught stock may need 10% less.

N.B. Calm and routine – save food.

4. Check the environment
Feed extra under bad conditions both in field or in stable, e.g. cold stable, thin bedding, thin rug. A cold horse needs extra energy to keep warm.

5. Check for parasites
Feed only the horse. The commonest parasites are worms, especially round white worms in foals, red worms in all other stock.

6. Check the horse's efficiency as a converter of food
Horses reared on worm infested pastures may have permanently damaged guts and will always need extra care with their nutrition.

Horses with sharp teeth and sore mouths will not chew their food properly for good digestion.

7. Check that the horse has plenty of fresh water
Lack of water reduces capacity and digestion.

8. Check food quality and container hygiene
Mouldy hay, musty corn, tainted food, dirty manger; all depress appetite. Badly harvested, badly conserved, badly stored food loses quality, loses vitamins, loses appeal.

Food contaminated by vermin can carry disease.

9. Check that the horse is not lacking minerals or vitamins
Apart from salt, unless the horse is growing or under stress, it will not necessarily need supplements any more than humans do.

10. Check that the horse enjoys his food.

460   *Appendix I*

Table AI.1   Guidelines for estimating horse's bodyweight.

Height (hh)	Type	Approximate weight			Girth (cm)
		(kg)	(lbs)	(Other)	
10	Pony	200	440		135
13	Foal/Weaner	200	440	4 cwt	
12	Pony	300	660		150
13	Pony	350	770	7 cwt	160
14	Horse Yearling/ Pony	400	880		170
14.2	Pony	450	990		175
15	Hack	450	990		175
14.2	Cob	500	1,100	½ tonne	184
16	Thoroughbred	550	1,200		190
16	Hunter	600	1,320		196
16	Hunter	650	1,430		
16.2	Draught or Shire Horse	1,000	2,200	1 tonne	

Table AI.2   Nutritive value of some common foodstuffs.

	Crude protein (%)	Digestible energy (MJ/kg)
Cereals		
Oats	10	11–12
Barley	9.5	13
Maize	8.5	14
Protein		
Soya meal	44	13.3
Dried milk	36	18
Linseed	22	18.5
Field beans	26	16
Grass meal	12–18	13
Intermediate foods		
Wheatbran	15.5	11
Sugar beet pulp	7	10.5
Hays		
Good grass hay	9–10	9
Av. grass hay	4.5–8	7–8
Poor grass hay	3.5–6	7

Note: this is only a guide and a lot of variation is found in practice.

Appendix II: Interval Training to Novice One-day-event Fitness: A Detailed 12-week Schedule

Throughout the fitness programme the horse should be turned out for a couple of hours whenever possible, particularly on rest days. All hacks should be for a minimum of one hour.

Week 1
   Day 1: 20 minute walk
   Day 2: 30 minute walk
   Day 3: 40 minute walk
   Day 4: 50 minute walk
   Day 5: 60 minute walk
   Day 6: 60 minute walk
   Day 7: Rest day

Week 2
   Day 1: 1 hour 10 minute walk
   Day 2: 1 hour 20 minute walk
   Day 3: 1 hour 30 minute walk
   Day 4: 1 hour 40 minute walk
   Day 5: 1 hour 50 minute walk
   Day 6: 2 hour walk
   Day 7: Rest day

Week 3
   Day 1: 2 hour hack including one 400 m (1 minute 50 seconds) trot
   Day 2: 2 hour hack including two 400 m trots
   Day 3: 2 hour hack including three 400 m trots
   Day 4: 1 hour 30 minute hack including two 800 m (3 minute 40 seconds) trots
   Day 5: 1 hour 30 minute hack including three 800 m trots; check recovery

Day 6: 1 hour 15 minute hack including two 1100 m (5 minute) trots

Day 7: Rest day

Week 4

Day 1: 1 hour 30 minute hack including three 5 minute trots; check recovery

Day 2: As Day 1

Day 3: 1 hour walk plus 20 minutes schooling

Day 4: As Day 1

Day 5: 1 hour walk plus 20 minutes schooling

Day 6: As Day 1

Day 7: Rest day

Week 5

Day 1: 1 hour 30 minute hack including three 5 minute trots and one 1 minute canter (400 m at 400 mpm); check recovery. The canter work may be done in the school.

Day 2: 1 hour walk plus 20 minutes schooling, including pole work

Day 3: 1 hour walk plus 30 minutes schooling

Day 4: 1 hour 30 minute hack including three 5 minute trots and two 1 minute canters; check recovery

Day 5: 1 hour walk plus 30 minutes schooling, including small jumps

Day 6: 1 hour 30 minute hack including three 5 minute trots and three 1 minute canters; check recovery. Alternatively, a dressage competition

Day 7: Rest day

Week 6

Day 1: 1 hour 30 minute hack including three 5 minute trots and two 2 minute canters (800 m at 400 mpm); check recovery

Day 2: 1 hour walk plus 40 minutes schooling, including pole work

Day 3: 1 hour walk plus 40 minutes schooling, including small jumps

Day 4: 1 hour 30 minute hack including three 5 minute trots and three 2 minute canters; check recovery

Day 5: 1 hour walk plus 40 minutes schooling

Day 6: 1 hour 30 minute hack including three 5 minute trots and

two 3 minute canters (1200 m at 400 mpm); check recovery.
Alternatively, a small show-jumping competition

Day 7: Rest day

Week 7

Interval training begins in earnest and the 4-day schedule is adhered to as far as possible.

Day 1: Hack
Day 2: 1 hour hack plus 40 minutes schooling
Day 3: 1 hour hack plus 45 minutes schooling and jumping
Day 4: 45 minute hack plus three 3 minute canters at 400 mpm with 3 minute walk between; check recovery
Day 5: Hack
Day 6: 1 hour hack plus 40 minutes schooling
Day 7: A dressage or show jumping competition

Week 8

Day 1: 45 minute hack plus one 3 minute canter and two 4 minute canters at 400 mpm with 3 minute walk between; check recovery
Day 2: Rest day
Day 3: 1 hour hack plus 40 minutes schooling
Day 4: 1 hour hack plus 45 minutes schooling and jumping
Day 5: 45 minute hack plus three 4 minute canters at 400 mpm with 3 minute walk between; check recovery
Day 6: Hack
Day 7: 1 hour hack plus 40 minutes schooling

Week 9

Day 1: 1 hour hack plus 45 minutes schooling and jumping
Day 2: 45 minute hack plus two 4 minute canters and one 5 minute canter at 400 mpm with 3 minute walk between; check recovery
Day 3: Rest day
Day 4: 1 hour hack plus 40 minutes schooling
Day 5: 1 hour hack plus 45 minutes schooling and jumping
Day 6: 45 minute hack plus one 4 minute canter and two 5 minute canters at 400 mpm with 3 minute walk between; check recovery
Day 7: Hack

Week 10

    Day 1: 1 hour hack plus 40 minutes schooling

    Day 2: 1 hour hack plus 45 minutes schooling and jumping

    Day 3: 45 minute hack plus three 5 minute canters at 400 mpm with 3 minute walk between; check recovery

    Day 4: Rest day

    Day 5: 1 hour hack plus 40 minutes schooling

    Day 6: 1 hour hack plus 45 minutes schooling and jumping

    Day 7: Cross-country schooling to replace canter work

Week 11

    Day 1: Hack

    Day 2: 1 hour hack plus 40 minutes schooling

    Day 3: 1 hour hack plus 45 minutes schooling and jumping

    Day 4: 45 minute hack plus one 5 minute canter at 400 mpm, two 4 minute canters at 400 mpm finishing with one 1 minute canter at 500 mpm with 3 minute walk between; check recovery

    Day 5: Rest day

    Day 6: 1 hour hack plus 40 minutes schooling

    Day 7: 1 hour hack plus 45 minutes schooling and jumping

Week 12

    Day 1: Hack

    Day 2: 45 minute hack plus one 5 minute canter at 400 mpm, one 4 minute canter at 400 mpm plus one 1 minute canter at 500 mpm, one 4 minute canter at 400 mpm plus one 1 minute canter at 550 mpm with 3 minute walk between; check recovery

    Day 3: Hack

    Day 4: 1 hour hack plus 40 minutes schooling

    Day 5: 1 hour hack plus 45 minutes schooling and jumping

    Day 6: FIRST HORSE TRIALS

    Day 7: Rest day

Index